THE RED BOOK

FACTS & FIGURES

IN VASCULAR SURGERY

Mr Abdullah Jibawi

MBBS MS FRCS AVS MD

Consultant Vascular, Endovascular and General Surgeon

DISCLAIMERS

The material included in this book was prepared by the author(s) in their personal capacity. The opinions expressed in this book are the authors' own and do not reflect the view of any health institution that the author(s) employed by or affiliated to.

The author makes no representation, express or implied, that the drug dosages or other therapeutic recommendations in this book are cor-rect. Readers must therefore always check the product information and clinical procedures with the most up-to-date published product information and data sheets provided by the manufacturers, and the most recent codes of conduct and safety regulations. The author(s) and the publisher do not
accept responsibility or legal liability for any errors in the text, or for the misuse or misapplication of material in this work. Except where otherwise stated, drug dosages and recommendations are for the non-pregnant adult who is not breastfeeding.

About the author
Mr. Abdullah Jibawi
MBBCh MS AVS FRCS DM

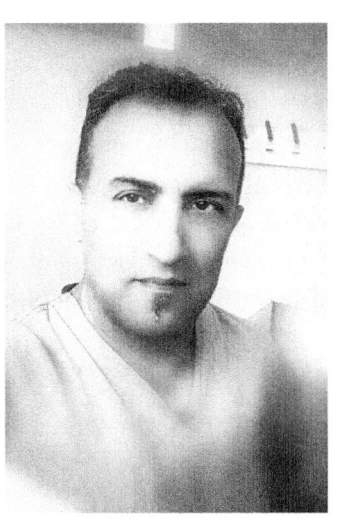

Abdulla Jibawi (AJ) is a consultant vascular surgeon with specialist experience of managing various aspects of common vascular diseases, such as diabetic foot disease, aortic surgery and varicose vein treatments. He has a special interest in stent graft design, complex wound management (using fish skin and low-level laser therapy), lymphoedema, and varicose veins (using sclerotherapy, laser and thermavein technologies).

Dr. Jibawi grew up in the city of Damascus, Syria, where he received a medical school degree (MBBS) and a higher degree (MS) in general and trauma surgery. Following this, he then moved to the UK where he gained training in general, vascular and endovascular surgery (FRCS). Dr. Jibawi was further trained as a vascular scientist with the Royal College of Surgeons of England and the Society for Vascular Scientists (AVS). He achieved his Doctorate under the supervision of Prof. Gary Collins (University of Oxford), Mr. Waquar Yusuf and Prof. Kevin Davies (University of Brighton). Dr. Jibawi was awarded an MD in the field of improving outcome in vascular surgery. Dr. Jibawi is currently a practicing consultant in the NHS, an instructor at various surgical courses (including Alpine FRCS course, ASiT MRCS course, and CCrISPs Course), and is the chief surgeon in the Surrey and London AJLyon clinic (ajlyon. co.uk).

Throughout his career, Dr. Jibawi has been deeply involved in evidence-based practice and applied research in the field of surgery. This interest has formed the basis for his Oxford book (Current Surgical Guidelines) and has influenced the current book. Dr Jibawi passionately believes that serving patients to the highest level of care requires surgeons to remain up-to-date with most recent guidelines and the evidence which underpins them. However, it has become increasingly challenging to achieve this level of knowledge amidst the huge amount of scientific literature published each day. Smooth and easy access to high level evidence is critical for both real life practice and trainees and candidates for the FRCS exam. Hence, there is a great need for a high quality, up-to-date reference book which can feed into the daily practice. This resource can provide users with the most important and relevant information from the wealth of novel scientific research available.

With this in mind, Dr Jibawi has synthesised his own expertise and contemporary scientific evidence to provide a useful and meaningful reference text for physicians and trainees. The current work aims to provide valuable foundation for the daily practice of all vascular surgeons.

About the Book

"There comes a time when for every addition of knowledge you forget something that you knew before. It is of the highest importance, therefore, not to have useless facts elbowing out the useful ones."
Arthur Conan Doyle, A Study in Scarlet"

The contents of this book have been extensively used in teaching vascu- lar trainees (juniors and seniors) and examining trainee knowledge through the exit exam (FRCS). Moreover, the information and ideas contained within the text have enriched discussions between senior consultant colleagues during multidisciplinary meetings (MDTs). Therefore, the style of presenting information has evolved over time to reflect the practicality, depth of discussion, and maturity of such interactions.

Chapters 1 to 16 are concerned with the evidence, statistics, facts and figures of a given topic in the spectrum of vascular diseases. The most up-to-date guidelines have been summarised concisely at the beginning of the chapter. This summary is followed by a thorough but concise one-page summary of high-quality scientific evidence related to the subject matter. Systematic reviews, meta-analyses, and major trials published in relation to that topic have been included and summarised. It is in light of those results that a well-informed decision, encompassing all contemporary and relevant research, can be made in relation to any clinical situation. The contents of each chapter will support optimal decision making in real-life practice.

Chapter 17 moves the book in a different direction. This chapter explores some of the anatomical 'treasures' which I discovered through the Welcome Trust (wellcome.ac.uk). The 'dormant' surgical arts have been sketched with the highest attention to details by outstanding clinicians, surgeons, medical students, and others throughout the eighteenth century. Therefore, I believed it was my job to thoroughly explore the collection and identify the pieces that may significantly enhance the experience of practising surgeons. Throughout this process, I have applied suitable filters and annotated main anatomical landmarks for presentation in a printable format. This has given these historical treasures the spirit of life they have long deserved. Each piece has been annotated with appropriate disclaimer to reflect its suitability to be used and presented within this book.

Chapter 17 also includes an alternative form of sketch: vascular operation sketches. These sketches has been created entirely by myself, and were inspired by real-life cases I have performed or been directly involved in. My sketches also draw inspiration from previously published operative sketches presented by other surgeons and artists in surgical text-books. Of particular note is the time I spent with a colleague of mine, Mr. Islam Ahmed, who is a gifted surgeon and a talented artist. I optimised many of my sketches, and operations, during the period spend with Islam. The purpose of this second section of the chapter is NOT to provide a detailed step-by-step surgical technique book. Instead, in line with the spirit of this book, I have focused on the facts and figures related to each operation. Each procedure is accompanied by few statistics which reflect the key aspects; these include, success rate, complications, and other points which are invaluable for good decision making of both clinicians and patients. It is, of course, possible to use the sketches in teaching junior students and patients in clinic; nevertheless, this is a 'secondary' outcome and is certainly welcomed!

Finally, I have included two appendices to complete the set of facts and figures needed in busy daily life. The first appendix includes facts and figures related to haemodynamic and ultrasonography. The second includes more information about available endovascular tools and charts. Appendix two is intended to provide the busy surgeon with reference charts to navigate their way through the endovascular field, especially in endovascular repair of ruptured aneurysms and in treating incidental remote lesions in hybrid procedures.

I hope the book will be to my colleagues and junior's satisfaction.

All feedback is very welcome!

CONTENTS

Chapter1 Natural History and Prevention

Chapter 2 Vascular Assessment & Perioperative Care

Chapter 3 Abdominal Aortic Aneurysms

Chapter 4 Thoracic Aortic Pathologies

Chapter 5 Visceral Arteries Aneurysms

Chapter6 Venous Diseases

Chapter 7 Lymphoedema

Chapter 8 Intermittent Claudication

Chapter 9 Critical Limb-Threatening Ischaemia

Chapter 10 Acute Limb Ischaemia (ALI)

Chapter 11 Diabetic Foot Disease

Chapter 12 Minor & Major Amputations

Summary of Current Surgical Guidelines for Lower Limb Am-

Chapter13 Revision Vascular Suregry

Chapter 14 Carotid & Vertebral Arteries Diseases

Chapter15 Acute Mesenteric Ischaemia

Chapter 16 Miscellaneous

Chapter17 Atlas of Vascular Anatomy and Surgical Techniques Facts and Figures

Toe amputation

Appendices

CHAPTER 1
NATURAL
HISTORY AND
PREVENTION

Prevalence of PAD in normal population

EDINBURGH ARTERY STUDY 1991

AT A GLANCE
- A questionnaire-based randomised study
- 1592 participants randomly selected
- Sensitivity 91%; Specificity 99

MAIN RESULTS
- Symptomatic PVD disease prevalence based on objective testing: 3% to 10%, increasing to 15% to 20% for age >70.
- Within 5-yrs from PVD diagnosis:
  » 2-4% sustain non-fatal MI or Stroke in 1st yr then 1-2%/yr thereafter
  » 25% die from a cardiovascular disease.
- In the BASLE STUDY - 5% of symptomatic IC remain stable; 25% deteriorate clinically, mostly 1st yr (7%–9%) then 2-3%/yr. Only 5% affect QoL and need to consider intervention. 1-2% require amputation.

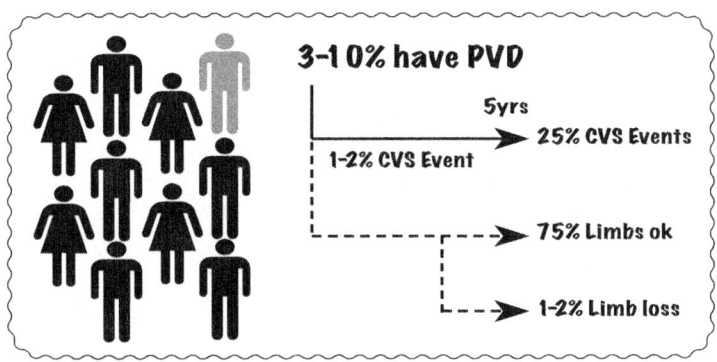

REFERENCES:
- Edinburgh Artery Study. Int J Epidemiol. 1991. PMID: 1917239
- Da Silva, A., and L. K. Widmer. Occlusive peripheral artery disease.Early diagnosis, incidence, course, significance. Hans Huber, Bern, Stuttgart, Vienna (1980): p1-97. see PMID: 6676932

Risk of PAD development over years

THE REACH REGISTRY 2006

AT A GLANCE
- Registry for 67888 patients >45yr-olds.
- Data on spectrum of disease progression, outcomes & patterns of treatment in the 21st century

MAIN RESULTS
- Death, MI or stroke occur in 4-6% of patients with symptomatic atherosclerosis in 1yr if one disease location
- Hospitalisation occurs in 15-20% of those patients.

REFERENCES:
- The Reach Registry. Am Heart J. 2006. PMID: 16569533.

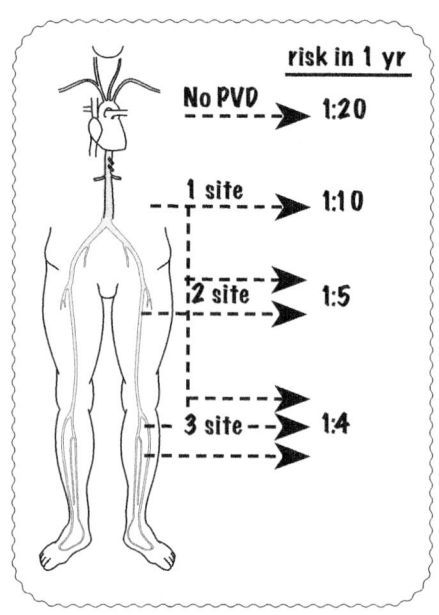

risk in 1 yr

No PVD ----> 1:20

1 site ----> 1:10

2 site ---> 1:5

3 site ---> 1:4

Concomittent CVS diseases with PAD

THE REACH REGISTRY 2006

AT A GLANCE

- Registry for 67888 patients >45yr-olds.
- Data on spectrum of disease progression, outcomes & patterns of treatment in the 21st century

MAIN RESULTS

- see page „The RE-ACH registry 2006" on page 32

REFERENCES:

- The Reach Registry. Am Heart J. 2006. PMID: 16569533.

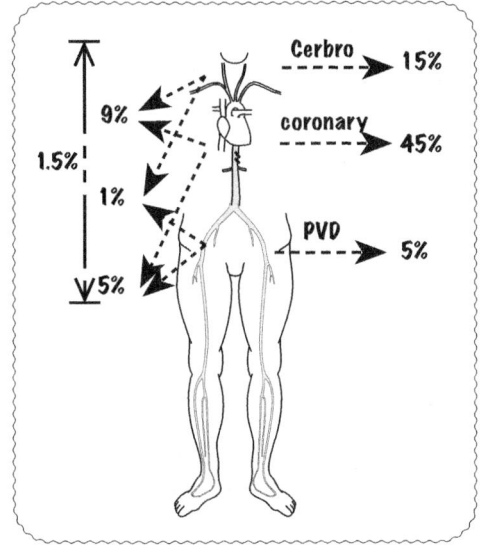

Change of ABI over time

THE CARDIOVASCULAR HEALTH STUDY 1991

AT A GLANCE
- Cohort study of for 5888 patients (male and femal) >65yr-olds.
- Comparing pts with low vs. normal ABI over time.

MAIN RESULTS
- Overall, ABI declined by 9.5% over 6 years of follow-up (0.33 for cases with PVD vs. 0.02 in non-PVD cases).
- Predictors of ABI decline are:
  - » age (x1.96)
  - » current cigarette use (x 1.74)
  - » hypertension (x 1.64)
  - » diabetes (x1.77)
  - » higher LDL (x 1.60)
  - » lipid-lowering drug use (x1.74)

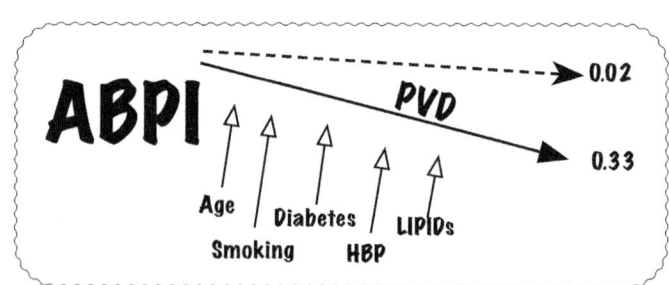

REFERENCES:
- The Cardiovascular Health Study Ann Epidemiol. 1991. PMID: 1669507

Progress of patients with IC

THE BASLE STUDY 1980

AT A GLANCE

- several observational follow-ups.

MAIN RESULTS

- 2/3 of patients surviving at 5 years reported no limiting intermittent claudication (i.e. their symptoms had resolved),
- 63% had angiographic progression of PAD disease.
- 1/4 of pts with intermittent claudication have symptoms that worsen over time.
- 5% deteriorate sufficiently to merit revascularisatio
- only 1–2% will require a major amputation. See also TASC review

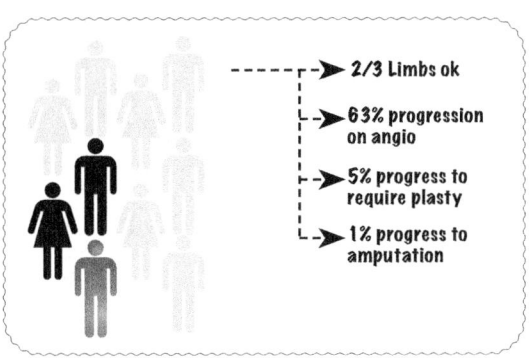

2/3 Limbs ok

63% progression on angio

5% progress to require plasty

1% progress to amputation

REFERENC-   ES:
- Da Silva, A., and L. K. Widmer. Occlusive peripheral artery disease. Early diagnosis, incidence, course, significance. Hans Huber, Bern, Stuttgart, Vienna (1980): p1-97. see PMID: 6676932

Risk factors for PAD

THE **NHANES** STUDY **2004**

AT A GLANCE

- National Health and Nutrition Examination Survey (1999–2000)
- US-Based, age- and gender-adjusted with logistic regression analyses.

MAIN RESULTS

- Black race/ethnicity (OR 2.83), current smoking (OR 4.46), diabetes (OR 2.71), hypertension (OR 1.75),
- Hypercholesterolaemia (OR 1.68) and poor kidney function (OR 2.00).
- The Atherosclerosis Risk in Communities (ARIC) study: Database showed similar profile.

REFERENCES:

- The NHANES study. Circulation. 110, 2004. PMID: 15262830

Risk factors for PAD

THE FRAMINGHAM HEART STUDY 2008

AT A GLANCE
- 8491 participants (mean age, 49 years; 4522 women) attended a routine examination between 30 and 74 years of age and were free of CVD.

MAIN RESULTS
- Over 12 years of follow-up, 1174 participants (456 women) developed a first CVD event.
- All traditional risk factors evaluated predicted CVD risk (multivariable-adjusted P<0.0001).
- In women, age (x10), total cholesterol (x3.4), HDL (x0.5), high sBP (x16), smoking (x1.7) and diabetes (x2).
- In men, age (x21), total cholesterol (x3), HDL (x0.4), high sBP (x7), smoking (x1.9) and diabetes (x1.8).
- A general cardiovascular risk profile (https://foh.psc.gov/calendar/crp.html) is widely available in the USA.

REFERENCES:
- Circulation. 2008;117:743-753. PMID: 18212285

Risk of Disease Progression in PAD

A META-ANALYSIS 2016

AT A GLANCE
- 35 studies (sample size varied between 109 and 16,440 subjects).

MAIN RESULTS
- Age ranged from 56 to 81 years and mean follow up was 6.3 years.
- Symptomatic PAD subjects had higher 5 year cumulative CV mortality than the reference population, 13% versus 5%.
- During follow up, approximately 7% of APAD patients progressed to IC, and 21% of IC patients were diagnosed as having critical limb ischemia, with 4-27% undergoing amputations.

REFERENCES:
- Eur J Vasc Endovasc Surg. 2016 Mar;51(3):395-403. PMID: 26777541

SMOKING

Effectiveness of NRTs in Smoking Cessation

A SYSTEMATIC REVIEW AND META-ANALYSIS 2006

AT A GLANCE

- 70 trials of NRT versus control at 1 year included.

MAIN RESULTS

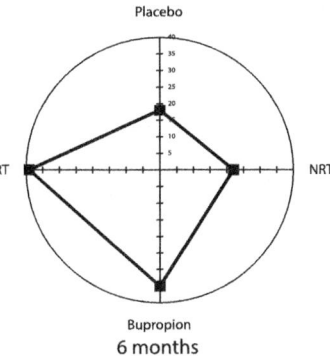

Placebo

Bupropion+NRT — NRT

Bupropion
6 months

- NRT vs. control - Odds Ratio [OR] 1.71 (P =< 0.0001).
- Placebo-controlled trials (OR 1.78), NRT gum (OR 1.60), and patch (OR 1.63).
- NRT reduced smoking at 3 months (OR 1.98).
- Bupropion vs controls: more effective at 1 year (OR1.56) and at 3 months (OR 2.13).
- Bupropion vs. NRT - more effective at 1 year (OR 1.14). Varenicline vs. placebo: superior at 1 year (OR 2.96) and 3 months (OR 3.75).
- Varenicline vs. bupropion at 1 year (OR 1.58) and at 3 months (OR 1.61).
- Varenicline superior to NRT when compared to placebo controls (OR 1.66) or to all controls at 1 year (OR 1.73).

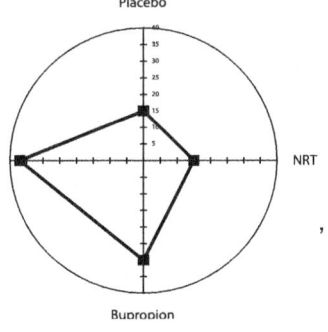

Placebo

Bupropion+NRT — NRT

Bupropion

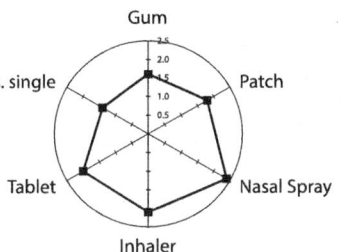

Gum

Cobined vs. single — Patch

Tablet — Nasal Spray

Inhaler

- Adverse events were not systematically different across studies.

REFERENCES:

- BMC Public Health. 2006 Dec 11;6:3000. PMID: 17156479

Vareniciline for smoking cessation

A COCHRANE REVIEW 2007

AT A GLANCE

- Nicotine receptor partial agonists for smoking cessation.
- 6 trials (4924) participants included.

MAIN RESULTS

- Pooled odds ratio (OR) for continuous abstinence at 12 months for varenicline vs. placebo - 3.22
- Pooled OR for varenicline vs. bupropion - 1.66
- Main adverse effect of varenicline is nausea (mostly mild to moderate) and usually subsided over time.
- Varenicline beyond the 12-week - the drug well-tolerated and effective during long-term use.

REFERENCES:

- Cochrane Database Syst Rev. 2007 Jan 24;(1):CD006103. PMID: 17253581.

Genetic predisposition to smoking & CVS Diseases

A META-ANALYSIS 2020

AT A GLANCE

- 361 single-nucleotide polymorphisms (SNPs) associated with smoking initiation were identified
- Association between SNPs and cardiovascular diseases were studied using UK Biobank study (N = 367 643 individuals), CARDIoGRAMplusC4D consortium (N = 184 305 individuals), Atrial Fibrillation Consortium (2017 dataset; N = 154 432 individuals), and Million Veteran Program (MVP; N = 190 266 individuals).

MAIN RESULTS

- Genetic predisposition to smoking initiation was most strongly and consistently associated with higher odds of:
  - » coronary artery disease
  - » heart failure
  - » abdominal aortic aneurysm
  - » ischaemic stroke
  - » transient ischaemic attack
  - » peripheral arterial disease
  - » arterial hypertension
  - » deep vein thrombosis and pulmonary embolism.
- Limited evidence of causal associations of smoking initiation was found with thoracic aortic aneurysm.

REFERENCES:

- Eur Heart J. 2020 Apr 16;ehaa193. PMID: <u>32300774</u>

Electronic Cigarettes and Cardiovascular Risk

SYS REVIEW 2019

AT A GLANCE
- 23 studies included in this review (see table 1 in original article).

MAIN RESULTS
- Many studies have shown ↑ heart rate, ↑ arterial stiffness, ↑ odds of having a myocardial infarction, ↑ platelet aggregation, ↑ general health scores, ↑ breathing difficulty scores, ↑ higher proportion of self-reported chest pain, ↑ risk of thrombogenesis and ↑ platelet function.
- Despite that, other studies did not persistently confirm the fi - dings and epidemiological data mostly suggest that the use of electronic cigarettes appears to be safer than that of traditional tobacco cigarettes.

REFERENCES:
- Eur Cardiol. 2019 Dec 18;14(3):151-158. PMID: 31933682

HYPERTENSION

Blood Pressure Lowering for Prevention of CVS risk

SYS REVIEW & META-ANALYSIS

AT A GLANCE

- 123 studies (613,815 participants) included.

MAIN RESULTS

- There is relative risk reductions proportional to the magnitude of the blood pressure reductions achieved.
- Every 10 mm Hg reduction in sBP significantly reduced the risk of major cardiovascular disease events (relative risk [RR] 0·80), coronary heart disease (0·83), stroke (0·73), and heart failure (0·72) , 0·67-0·78)
  - ▷ This also led to a significant 13% reduction in all-cause mortality.
  - ▷ The effect on renal failure was not significant.
- β blockers were inferior to other drugs for the prevention of major cardiovascular disease events, stroke, and renal failure.
- Calcium channel blockers were superior to other drugs for the prevention of stroke.
- For the prevention of heart failure - calcium channel blockers were inferior and diuretics were superior to other drug classes.

REFERENCES:

- Lancet. 2016 Mar 5;387(10022):957-967. PMID: 26724178

Blood Pressure Variability and CVS risk

Sys Review & Meta-Analysis

At a glance
- 46 separate analyses identified.
- Results from 23 analyses were excluded from main analyses owing to high risks of confounding.

Main Results
- Increased long term variability in sBP was associated with risk of all cause mortality (hazard ratio 1.15), CVS mortality (1.18), CVS disease events (1.18), coronary heart disease (1.10) and stroke (1.15).
- Increased mid-term and short term variability in daytime sBP were also associated with all cause mortality (1.15).

References:
- BMJ. 2016 Aug 9;354:i4098. PMID: 27511067

Blood Pressure Targets and CVS risk

COCHRANE SYS REVIEW

AT A GLANCE
- 6 RCTs (9484 participants) included.
- Mean follow-up was 3.7 years.

MAIN RESULTS
- No change in total mortality (risk ratio (RR) 1.06)) or cardiovascular mortality (RR 1.03).
- No differences in serious adverse events or total cardiovascular events (including myocardial infarction, stroke, sudden death, hospitalization, or death from congestive heart failure).
- Studies reported more participant withdrawals due to adverse effects in the lower target arm (RR 8.16).
- Blood pressures were lower in the lower target group by 8.9/4.5 mmHg.
- More drugs were needed in the lower target group.

REFERENCES:
- Cochrane Database Syst Rev. 2018 Jul 20;7(7):CD010315.. PMID: 30027631

Blood Pressure Reduction and CVS risk

Sys Review & Meta-Analysis

At a glance
- 42 trials (144 220 patients) included.

Main Results
- In general, there were linear associations between mean achieved sBP and risk of CVS disease and mortality
- The lowest CVS risk was achieved at sBP of 120 to 124 mm Hg
  - Hazard ratio (HR) for major CVS disease was 0.71
- For sBP of 140 to 144 mm Hg -
  ▷ HR of 0.46 compared with those with a mean achieved SBP of 150 to 154 mm Hg
  ▷ HR of 0.36 compared with those with a mean achieved SBP of 160 mm Hg or more.
- For sBP of 120 to 124 mm Hg -
  ▷ HR for all-cause mortality is 0.73 compared with those with SBP of 130 to 134 mm Hg.
  ▷ HR of 0.59 compared with those with a mean achieved SBP of 140 to 144 mm Hg.
  ▷ HR of 0.51 compared with those with a mean achieved SBP of 150 to 154 mm Hg
  ▷ HR of 0.47 compared with those with a mean achieved SBP of 160 mm Hg or more..

References:
- JAMA Cardiol. 2017 Jul 1;2(7):775-781. PMID: 28564682

Intensive Blood Pressure Reduction and CVS risk

SYS REVIEW & META-ANALYSIS

AT A GLANCE
- 19 trials (44,989 participants) included.
- 2496 major cardiovascular events were recorded during a mean 3·8 years of follow-up.
- Patients in the more intensive blood pressure-lowering treatment group had mean blood pressure levels of 133/76 mm Hg vs. 140/81 mm Hg in the less intensive treatment group.

MAIN RESULTS
- Intensive blood pressure-lowering treatment achieved RR reductions for major cardiovascular events (14%), myocardial infarction (13%), stroke (22%), albuminuria (10%), and retinopathy progression (19%).
- More intensive treatment had no clear effects on heart failure (15%), cardiovascular death (9%), total mortality (9%), or end-stage kidney disease (10%).
- Additional blood pressure lowering had a clear benefit even in patients with systolic blood pressure lower than 140 mm Hg.
- Severe hypotension was more frequent in the more intensive treatment regimen (RR 2·68), but the absolute excess was small (0·3% vs 0·1% per person-year for the duration of follow-up).

REFERENCES:
- Lancet. 2016 Jan 30;387(10017):435-43. PMID: 26559744

HYPERLIPIDEMIA

Hyperlipidaemia - in a nutshell

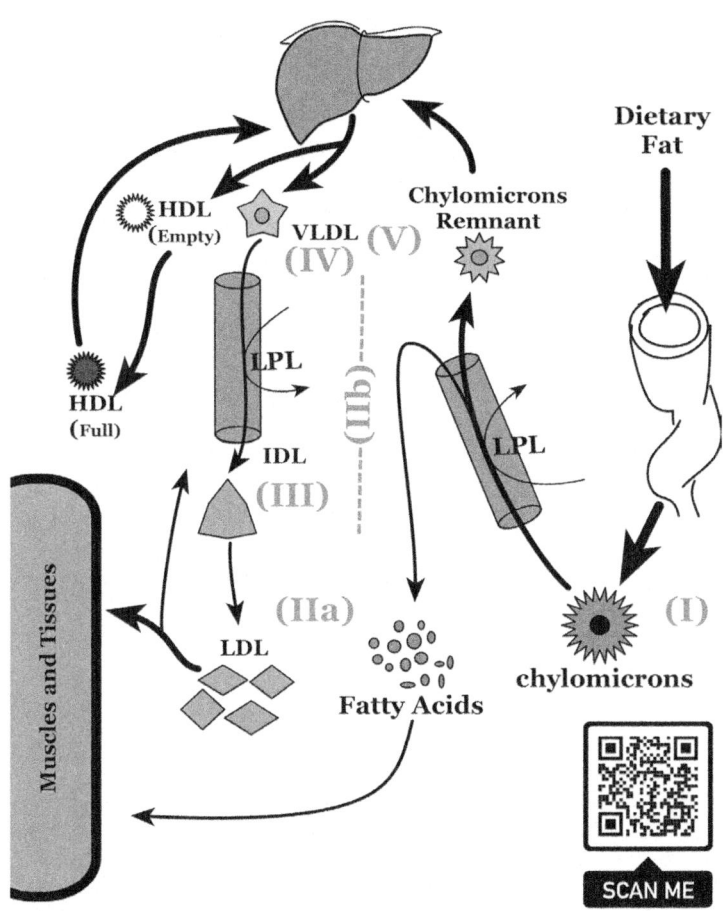

KEY FACTS AND FIGURES

- There are five main types: I (Chylomicrons), IIa(LDL also called familial hypercholesterolemia), IIb(LDL+VLDL), III (IDL also known as Familial dysbetalipoproteinemia), IV (VLDL also known as Familial hypertriglyceridemia), V (VLDL + chylomicrons).
- Primary hyperlipidaemia is usually due to genetic causes (such as a mutation in a receptor protein), while secondary hyperlipidemia arises due to other underlying causes such as diabetes.

Effect of Statins Therapy in CLTI patients

SYS REVIEW & META-ANALYSIS 2020

AT A GLANCE

- 19 studies (26,985 patients) included.

MAIN RESULTS

- Patients treated with statins were:
  - ▷ 25% less likely to undergo amputation (HR 0.75);
  - ▷ 38% less likely to have a fatal event (HR 0.62)
  - ▷ increased overall patency rates.
  - ▷ lower incidence of major adverse cardiac or cerebrovascular events (MACCE).

REFERENCES:

- Vasc Med. 2020 Apr;25(2):106-117. PMID: 31964311

Lipid Lowering for PAD patients

COCHRANE SYS REVIEW 2007

AT A GLANCE
- 18 trials (10,049 participants) included.

MAIN RESULTS
- Pooled results indicated that lipid-lowering therapy had no statistically significant effect on overall mortality (Odds Ratio (OR) 0.86) or on total cardiovascular events (OR 0.8).
- Subgroup analysis which excluded PQRST trial showed that lipid-lowering therapy significantl reduced the risk of total cardiovascular events (OR 0.74).
- Use of simvastatin in people with a blood cholesterol >/= 3.5 mmol/litre (HPS) showed the greatest evidence of effectiveness.
- Improvement in total walking distance (Weighted Mean Difference (WMD) 152 m) and pain-free walking distance (WMD 89.76 m) was noted.
- No significant impact on ankle brachial index (WMD 0.04).

REFERENCES:
- Cochrane Database Syst Rev. 2007 Oct 17. PMID: 17943736

Triglyceride Lowering & Reduction of CVS Risk

SYS REVIEW AND META-ANALYSIS 2019

AT A GLANCE

- A total of 197 270 participants from 24 trials of nonstatin therapy included.

MAIN RESULTS

- For non-high-density lipoprotein cholesterol: risk ratio (RR) per 1-mmol/L reduction in non-high-density lipoprotein cholesterol was 0.79. RR was 0.80 per 1-mmol/L reduction in LDL-C and 0.84 per 1-mmol/L reduction in triglycerides.
- When REDUCE-IT trial was removed, the RRs became 0.79 per 1-mmol/L reduction in LDL-C and 0.91 per 1-mmol/L reduction in triglycerides.
- For each 1 g/d eicosapentaenoic acid (Omega-3) administered, there was associated 7% relative risk reduction in major vascular events (RR, 0.93).
- There was no significant association between dose of docosahexaenoic acid and the relative risk reduction in major vascular events.

REFERENCES:

- Circulation. 2019 Oct 15;140(16):1308-1317. PMID: 31530008

Antiplatelets

Benefits of low dose Aspirin

THE ANTIPLATELET TRIALISTS' COLLABORATION META-ANALYSIS 2009

AT A GLANCE
- A meta-analysis from the Antiplatelet Trialist Collaboration.

MAIN RESULTS
- Low-dose aspirin was persistently associated with reduced risk of non-fatal MI, non-fatal stroke and vascular death in high-risk patients, including those with intermittent claudication.

REFERENCES:
- Lancet 2009;373:1849–60. PMID: 19482214

Clopidogrel vs. Aspirin for Secondary Prevention

THE CAPRIE TRIAL 1996

AT A GLANCE

- 19 185 patients with CVS disease randomised to clopidogrel (75 mg once daily) vs. aspirin (325 mg once daily).
- Looking at reducing the risk of a composite outcome cluster of ischaemic stroke, myocardial infarction, or vascular death.
- Relative safety was also assessed.

MAIN RESULTS

- Clopidogrel results in relative reduction in the risk of MI, ischaemic stroke and vascular death by 8.7% (P = 0.04) - mean follow-up of 1.9 years.
- The absolute risk reduction is 0.51%, and NNT is 196 to avoid one ischaemic event.
- [In the sub-analysis, the risk reduction reaches 22% for patients with PAD].

REFERENCES:

- Lancet. 1996. PMID: 8918275

Dual antiplatelet vs. Aspirin for Prevention

THE CHARISMA TRIAL 2006

AT A GLANCE

- 19,185 patients with CVS disease randomised to clopidogrel (75 mg once daily) and aspirin (325 mg once daily).
- Composite outcome cluster was ischaemic stroke, myocardial infarction, or vascular death.
- Relative safety was also assessed.

MAIN RESULTS

- Clopidogrel results in relative reduction in the risk of MI, ischaemic stroke and vascular death by 8.7% (P = 0.04) - mean follow-up of 1.9 years.
- The absolute risk reduction is 0.51%, and NNT is 196 to avoid one ischaemic event.
- [In the sub-analysis, the risk reduction reaches 22% for patients with PAD]

REFERENCES:

- N Engl J Med. 2006. PMID: 16531616

Antiplatelets or Anticoagulants for protection

THE ACTIVE W TRIAL 2006

AT A GLANCE

- Randomised controlled trial - Atrial fibrillation Clopidogrel Trial with Irbesartan for prevention of Vascular Events [ACTIVE W]). .

MAIN RESULTS

- Clopidogrel plus Aspirin is inferior to oral anticoagulation for preventing vascular events in atrial fibrillation.
- Warfarin + Aspirin were not more effective than Aspirin alone in preventing major CV events in this setting.

REFERENCES:

- Lancet. 2006. PMID: 16765759.

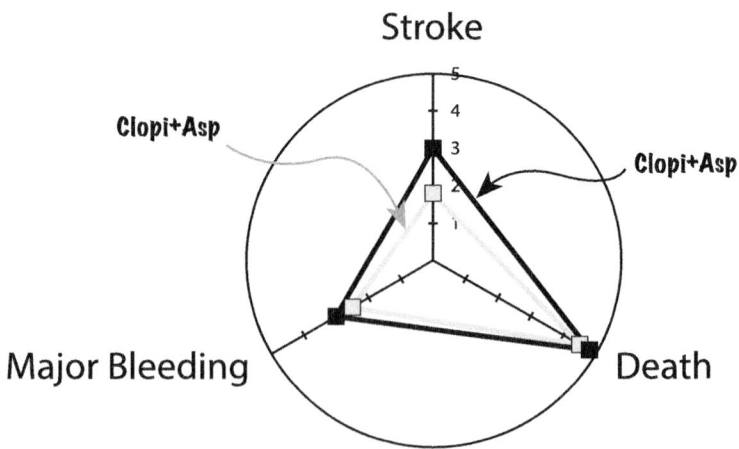

Dual vs. Mono-Antiplatelets in Prosthetic grafts

THE CASPAR TRIAL 2010

AT A GLANCE

- Patients undergoing unilateral, below-knee bypass graft were enrolled 2 to 4 days after surgery for clopidogrel 75 mg/day plus ASA 75 to 100 mg/day or placebo plus ASA 75 to 100 mg/day for 6 to 24 months.
- Primary endpoint - index-graft occlusion or revascularization, above-ankle amputation, or death.
- Primary safety endpoint - severe bleeding.

MAIN RESULTS

- Primary endpoint occurred in 149 of 425 patients in the clopidogrel group vs 151 of 426 patients in the placebo (plus ASA) group (hazard ratio [HR], 0.98).
- Primary endpoint significantl reduced by clopidogrel in prosthetic graft patients (HR, 0.65) but not in venous graft patients (HR, 1.25).
- Total bleeds - more frequent with Clopidogrel. But no significan difference between the rate of severe bleeding in the clopidogrel and placebo (plus ASA) groups (2.1% vs 1.2%).

REFERENCES:

- J Vasc Surg. 2010. PMID: 20678878

EXERCISE PROGRAMMES

Usefulness of Supervised Exercise Programme

META ANALYSIS 1995

AT A GLANCE
- 21 comparative studies included.

MAIN RESULTS
- Best programme: duration greater than 30 minutes per session, frequency of at least three sessions per week, walking used as the mode of exercise, use of near-maximal pain during training as claudication pain end point, and program length of greater than 6 months.
- The distance (mean +/- SD) to onset of claudication pain increased 179% (P < .001), and the distance to maximal claudication pain increased 122% (P < .001).

REFERENCES:
- JAMA. 1995. PMID: 7674529

Supervised vs. Unsupervised Exercise for IC

COCHRANE SYS REVIEW AND META ANALYSIS 2013

AT A GLANCE

- 14 comparative studies included (1002 candidates).

MAIN RESULTS

- Supervised programme has an overall effect size of 0.69 and 0.48 at 3 and 6 months, respectively. This translates to an increase in walking distance of approximately 180 meters that favoured the supervised group.
- Supervised exercise was still beneficial for maximal and pain-free walking distances at 12 months, but it did not have a significant effect on quality of life parameters.
- Unsupervised exercise has less or no benefits for IC compared to supervised ones.

REFERENCES:

- Cochrane Sys Rev - 2013. PMID: 23970372

MEDICATIONS

FOR

CLAUDICATION

Vasoactive drugs for IC

A Cochrane Sys Review and Meta Analysis 2014

At a glance
- 15 double-blind, RCTs (5718 pts) comparing cilostazol vs. pentoxifylline vs. placebo.

Main Results
- For initial claudication distance (ICD - the distance walked on a treadmill before the onset of calf pain) there was an improvement in the cilostazol vs. placebo (31 m vs. 20 m. P <0.005).
- Absolute claudication distance (ACD - the maximum distance walked on a treadmill) significantly increased in participants taking cilostazol 100 mg and 50 mg twice daily vs. placebo (43 m vs. 32 m; P <0.005)
- Cilostazol has higher odds of headache, diarrhoea, abnormal stool, dizziness and palpitations

References:
- Cochrane Database Syst Rev. 2014. PMID: 25358850

Vasoactive drugs for IC 2

Sys Reviewes 2003-2015

At a glance

- Omega-3 fish oil reduces re-infarction rate following MI. Cochrane Syst Rev 2004
- Atrovestatin 80mg/d improves claudication distance. Circulation 2003; 108: 1481-6
- Iloprost for severe IC:
  - » Meta-analysis of RCTs. Beneficial effect - 55% leg saving vs. 35% with no iloprost. Int Angio 1994
  - » RCT for critical limb ischaemia for thromboangitis obliterans. Complete pain relief in 63% vs. 28% at 6mo. Lancet 1990
- Cell therapy – Detailed analysis of recent literature data confirmed the beneficial role of cell therapy in reducing the rate of major amputations, improving distal perfusion, increasing walking distance, reducing pain, improving ABI and TcPO2, and improving overall ischemic symptoms in patients with CLI and their quality of life.

References:

- Syst Review. Stem Cells Int. 2015; 2015: 931420

Spinal cord stimulation for Ischaemic Leg

COCHRANE SYS REVIEW AND META ANALYSIS 2013

AT A GLANCE

- A Spinal Cord Stimulator (SCS) is an implantable neuromodulation device that is used to send electrical signals to selected areas of the spinal cord for the treatment of certain conditions (mainly pain).
- This is a review of Six studies (450 pts) using SCS in patients suffering from inoperable chronic critical leg ischaemia with a proposed amputation of the leg.

MAIN RESULTS

- Limb salvage after 12 months was significantly higher in the SCS group (risk ratio (RR) 0.71).
- Significant pain relief occurred in both treatment groups, but was more prominent in the SCS group where the patients required significantly less analgesics.
- In the SCS group, significa tly more patients reached Fontaine stage II than in the conservative group (RR 4.9).
- No significantly different effect on ulcer healing was observed with the two treatments.
- SCS complication rate 17% and number needed to harm is 6.

REFERENCES:

- Cochrane Database Syst Rev. 2013. PMID: 23450547

Lumbar Sympathectomy for Ischaemic Leg

COCHRANE SYS REVIEW 2010 & 2016

MEDICINA CLINICA 2010 REVIEW

- Four clinical trials and four observational studies included.
- Sympathectomy did not show significant differences for mortality, amputations and grade of intermittent claudication.
- When it was assessed regarding local anaesthetics or prostaglandin-E1, differences were not detected.
- Chemical sympathectomy showed better results than surgical sympathectomy in hospital stance.

COCHRANE DATABASE SYST REV. 2016

- No RCTs identified that allow to avoid selection bias (i.e. that include objective assessment of peripheral perfusion).
- No study was eligible for inclusion in the review.

REFERENCES:

- Medicina Clinica. 2010. PMID: 20022613
- Cochrane Database Syst Rev. 2016. PMID: 27959471

Intense Antithrombotic Therapy for PAD

SYS REVIEW AND META-ANALYSIS 2020

AT A GLANCE

- 7 RCTs (30,447 patients) included.
- Patients randomised to more vs. less intense antithrombotic therapy:
  ▷ more vs. less intense single-antiplatelet therapy (SAPT)
  ▷ dual-antiplatelet therapy vs. SAPT
  ▷ dual antithrombotic therapy vs. SAPT
  ▷ oral anticoagulant.
- Median follow-up of 24 months.

MAIN RESULTS

- More vs. less intense antithrombotic therapy or placebo significantly reduced the risk of limb revascularization (relative risk (RR) 0.89), limb amputation (RR 0.63), and stroke (RR 0.82).
- No statistically significant effect on the risk of myocardial infarction, all-cause, and cardiovascular death.
- Risk of major bleeding increased (RR 1.23).

REFERENCES:

- Eur Heart J Cardiovasc Pharmacother. 2020 Apr 1;6(2):86-93. PMID: 31392312

Marine Omega-3 Supplementation and CVS Disease

A META-ANALYSIS 2019

AT A GLANCE

- 13 trials included.
- Outcome measured were myocardial infarction, coronary heart disease (CHD) death, total CHD, total stroke, CVD death, total CVD, and major vascular events.
- A meta-regression was conducted to estimate the dose-response relationship between marine omega-3 dosage and risk of each prespecified outcome

MAIN RESULTS

- Marine omega-3 supplementation was associated with significantly lower risk of myocardial infarction (rate ratio [RR]: 0.92), CHD death (RR: 0.92), total CHD (RR: 0.95), CVD death (RR: 0.93), and total CVD (RR: 0.97).
- After including REDUCE-IT trial, inverse associations for all outcomes were strengthened.
- Statistically significant linear dose-response relationships were found for total CVD and major vascular events in the analyses with and without including REDUCE-IT. Risk reductions appeared to be linearly related to marine omega-3 dose.

REFERENCES:

- J Am Heart Assoc. 2019 Oct;8(19):e013543. PMID: 31567003

CHAPTER 2
VASCULAR ASSESSMENT & PERIOPERATIVE CARE

Duplex vs CTA vs MRA for IC Assessment

META ANALYSIS 2007

AT A GLANCE

- 13 studies included.

MAIN RESULTS

- Detection of stenosis > 50% in the whole leg: contrast-enhanced (CE) MRA (14 studies) had the highest diagnostic accuracy (sensitivity 92- 99.5%; specificity 64-99%)
- Two-dimensional (2D) time-of-flight (TOF) MRA (11 studies): less accurate; sensitivity 79 to 94% and specificity 74 to 92%
- DUS (28 studies): sensitivity ranging 80 to 98% and specificity 89 to 99%.
- In the 55 studies identified for adverse events, MRA had highest reported proportion. The most severe adverse events were more common in patients undergoing CA.

REFERENCES:

- Health Technol Assess. 2007. PMID: 17462170.

DSA vs. CT angiography for PAD Assessment

RANDOMISED TRIAL 2005

AT A GLANCE

- 145 patients: 72 randomly allocated to DSA and 73 to CT angiography.
- Outcomes measures: therapeutic confidence assessed by physicians (on a scale from 0 to 10), need for additional imaging, health-related quality of life at 6-month follow-up, diagnostic and therapeutic costs, and costs for a hospital stay.

MAIN RESULTS

- Physician confidence in making a correct therapeutic choice was significantly higher at DSA (mean confidence score, 8.2) than at CT angiography (mean score, 7.2; P < .001).
- No significant quality-of-life di ferences were found.

REFERENCES:

- Radiology. 2005. PMID: 16244280

PERIOPERATIVE CARE

Supplemental Preoperative Anti-MRSA Antibiotics

RANDOMISED TRIAL 2015

AT A GLANCE

- Prospective randomized double-blinded trial comparing 2 anti-MRSA agents with supplemental coverage of cefazolin before lower extremity revascularization.
- The study included 178 patients undergoing bypass surgery.

MAIN RESULTS

- The addition of either vancomycin or daptomycin to standard cephalosporin prophylaxis had a similar effect: surgical site infection rates of 8.2 and 11.8 respectively.
- Vancomycin appeared to reduce the rate of Gram positive bacterial infections.

REFERENCES:

- Ann Surg 2015; 262: 495–501

Preventing delirium in elderly patients after non-cardiac surgery

RANDOMISED TRIAL 2016

AT A GLANCE

- Randomised, double-blind, placebo-controlled trial.

MAIN RESULTS

- Intravenous dexmedetomidine given to patients over 65 in the first 24 hours who are admitted to ITU following a major surgery can significantly reduce the risk of delirium (9% vs 23%, P<0.0001)

REFERENCES:

- Lancet 2016; 388: 1893–1902

Frailty Factors and Outcomes in Vascular Surgery

SYS REVIEW AND META-ANALYSIS 2019

AT A GLANCE
- 53 studies included in the review
- Only 8 were both good quality.
- Eighteen studies (62,976 patients) provided data for the meta-analysis.

MAIN RESULTS
- Frailty was associated with increased age (MD 4.05 years), female sex (RR 1.32), and lower body mass index (MD -1.81).
- Frailty was associated with 30-day mortality [adjusted OR (AOR) 2.77), postoperative complications (AOR 2.16), and long-term mortality (HR 1.85).
- Sarcopenia was not associated with any outcomes.

REFERENCES:
- Ann Surg. 2019 Oct 22. PMID: 31651536

CHAPTER 3
ABDOMINAL
AORTIC
ANEURYSMS

Summary of Current Surgical Guidelines for Abdominal Aortic Aneurysms

► NICE Guidelines 2020 (UK)
➡ ESVS Clinical Practice Guidelines 2020 (EU)
→ Society For Vascular Surgery Guidlines 2017 (USA)

On Screening and Prevention -

- A screening programme for AAA should be setup for all men aged 65 (➡I; ►age 66 in the UK).
  - » Patients with AAA > 3 cm should be enrolled into a surveillance programme (➡I,→2): every 3 yrs for 3-3.9cm; annually for 4-4.9cm; and every 3-6 months for >5cm (➡I).
  - » Consider men with an aorta 2.5-2.9 cm in diameter at initial screening for rescreening after 5-10 years (➡IIb, →2).
  - » Patients with a first degree relative with AAA should be considered for a screening ultrasound scan (→2), at interval of 10 years, begining at age 50 (➡IIb).
  - » Patients with a true peripheral aneurysm should be considered for AAA surveillance at 5-10 yr intervals.
  - » Females aged 70 yrs or older should be considered for a scan (if AAA not excluded before) if they have another risk factor such as COPD, hypertension, or family history of AAA (►R).
- No need to review a patient with incidental AAA finding if they have very limited life expectancy (➡I).
- Advise all patients to stop smoking (➡I, ►R), for at least 2 weeks if a repair is considered (→1). Ensure they receive appropriate help to support this. Ensure blood pressure is well controlled (►R).
- There are currently no approved medical therapies that can be used to reduce the expansion of AAA, and none should be advised to patients (➡III,→2). Alternatively, encourage a healthy life style (improved diet and ample excercise) (➡IIa).
- Where the patient is not a good candidate for surgery when their AAA reaches 5.5cm, consider continuing the surveillance and aim to optimise their medical condition. Consider whether a procedure has become more suitable (risk:benefit ratio) if they reach a higher threshold (for example 7cm) (➡IIa).

On Diagnosis -
- Offer an USS if AAA is suspected on physical exam (▶R).
- Use ultrasound scan as a first line modality for diagnosis and surveillance of small AAA (➡I). Use anterio-posterior plane and be consistent in calipre placement (➡IIa). Report the inner-to-inner maximum anterior-posterior aortic diameter (▶R).
- Once a decision to consider AAA repair is made, a CTA scan is recommended (➡I, ▶R). Use a dedicated softeware to make your measurements and uphold consistency (➡IIa).

Indications for Treatment -
- Consider elective repair for all suitable men with AAA ≥ 5.5 cm (➡I, ▶R).
- Consider elective repair for all suitable women with AAA ≥ 5 cm (➡IIb, →2, ▶Be aware that AAAs are more likely to rupture in women than men).
- Consider the repair option (and not observation only) in patients with small (4-5.4cm) aneurysms who require chemotherapy, radiotherapy, or solid organ transplantation. A shared decision-making approach regarding treatment options is required (→2).
- Aim to repair a threshold AAA within 8 weeks from diagnosis (➡I).
- Consider fast tracking patients with AAA expanding ≥ 1cm/yr (➡IIa, ▶R).
- Do not screen for unknown carotid artery disease prior to AAA repair (➡III). Do not routinely perform a prophylactic carotid endarterectomy for asymptomatic patients prior to AAA (➡III). Only treat the carotid prior to AAA repair if the patient has been symptomatic in the last 6 months (➡IIa).
- Do NOT offer AAA repair for patients with limited (2-3 yrs) life expectancy (➡III).
- Do NOT base your decision to proceed (or not) on any one risk assessment tool (▶R). Instead, use objective testing and specialist opinion instead. The Vascular Quality Initiative

(VQI) perioperative mortality risk score can be considered to inform the patient where appropriate (→2).

OPTIMISATION FOR TREATMENT -
• Once the repair is indicated, refer patients with poor functional capacity or significant risk factors for cardiac workup and optimisation (➡I). Patients with stable coronary artery disease do not need routine revascularisation (➡III). However, unstable coronary disease should be considered for prophylactic preoperative coronary revascularisation (➡IIa).
• Do NOT stop dual antiplatelets after interventional coronary revascularisation to perform AAA repair. Either wait for patients to move onto monotherapy, or consider EVAR under dual antiplatelets (➡IIb).
• Consider checking pulmonary function tests (excluding chest X-ray), renal function tests, nutritional assessment (via serum albumin measurements) prior to surgery (➡I-IIa).
• Do NOT commence patients on β blockers (if not already been on) prior to AAA repair (➡III, ►R). If β blockers are considered of high importance (for example, to treat multiple comorbidites), commence well in advance (→2).
• Commence statins where possible (ideally at least 4 weeks prior) (➡I). Do NOT stop monotherapy antiplatelets prior to surgery (➡I). Do NOT offer remote ischaemic preconditioning to people having AAA repair (►R).
• Commence overnight hydration for non-dialysis patients with renal insufficiency (→1). Maintain hydration (with normal saline or 5% dextrose/sodium bicarbonate) in the perioperative period if EVAR is performed (→1). Hold Metformin before using the contrast if eGFR is <60 mL/min (up to 48h if eGFR <45). Restart Metformin 48h postprocedure if renal functions remain relatively stable (→1).
• In patients with a history of heparin-induced thrombocytopenia, consider using alternative thrombin inhibitor such as bivalirudin or argatroban (→1).

ELECTIVE AAA REPAIR -
• In open AAA repair:

» In patients with <u>long</u> (>10-15 yrs) life expectancy, open abdominal aortic aneurysm repair should be considered as the preferred treatment modality (➡️IIa).

» Consider perioperative epidural analgesia before open repair (➡️IIa, ▶R).

» Consider transverse abdominal incision for patients with significant pulmonary disease (→2).

» Consider cell salvage and retransfusion during surgery (➡️IIa).

» Ensure proximal anastomosis as close to renal artery as possible (➡️I,→1).

» Consider a straight tube graft if no significant iliac disease exists (→1).

» Preserve blood flow to at least one internal iliac artey after finishing the repair ➡️I,→1).

» Only consider inferior mesenteric artery re-implantation in selected cases of suspected insufficient perfusion of pelvic organs with risk of colonic ischaemia (➡️IIb,→1).

» Consider prophylactic mesh insertion during abdominal closure only in high risk patients for incisional hernia (➡️IIb).

» Consider concomitant open surgical treatment of aneurysm and other pathologies (cholecystitis, tumours) if aneurysm not suitable for EVAR (→2).

• In EVAR:

» Ensure radiation safety all the time (➡️I).

» Consider preserving large accessory renal artery (>3mm) or accessory arteries feeding large proportion of kidney (➡️IIb,→2).

• Consider angioplasty and stenting of symptomatic renal artery stenosis or SMA stenosis BEFORE doing EVAR or open repair (→2).

» Preserve blood flow to at least one internal iliac artey (➡️IIb,→1).

• A branched endograft should be considered to achieve this if need be(→1).

• If both internal iliacs need to be occluded, consider sta-

ging this by at least 1-2 weeks (→1).
  - » Do NOT use novel techniques/concepts unless implemented within a proper research framework (➡III).
  - » In most patients with suitable anatomy and <u>reasonable</u> life expectancy, EVAR should be considered as the PREFERRED treatment modality (➡IIa). This applies specificall for patients who have abdominal co-pathology (hostile abdomen, horseshoe kidney or a stoma), anaesthetic risks and/or medical comorbidities, or other considerations, specific to and discussed with the person, that may render open surgery a less suitable option (▶R).

REPAIRING RUPTURED AAA -
- Preparation and decision making -
  - » Evaluate a timeframe of 90min of door-to-intervention (→G).
  - » Obtain thoracoabdominal CTA for stable (➡I) and even relatively unstable (➡IIa) patients with suspected ruptured AAA.
  - » Do NOT repair symptomatic non-ruptured AAA urgently. If possible, repair under more elective conditions (➡I). Consider monitoring those patients in an intensive care unit (ICU) setting with blood products available (→1).
  - » In patients with ruptured abdominal aortic aneurysm and suitable anatomy, endovascular repair is recommended as a <u>firs</u> option (➡I, ▶R, →1). This is especially for men over 70 and women of any age (▶R). Highly consider open repair for men under 70 (▶R).
  - » Use permissive hypotension preferably in conscious patients (➡I,→1).
  - » Do NOT base a palliative decision on age or a scoring system (➡III, ▶R).
- Technique recommendations -
  - » Where possible, use local anaesthetic as a first choice for access to stabilise the patient (with a balloon) or for performing EVAR (➡IIa, ▶R).
  - » Always consider using aortic balloon to stabilise unstable patients undergoing open or EVAR repairs (➡IIa).

» IN EVAR for ruptured AAA -
  • Consider bifurcated graft as a first choice whenever suitable over aorto-uniiliac devices (➨IIa).
  • An over sizing of around 30% may be required.
» Use of intraoperative Heparin remains controversial. Heparin use is perhaps optimal when administered after controlling the aneurysm. Similarly, use mechanical VTE prophylaxis untill risk of bleeding reduces.
• Follow up -
  » Consider using NGT intraoperatively, but only if nausea and distension present postoperatively (→1).
  » Monitor intra-abdominal pressure post open and EVAR repair and act quickly where needed (➨I, ▶R).
    • Perform decompressive laparotomy where medical treatment fails and pressure remains high (>20mmHg), in case of organ failure or if the pressure is very high (>30mmHg) (➨I). Consider using vacuum-assisted closure to manage the wound (➨IIa).

MANAGING LONG TERM OUTCOME -

• Optimise patient atherosclerosis risk factors for all AAA-repaired candidates (➨I). The current average survival is 9 years.
• Treat para-anastomotic aneurysm with endovascular (proximal) or open approach.
• Check and treat any kink or occlusion of graft limb immediately (➨I).
• Inform patients of possible sexual dysfunction following open (53% in one year) and EVAR (17% when covering one internal iliac artery, and 24% when covering both).
• Consider surveillance of patients following OPEN repair every 5 years, using CT or MRI (➨IIb,→2).
• Consider surveillance programme for patients following successful deployment of EVAR, based on their individual risk for EVAR-related complications (▶R):
  » Consider using CTA or colour duplex ultrasound scan for surveillance (▶R), but do not exclude endoleaks based on duplex only (▶R).
  » Consider imaging (with CTA) in 30 days postoperatively

($\rightarrow$I,$\rightarrow$I).

» Low risk group (no endoleak, anatomy within IFU, adequate overlap and seal of ≥10 mm proximal and distal stent graft apposition to arterial wall): consider limited follow up with repeated CT scan in 1 yr ($\rightarrow$I) or 5 years ($\rightarrow$IIb).

» Intermediate risk group (adequate overlap and seal, but presence of Type II endoleak:

• Consider DUS at 6 ($\rightarrow$2) or 12 months ($\rightarrow$IIb) intervals for 24 months then annually thereafter ($\rightarrow$2).

• Patients with sac shrinkage ≥1 cm (even in the presence of a Type II endoleak) can be regarded as low risk.

• If sac increases in size, continue annual surveillance, or (if sac increasing ≥ 1cm per yr) treat as high risk ($\rightarrow$IIb, ▶R).

• Consider further investigations for type 5 endoleak, i.e. continued AAA expansion without radiographic evidence of a leak site (▶R,$\rightarrow$2).

» High risk group (presence of Type I or III endoleak, inadequate overlap or seal < 10 mm).

• Always consider reintervention for type I, III and kinking ($\rightarrow$IIb, ▶R). Consider using open repair if endovascular intervention fails ($\rightarrow$2).

• Consider intervention for type II if sac is expanding (▶R,$\rightarrow$1). Repeat scans as required and re-evaluate.

Managing Juxta-renal AAA -

• Consider repair when the 5.5cm threshold is reached ($\rightarrow$IIb). consider using open repair or complex endovascular repair based on patient's features and large centre team experience ($\rightarrow$IIa).

• Fenestrated EVAR are currently the prefered first method, where feasible ($\rightarrow$IIa). Ensure the patient is fully aware of the lack of clarity regarding perioperative survival or long-term outcomes, as compared with open surgical repair (▶R).

• Alternatively (especially in emergency setting), consider

using parallel graft technique (<u>Chimneys</u>) (➡️IIb). Apply same principles for ruptured cases (➡️IIb).

- Do NOT use other methods as a first line or outside of a research programme (➡️III).
- Follow up patients more extensively, with annual CTA for example (➡️I).

MANAGING ILIAC ARTERY ANEURYSM -

- Consider repairing common, external or internal iliac aneurysms when reaching 3.5cm or above (➡️IIB). They rarely ruptured when <4 cm and most ruptured cases are usually present from size >5cm.
- Enter patients with iliac aneurysm into surveillance programme. For example, every three years for a diameter 2.0-2.9 cm, and annually for 3.0-3.4 cm.
- Consider endovascular repair as a first option, where possible (➡️IIb). Always strive to keep at least one internal iliac artery in open or endovascular repair (➡️I), or at least preserve the distal collateral circulation to pelvis (➡️I).
- Follow up patients using the same AAA follow up principles.

MANAGING MYCOTIC ANEURYSM -

- By definition, mycotic aneurysms (or primary infected aortic aneurysms) result from septic emboli to the aortic vasa vasorum, by haematogenous spread or by direct extension, leading to an infectious degeneration of the arterial wall and aneurysm formation.
- Diagnosis should combine clinical, laboratory, and imaging parameters (➡️I).
- Start IV antibiotics against Staph aureous and G -ve rods (➡️I). Consider continuing antibiotics for 6-12 months (➡️IIa).
- Repair of the aneurysm should be considered regardless of the size (➡️I). Use EVAR or open surgery as appropriate, both are acceptable (➡️IIa).

MANAGING INFLAMMATORY ANEURYSM -

- By definition, inflammatory AAA is the unusually thickened aneurysm wall, associated with shiny white peri-aneurysmal and retroperitoneal fibrosis, and dense adhesions of adjacent intra-abdominal structures.

- Aetiology remains widely unknown. Autoimmunity is likely to be involved.
- Adjacent organs might be entrapped. Other parts of the aorta may also be involved.
- Acute phase reactants (ESR, CRP) alone are not reliable for management and follow up.
- Consider using anti-inflamm tory medications (➡️IIa). These include corticosteroids, immunosuppressive agents (azathioprine and methotrexate), and tamoxifen.
- Consider surgical repair using same criteria as elective AAA: 5.5cm diameter, with suitable anatomy, use EVAR where possible (➡️IIs).
- Consider using a retroperitoneal approach for open infla - matory aneurysm repair, a horseshoe kidney, or an aortic aneurysm in the presence of a hostile abdomen (→1).

MANAGING ACUTE AORTIC SYNDROME (AORTIC ULCER, PSEUDOANEURYSM, INTRAMURAL HAEMATOMA, LOCAL DISSECTION, AND SACCULAR ANEURYSM)-

- Optimise medical management, including blood pressure, in all acute aortic syndrome cases (➡️I).
- Apply serial imaging surveillance for uncomplicated aortic ulcers, intramural haematoma, and local dissection (➡️I). Once symptomatic or complicated, a repair is indicated (➡️I). Consider endovascular approaches where possible (➡️IIa).
- Consider early intervention for saccular AAA (➡️IIb,→2).

MANAGING CONCOMITTENT MALIGNANCY -

- Do not repair AAA prophylactically when below threshold (➡️III).
- A staged repair, starting with EVAR (where possible) to the large or symptomatic AAA, is recommended (➡️I).
- Consider prolonged (up to 4 weeks) prophylactic LMWH postoperatively (IIa).

Long-term outcome from EVAR I Trial

A 15-YR FOLLOW UP RESULTS OF RANDOMISED TRIAL 2016

AT A GLANCE
- The EVAR trial 16 previously reported aneurysm-related mortality and total mortality up to 10 years of follow-up. This is a 15 years follow up analysis.

MAIN RESULTS
- EVAR has an early survival benefit but an inferior late survival compared with open repair (Early gain but late pain).
- At 0–6 months after randomisation, EVAR pts had lower mortality (adjusted HR 0.61).
- Beyond 8 years of follow-up, open-repair had a significantl lower mortality (adjusted HR 1.25)
- Aneurysm-related mortality in EVAR group after 8 years was mainly attributable to secondary aneurysm sac rupture (Adjusted HR 5.82), and increased cancer mortality also observed in the EVAR group (Adjusted HR 1.87)
- Rate of reinterventions remained higher in EVAR throughout follow-up (1st one could occur after 5 years).

REFERENCES:
- Lancet. 2016 Nov 12; 388 (10058): 2366-2374. PMID: 27743617

Surgery for small (4-5.5cm) asymptomatic AAA

A COCHRANE SYS REVIEW 2015

AT A GLANCE

- Systematic Review of Four trials (3314 pts): UK Small Aneurysm Trial (UKSAT), the Aneurysm Detection and Management (ADAM) trial, the Comparison of Surveillance Versus Aortic Endografting for Small Aneurysm Repair (CAESAR) trial, and the Positive Impact of Endovascular Options for treating Aneurysms Early (PIVOTAL) trial.

MAIN RESULTS

- No advantage of early repair for small AAA.
- Early survival benefit (i.e. no operative death) is clear in surveillance group but no significa t differences in long-term survival (adjusted hazard ratio (HR) 0.76-1.21
- Mortality at one year (CAESAR and PIVOTAL only) and six years (UKSAT and ADAM only) revealed a non-significant association (Peto odds ratio at one year 1.15, and at six years 1.11).

REFERENCES:

- Cochrane review 2015. PMID: 25927098

AAA Screening Recommnedations

A Sys Review Of Guidelines

At a glance
- Seven guidelines included.

Main Results
- All seven guidelines contained a recommendation for one-time screening of elderly men by ultrasonography to select AAAs ≥ 5.5 cm for elective surgical repair.
- Four guidelines, of which three were less rigorously developed, contained disparate recommendations on screening of women and middle-aged men at elevated risk.
- There was no agreement on the management of smaller AAAs.

References:
- J Vasc Surg. 2012 May;55(5):1296-1304. PMID: 21324630

Factors Affecting Growth and Rupture of Small AAA

A SYS REVIEW 2012

AT A GLANCE
- 18 studies included (15 475 people).

MAIN RESULTS
- Mean aneurysm growth rate was 2.21 mm/year, independent of age and sex.
- Growth rate was increased in smokers (by 0.35 mm/year) and decreased in patients with diabetes (by 0.51 mm/year).
- Mean arterial pressure had no effect and antihypertensive or other cardioprotective medications had only small, non-significant effects on aneurysm growth.
- Calendar year of enrollment was not associated with growth rate.
- Rupture rates were almost fourfold higher in women than men, double in current smokers, and increased with higher blood pressure.

REFERENCES:
- Br J Surg. 2012 May;99(5):655-65. PMID: 22389113

EVAR or Open for elective AAA

A META-ANALYSIS OF RCTs 2013

AT A GLANCE

- 4 key RCTs and 2 large datasets included
- Total of 1393 EVAR+1390 Open cases with elective AAA:
  - » French Anévrysme de l'aorte abdominale trial
  - » Chirurgie versus Endoprothèse (ACE) trial
  - » Open Versus Endovascular Repair (OVER) Veterans Affairs Cooperative Study
  - » UK EndoVascular Aneurysm Repair (EVAR1) trial
  - » Dutch Randomized Endovascular Aneurysm Management (DREAM) trial.
- Additionally, over 50,000 cases from non-randomised trials analysed.

MAIN RESULTS

- EVAR patients had significan ly lower 30-day or in-hospital mortality rate (1·3% vs. 4·7% for open; odds ratio (OR) 0·36).
- By 2-year: no difference in all-cause mortality (14·3 versus 15·2%; OR 0·87), and no significant difference in aneurysm-related mortality.
- After at least 4 years: no difference (35 versus 34%; OR 1·11).
- A significantly higher proportion of patients undergoing EVAR required reintervention (P = 0·003) and suffered aneurysm rupture (P < 0·001).

REFERENCES:

- Br J Surg. 2013 Jun;100(7):863-72. PMID: 23475697

EVAR or Open for elective AAA

A Cochrane Sys Review 2014

At a glance

- 5 key RCTs (4 EVAR vs Open and 1 EVAR vs No intervention)-
- Total of 2790+404 pts: ACE, OVER, EVAR1, DREAM, and EVAR2.

Main Results

- EVAR patients had significan ly lower 30-day or in-hospital mortality rate (1·4% vs. 4·2% for open; odds ratio 0·33).
- Up to 4 years: no difference in mortality (16% versus 17%; OR 0.92).
- Similar incidences of cardiac deaths (OR 1.14), and fatal stroke (OR 0.81).
- Long-term reintervention rate significantly higher in EVAR (OR 1.98) – This should be interpreted with caution due to significant heterogeneity.
- Operative complications, health-related quality of life and sexual dysfunction were generally comparable between the EVAR and OSR groups.
- Pulmonary complications occurred more in open surgery (OR 0.36).

References:

- Cochrane Database Syst Rev. 2014 Jan 23;(1):CD004178. PMID: 24453068

Health-related Quality of Life Outcome for EVRA vs. Open for elective AAA

A Sys Review & Meta-Analysis 2015

At a glance
- 18 studies - total of 13,281 pts.

Main Results
- SF-36 general health scores: higher for EVAR at 3, 6, and 12 months.
- SF-36 physical functioning scores: higher for EVAR at 6 months but advantage lost at 12 months.
- SF-36 social functioning scores: higher for EVAR at 12 months.
- SF-36 component summary scores: not significantly di erent.
- EVAR was associated with a better EQ-5D score at 3, 6, and 12 months, but not at 24 months of follow-up.

References:
- J Vasc Surg. 2015 Aug;62(2):491-8. PMID: 26211382

EVAR or Open for ruptured AAA

A Cochrane Sys Review 2017

At a glance
- 4 RCTs included
- Total of 868 patients with rAAA: AJAX (Amesterdam), IMPROVE (UK), Hincliffe (2006), and ECAR (France).

Main Results
- No difference in 30-day mortality between rEVAR and open repair.
- Not enough information was provided on complications to make a well-informed conclusion, although it is possible that eEVAR is associated with a reduction in bowel ischaemia.
- Long-term data were lacking for both survival and late complications.

References:
- Cochrane Database Syst Rev. 2017 May 26. PMID: 28548204

EVAR or Open for ruptured AAA

A META-ANALYSIS 2015

AT A GLANCE

- 3 RCTs included - total of 836 patients with rAAA: AJAX (Amesterdam), IMPROVE (UK), and ECAR (France).

MAIN RESULTS

- Mortality rate: 32% for EVAR vs. 34% for open at 30 days, and 35% and 38% respectively at 90 days.
- No evidence of significant heterogeneity in the odds ratios between trials.
- No significant effect modification with age or Hardman index, but early benefit from E AR for women.
- Discharge from the primary hospital was faster after EVAR (hazard ratio 1.24).

REFERENCES:

- Br J Surg. 2015 Sep; 102(10): 1229–1239. PMID: 26104471

Diagnosis for Aortic Graft Infection (AGI)

A COLLABORATIVE CRITERIA 2016

AT A GLANCE

- Expert review form the Management of Aortic Graft Infection Collaboration [MAGIC].

MAIN RESULTS

- AGI is suspected where 1 Major + >2 minor same-category criteria. Diagnosis is made with 1 Major + 1 minor different-category criteria.
  1. Clinical/surgical – major: intraoperative peri-graft pus or direct communication with nonsterile site (fistulae, exposed grafts, mycotic aneurysm); minor - localized AGI features or fever where AGI is most likely.
  2. Radiological - major perigraft gas volume, perigraft gas (>7wk) or fluid ≥3 mo); minor - other CT features; or evidence from alternative imaging.
  3. Laboratory - major isolation of microorganisms from perigraft aspirates or explanted grafts; minor - +ve blood cultures or inflammatory indices with no alternative source

REFERENCES:

- Eur J Vasc Endovasc Surg (2016) 52, 758e763. PMID: 27771318

Transverse vs. Midline Incisions

A COCHRANE SYS REVIEW 2005

AT A GLANCE

- All prospective randomised trials comparing midline with transverse incisions for abdominal surgery included.
- Caesarian sections were excluded.

MAIN RESULTS

- Despite the limitations, and potentially significant biases related to methodological quality, evidence suggests that a transverse or oblique incision may be less painful than a midline.
- Transverse incision have less impact on pulmonary function than a midline incision, particularly in the early postoperative period.
- There was no difference seen in early or late postoperative complications
- Recovery times were similar.

REFERENCES:

- Cochrane Database Syst Rev. 2005 Oct 19;(4):CD005199. PMID: 16235395

Percutaneous EVAR

A Cochrane Sys Review 2017

At a glance
- 2 RCT - total of 181 patients: percutaneous vs. standard femoral artery access.

Main Results
- No significant difference in mortality between groups (one mortality occurring overall in percutaneous group).
- No wound infections occurred in the cut-down femoral artery access group or the percutaneous group across either study (moderate-quality evidence).
- No difference in major complication rate or in bleeding complications and haematoma between groups.
- Only one study reported long-term complication rates at six months, with no differences between groups.
- Surgery time: significantly faster in percut group (mean difference -31.46 minutes
- One study reported duration of ITU (intensive treatment unit) and hospital stay, with no difference found between groups.

References:
- Cochrane Database Syst Rev. 2017 Feb 21;2. PMID: 28221665

Treatment for Type II Endoleak

Sys Review & Meta-Analysis 2018

At a glance
- 59 studies (1073 patients) included.
- Investigating the clinical outcomes of different type II endoleak treatments in patients with a persistent type II endoleak after EVAR.

Main Results
- Peri-operative complications: 3.8%.
- AAA related mortality: 1.8%
- Overall technical success: 87.9%
- Overall clinical success: 68.4%
- Decrease or stable sac, with or without resolution, was achieved in 78.4% .
- Little evidence supporting the efficacy of secondary intervention for type II endoleaks after EVAR.

References:
- Eur J Vasc Endovasc Surg. 2018 Dec;56(6):794-807. PMID: 30104089

Juxta-renal Aneurysm Repair

SYS REVIEW & META-ANALYSIS 2019

AT A GLANCE

- 214 studies (1506 endovascular, 3615 open) included.

MAIN RESULTS

- Patients undergoing endovascular repair were older, more likely to be men, and more likely to have diabetes, coronary artery disease, and chronic kidney disease.
- Endovascular repair was associated with significantly decreased 30-day mortality (OR, 0.50). This remained significant when including only fenestrated EVAR (OR, 0.55).
- Endovascular repair resulted in a significantly decreased incidence of acute renal failure (OR, 0.50), increased incidence of spinal cord ischemia (OR, 3.14), a decreased incidence of bowel ischemia (OR, 0.50), and decreased length of stay (mean difference, -5.99 days).
- Long-term survival (1-7 years of follow-up) - 8 studies found no significant differences between groups; one study found improved long-term survival in the open repair group.
- Reinterventions during follow-up were increased in the endovascular group.

REFERENCES:

- J Vasc Surg. 2019 Dec;70(6):2054-2064.e3. PMID: 31327612

CHAPTER 4
THORACIC
AORTIC
PATHOLOGIES

DESCENDING AORTIC DISSECTION AND ACUTE AORTIC SYNDROME

TEVAR vs. Best Med Therapy for Aortic Dissection

NATIONAL INPATIENT SAMPLE (NATIONAL DATABASE) 2014

AT A GLANCE
- 4706 pts studied
- Treatment options included TEVAR (504) and medical management (4202).

MAIN RESULTS
- Adjusted in-hospital mortality was similar for both the groups (8.5% and 10.3% for TEVAR and medical management respectively, P = .224).
- TEVAR carried higher risk of stroke (odds ratio [OR] = 1.61) and prolonged LOS (12 vs 5.6 days), with patients less likely to be discharged home (OR 0.73).
- When stratified by age, outcomes were similar between the 2 groups.

REFERENCES:
- Endovasc Surg 2014; 48:230-3. PMID: 28221665

Management for Acute Type B Aortic Dissection

A Sys Review & Meta-Analysis 2014

At a glance

- Endovascular repair (TEVAR): 2,531 patients; open surgical repair: 1,276 patients; conservative medical management: 2,347 patients.

Main Results

- TEVAR -
  - » Pooled rate for 30-day/in-hospital mortality: 7.3%.
  - » Pooled estimates for cerebrovascular events, spinal cord ischemia (SCI) and total neurologic events were 3.9%, 3.1% and 7.3%, respectively.
- Open surgical repair -
  - » Pooled rate for 30-day/in-hospital mortality:19.0%.
  - » Pooled rate for cerebrovascular events was 6.8%, for SCI 3.3% and for total neurologic complications 9.8%.
- Acute uncomplicated type B dissection treated with conservative medical management -
  - » Pooled 30-day/in-hospital mortality rate was 2.4%.
  - » Pooled rate for cerebrovascular events was 1%, for SCI 0.8% and for overall neurologic complications 2%.

References:

- Ann Cardiothorac Surg. 2014 May; 3(3): 234–246. PMID: 24967162

TEVAR vs. Best Med Therapy for Aortic Dissection

SYS REVIEW 2018

AT A GLANCE

- A total of 1,960 patients (64.3 years; 75.8% male) included from six studies (one prospective and five retrospective).
- Study outcomes included short (1 month), intermediate (1 year), and mid-term (2-5 year) all-cause mortality.
- Additional outcomes included aortic dilation and rupture at 1 year.

MAIN RESULTS

- No difference observed in short-term (odd ratio [OR] 0.73), intermediate (OR 0.99), or mid-term all-cause mortality (OR 1.12).
- No difference in aortic dilation with either modality was noted at 1-year (OR 1.11).
- TEVAR was associated with a significantly lower 1-year risk of aortic rupture (OR 2.49).

REFERENCES:

- Catheter Cardiovasc Interv 2018 May 1;91(6):1138-1143. PMID: 29152822

TEVAR vs. Best Med Therapy for Aortic Dissection

SYS REVIEW 2018

AT A GLANCE
- 62 studies were eligible and analysed.

MAIN RESULTS
- Complicated cases treated acutely: 30-day or in-hospital mortality was 7.3% when managed by endovascular means, and 19.0% when subjected to open repair.
- Acute uncomplicated type B dissection - conservative management:
  » pooled 30-day or in-hospital mortality rate was 2.4%.
  » Survival rates at 5 years averaged at 60%.
  » Freedom from any aortic event ranged from 34.0% to 83.9%.
- Chronic complicated type B dissection:
  » Rates of stroke, paraplegia and operative mortality following endovascular repair ranged from 5% to 13%, 2% to 13% and 2 to 13%, respectively.
  » 5-year survival rates after open repair ranged from 60% to 90%.
- Chronic uncomplicated type B dissection:
  » 90% of patients survive initial hospitalization and were subjected to medical management. 5-year survival of 50-80%.
  » up to 20-55% of medically treated patients develop aneurysmal degeneration after 5 years with an unknown risk of rupture.

REFERENCES:
- J Vis Surg. 2018 Mar 23;4:59. PMID: 27175814

Predictors of Aortic Growth in Dissection

SYS REVIEW 2014

AT A GLANCE
- 18 articles (1698 pts) on natural history vs. risk factors of dissection reviewed.

MAIN RESULTS
- **Factors associated with increased aortic growth**:
  - » Age <60 years, white race, and Marfan syndrome
  - » High fibrinoge -fibrin degradation product level (≥20 μg/mL) at admission
  - » Aortic diameter ≥40 mm on initial imaging, fusiform dilated proximal descending aorta
  - » Proximal descending thoracic aorta false lumen (FL) diameter ≥22 mm, elliptic formation of the true lumen, patent FL, partially thrombosed FL, FL located at the inner aortic curvature, and saccular formation of the FL
  - » Presence of one entry tear, large entry tear (≥10 mm) located in the proximal part of the dissection
  - » Areas with ulcer-like projections
- **Factors associated with reduced aortic growth**:
  - » Tight heart rate control (<60 beats/min)
  - » Use of calcium-channel blockers
  - » Thrombosed FL, FL located at the outer aortic curvature
  - » Two or more entry tears
  - » Circular configuration of the true lume

REFERENCES:
- J Vasc Surg. 2014 Apr;59(4):1134-43. PMID: 24661897

Stenting vs. Medical Therapy in Dissection

THE ADSORBE TRIAL 2014

AT A GLANCE

- A randomized European study comparing endoluminal stent grafting (using GORE TAG device) and best medical therapy (BMT) to BMT alone in the treatment of acute uncomplicated type B aortic dissection.
- 31 patients were randomised to the BMT group and 30 to the BMT+TAG group.
- Patients had acute (<14d) aortic dissection

MAIN RESULTS

- No death in first 30days, but 3 cross overs from BMT to Stenting.
- At 1yr: 2 pts needed TEVAR from BMT. One death in BMT+Stent.
- Incomplete False lumen remained in 43% and 97% of BMT/Stent vs. BMT.
- True lumen increased in BMT/stent vs no change in BMT.
- Transverse diameter deceased in BMT/stent but unchanged in BMT
- Conclusion: Uncomplicated AD can be safely treated with the Gore TAG device. Remodelling with thrombosis of the false lumen and reduction of its diameter is induced by the stent graft, but long term results are needed.

REFERENCES:

- Eur J Vasc Endovasc Surg. 2014 Sep;48(3):285-91. PMID: 24962744

Stenting in Type B Acute Aortic Dissection

THE MEDTRONIC DISSESCTION TRIAL 2015

AT A GLANCE

- Prospective, nonrandomized, United States Food and Drug Administration-regulated, pivotal trial
- Fifty patients were enrolled. Mean age was 57 years.

MAIN RESULTS

- Rupture in 20%; malperfusion in 86%; Mean time from symptom onset to procedure 4.7 days
- Successful deployment and coverage of the primary entry tear - achieved in all. Two patients (4%) underwent open repair 5 and 56 days postprocedure for retrograde aortic dissections.
- 30d mortality - 8%; 12-month mortality was 15%.
- Spinal ischemia - 6%. Serious adverse events – (in 48%) within 12 months.
- In 12 months, true lumen diameter in stented region remained stable or increased.
- False lumen diameter remained stable or decreased in 22 patients and partially or completely thrombosed in 91%

REFERENCES:

- Ann Thorac Surg. 2015 Sep;100(3):802-8. PMID: 26209487

Stenting vs. Medical Therapy in Type B Aortic Dissection

THE INSTEAD-XL STUDY 2013

AT A GLANCE
- RCT
- 140 patients.

MAIN RESULTS
- All-cause mortality (11.1% vs 19.3%; P=0.13), aorta-specific mortality (6.9% vs 19.3%; P=0.04), and progression (27.0% vs 46.1%; P=0.04) after 5 years was lower with TEVAR than with optimal medical treatment alone.
- Both improved survival and less progression of disease at 5 years after elective TEVAR were associated with stent graft induced false lumen thrombosis in 90.6% of cases (P<0.0001).

REFERENCES:
- Circ Cardiovasc Interv. 2013 Aug;6(4):407-16. PMID: 23922146

Outcome of Stenting in Chronic Aortic Dissection

SYS REVIEW 2011

AT A GLANCE
- 17 studies (567 patients).

MAIN RESULTS
- Technical success rate - 89.9%
- Mid-term mortality was 9.2% with a median follow-up of 24 months.
- 8.1% pts developed endoleak, predominantly type I. Re-intervention rates ranged from 0- 60% (median follow-up of 31 mo).
- 7.8% of patients developed aneurysms of distal aorta or continued false lumen perfusion with aneurysmal dilatation.
- Rare complications included delayed retrograde type A dissection (0.67%), aorto-oesophageal fistula (0.22%) and neurological complications (paraplegia 0.45%; stroke 1.5%).

REFERENCES:
- Eur J Vasc Endovasc Surg. 2011 Nov;42(5):632-47. PMID: 21880515

Outcome of Open Repair in Chronic Aortic Dissection

SYS REVIEW 2011

AT A GLANCE

- 17 studies (567 patients).

MAIN RESULTS

- Technical success rate - 89.9%
- Mid-term mortality was 9.2% with a median follow-up of 24 months.
- 8.1% pts developed endoleak, predominantly type I. Re-intervention rates ranged from 0- 60% (median follow-up of 31 mo).
- 7.8% of patients developed aneurysms of distal aorta or continued false lumen perfusion with aneurysmal dilatation.
- Rare complications included delayed retrograde type A dissection (0.67%), aorto-oesophageal fistula (0.22%) and neurological complications (paraplegia 0.45%; stroke 1.5%).

REFERENCES:

- Eur J Vasc Endovasc Surg. 2011 Nov;42(5):632-47. PMID: 21880515

Outcome of Open Repair in Chronic Aortic Dissection

Sys Review 2014

At a glance
- 19 studies (970 patients).

Main Results
- Pooled short-term mortality - 11.1% overall, and 7.5% in the nine contemporary studies.
- Stroke, spinal cord ischemia, renal dysfunction, and reoperation for bleeding were 5.9%, 4.9%, 8.1%, and 8.1%, respectively, for the contemporary series.
- Absolute late reintervention - 13.3% (11.3% in contemporary series).
- Aggregated survival at 1-, 3-, 5-, and 10-years of all patients - 82.1%, 74.1%, 66.3%, and 50.8%, respectively.

References:
- Ann cardiothorac Surg. 2014 Jul;3(4):340-50. PMID: 25133097

Ruling out Aortic Dissection by using Risk Score+D-dimer

SYS REVIEW 2020

AT A GLANCE

- This review aims at validating the integration of aortic dissection detection risk score (ADD-RS) with D-dimer (DD) to rule out acute aortic syndrome.
- 4 articles (including a total of 3,804 patients)
- Aortic Dissection Detection Risk Score (ADD-RS):
  - » High-risk conditions
    - ◊ Marfan syndrome
    - ◊ Family history of aortic disease
    - ◊ Known aortic valve disease
    - ◊ Recent aortic manipulation
    - ◊ Known thoracic aortic aneurysm
  - » High-risk pain features: Chest, back, or abdominal pain:
    - ◊ Abrupt in onset
    - ◊ Severe in intensity
    - ◊ Ripping or tearing in quality
  - » High-risk exam features:
    - ◊ Pulse deficit or systolic B   differential
    - ◊ Focal neurologic deficit (with pain
    - ◊ Murmur of aortic insufficiency (ne   , with pain)
    - ◊ Hypotension or shock state

MAIN RESULTS

- Pooled sensitivity was 99.9% for ADD-RS = 0 and DD < 500 ng/mL, 98.9% for ADD-RS ≤ 1 and DD < 500 ng/mL, and 97.6% for ADD-RS ≤ 1 and DD < DDage-adj .
- Integration of ADD-RS = 0 or ≤ 1 with DD < 500 ng/mL shows consistently high sensitivity across studies, thus supporting reliability for diagnostic rule-out of AASs.

REFERENCES:

- Acad Emerg Med. 2020 Mar 18. PMID: 32187432

THORACIC AORTIC ANEURYSM

Open vs. TEVAR for Descending Thoracic Aneurysm

Sys Review & Meta-Analysis 2019

At a glance

- 14,580 patients were analysed in total of 13 articles
- 10,672 patients had open repair, and 3,908 patients had endovascular repair.

Main Results

- Patients undergoing open repair were younger, and had more elective repair
- Duration of intensive care and total hospital stay was much shorter in endovascular patients (4.5 vs. 8.5 days)
- Postoperative stroke was similar in both groups.
- Higher rate of paraplegia noted in open repair group
- Rate of renal failure and cardiac complications was higher in open repair group.
- Rate of vascular complications was much higher in the endovascular group of patients (5.29% vs. 1.17%).
- Operative mortality was higher in endovascular procedures (4.4% vs. 3.2%);
- The 1- and 5-year mortality showed no statistical difference between the endovascular and open repair groups (22.19%, vs. 24.04%, and 44.26% vs. 37.37%).

References:

- Ann Vasc Surg. 2019 Jan;54:304-315. PMID: 30081163

Open vs. TEVAR for Descending Thoracic Aneurysm

SYS REVIEW & META-ANALYSIS 2017

AT A GLANCE
- 22702 patients were analyzed in total of 27 articles.

MAIN RESULTS
- TEVAR had lower 30-day mortality in ruptured (OR, 0.58) and intact (OR, 0.6) aneurysms.
- Paraplegia or spinal cord ischemia (OR, 0.35) and pulmonary complications (OR, 0.41) were reduced in patients undergoing TEVAR
- Sstroke risk was not statistically significant
- Pooled mean difference in length of hospital and ICU stay was lower for TEVAR by -5.17 days
- Three studies showed that compared with open repair, a hybrid approach reduced hospital stay (pooled mean difference, -8.83 days) and ICU stay (pooled mean difference, -3.17 days).

REFERENCES:
- Vasc Surg. 2017 Oct;66(4):1258-1268. PMID: 28756047

Open vs. TEVAR for Reuptured Descending Thoracic Aneurysm

SYS REVIEW & META-ANALYSIS 2010

AT A GLANCE

- •28 studies (224 pts). 64% TEVAR vs 36% Open.

MAIN RESULTS

- TEVAR had significant lower 30-d mortality rate (19% vs 33%), and insignificant lower MI rate, stroke, and paraplegia.
- Late rupture occurred more commonly after TEVAR.
- Estimated 3-yr survival following TEVAR: 70%.

REFERENCES:

- J Vasc Surg. 2010 Apr;51(4):1026-32. PMID: 20347700

CHAPTER 5
VISCERAL
ARTERIES
ANEURYSMS

Basic Facts and Figures

AT A GLANCE

- Rare – renal 0.01% and splanchic 0.1-2%
- Treatment is generally indicated in:
  - » Symptomatic
  - » Aneurysms >2cm
  - » Progression of >0.5cm/yr
  - » Presence in pregnant women or childbearing age
  - » In pts having orthotpic liver transplantation
- Guidelines –
  - » American College of cardiology (level B evidence)
  - » European Society of Cardiology
- Trials –
  - » None. Only case series

Natural History for Visceral AAs

Study	Treatment	Outcome
Pitton 2015	253 patients with VAA	* mean overall size of VAAs was 16.1 ± 9.8 mm. * no difference between diameters of ruptured aneurysms vs. non-ruptured aneurysms (14.8 mm vs. 16.3 mm). *23% needed emergency treatment. Mortality 6%. *after >18mo FU: no aneurysm-related death. 30% death from other reasons.
Buck 2016	6234 renal artery aneurysm repairs between 1988 and 2011	* In-hospital mortality 1.8% endo vs. 0.9% open vs. 6% for nephrectomy *complication 11% endo vs. 13% open.
Klausner 2015	865 patients with renal AAs monitor for a mean of 49 months	* 75% asymptomatic. * symptoms: difficult-to-control hypertension, flank pain, haematuria, and abdominal pain. *Operation complication 10% * rupture occurred in 3 pts only. with no acute complications. *Aneurysm growth rate: 0.086 cm/y

Outcome of Treatment

STUDY	TREATMENT	OUTCOME
J Vasc Surg 2011	185 Cases in 176 pts. Endovascular treatment of visceral artery aneurysms and pseudoaneurysms. Location: splenic artery 35%, hepatic 30%, gastroduodenal 15%, pancreaticoduodenal 9%, superior mesenteric 3%, gastric 2%, celiac 2%, gastroepiploic 2%, inferior mesenteric 1%, middle colic artery 0.5%	*Initial intervention success rate: 98% *Bleeding was indication in 46% of cases. *Reintervention required in 3% within 30d. * Coiling used alone in 75% and in combination with at least one other technique in 11%. * 30d aneurysm-related mortality: 3.4%.
J Vasc Interv Radiol. 2012 Jul	50 Cases in 176 pts. *Elective coil embolization of splenic artery aneurysm (SAA) *A total of 63 SAAs treated (size, 13-97 mm; mean, 29 mm).	*Initial intervention success rate: 98% *Reintervention required in 9% within 125d. *splenic infarction: 9%. * 30d aneurysm-related mortality: 0%.
Koganemaru 2014	23 patients with visceral aneurysms	Success rate 96% Splenic infarct 4%
Balderi 2012	30 patients with true or false aneurysms	100% success rate 8pts had visceral ischaemia. 1pt died
Kunzle 2013	19 patients with emergency or elective visceral aneurysms	Mortality 11%. Stent patency rate 18% (28mo FU).

Outcome of Treatment 2

STUDY	TREATMENT	OUTCOME
Roberts 2015	47 patients with emergency bleeding visceral aneurysms	Success rate 83% Reintervention in 4% 30d Mortality 17%
Ghariani 2013	78 Visceral aneu-rysms in 60 pt. Open repair	Hospital Mortality 1.7% Reintervention 8% Survival rate 97% at 5yrs
Lakin 2011	128 patients with splenic AA. Open vs Endo vs Conserv.	*Mean size 2.9cm for endo, 4.4cm for Open and 1.7cm for conservative * operative mortality after rupture 28% *mean growth rate 0.2mm/yr *10-yr survival 90%.
Shukla 2015	181 patients re-paired: 77 ruptured, 104 intact	* rVAAs were smaller than the iVAAs (20.7 mm vs 27.5 mm * Endovascular 1st in 68% * Perioperative complication rate higher for rVAAs (13.7% vs 1% for iVAAs; P = .003), *mortality at 30 days (13% vs 0%). * mortality at 1 year: 33% vs 4.1%. reintervention rate higher for rVAAs: 7.7% vs 19.5% for iVAAs

Laparoscopic Repair for VAAs?

STUDY	TREATMENT	OUTCOME
Tiberio 2012	29 patients: 14 open and 15 laparoscopic repair of splenic AAs * All had aneurysmectomy with splenic artery ligature or direct anastomosis	* Conversion rate 14% *Laparoscopy associated with shorter procedures and lower morbidity (25 % vs. 64 %). *Laparoscopy associated with quicker resumption of oral diet, earlier drain removal, and shorter hospital stay.

Splenic Artery Aneurysm (SAA) Treatment Outcome?

SYS REVIEW 2014

AT A GLANCE

- 1321 with true SAA.

MAIN RESULTS

- Open (OP) repair 39%- Endovascular (EV) 30%- Conservative (CON) 32%.
- OP needed more in ruptured cases.
- OP had higher 30-day mortality than EV (5.1% vs 0.6%; P < .001).
- Minor complications occurred in a larger number of EV patients.
- EV required more reinterventions per year (3.2%) compared with OPEN (0.5%) and CONS (1.2%; P < .001).
- Late mortality rate higher in patients treated with CONS (4.9% vs 2.1% in OPEN and 1.4% in EV; P = .04).

REFERENCES:

- J Vasc Surg. 2014 Dec;60(6):1667-76. PMID: 25264364

CHAPTER 6
VENOUS
DISEASES

Summary of Current Surgical Guidelines for Venous insufficiency & Deep Venous diseases

▶ NICE GUIDELINES 2020 (UK)
➡ ESVS CLINICAL PRACTICE GUIDELINES 2015 (EU)
→ SOCIETY FOR VASCULAR SURGERY GUIDLINES 2011 (USA)

CHRONIC VENOUS INSUFFICIENCY (CVI):

ON DEFINITIONS AND INCIDENCE-

- CVI is the impairment of venous return in the lower limbs, presenting with a broad clinical spectrum, including varicose veins, skin changes, and venous ulceration.
- In most cases, CVI results from an obstruction to venous flo , dysfunction of venous valves, and/ or failure of the venous pump. This results in an abnormal direction of the venous blood flow from the deep to the superficial system, with resultant local tissue anoxia, inflammation, white cell trapping, and occasionally, necrosis. The resulting 'subcutaneous fibrosin panniculitis' obstructs further the proximal lymphatic and venous flo .
- CVI affects 7– 9% of population.
  ▷ Varicose veins affect 7% of men and 16% of women aged 18– 64 yrs.
  ▷ Telangiectasis and reticular veins occur in 80– 85% of both genders.
  ▷ Ankle oedema is present in 7% of men and 16% women.
  ▷ Venous leg ulcers (active or healed) occur in 1% of the population.
- Most venous leg ulcers require an average of 1yr to heal satisfactorily, 20% require >2yrs, and 66% of patients complain of episodes of ulceration for >5yrs.
- The cost of care for chronic venous disease accounts for ~1– 3% of the total health care budget in developed countries.
- Approximately one-third of patients show progression of disease over time, and in 95% of the patients the changes are noted after 6 months or more. The progression rate from varicose veins to CVI is estimated at 4% per year. (➡R)

ON RISKS AND PREVENTION -

- Risk factors for venous insufficiency include multiple pregnancies (RR×1.2 after two pregnancies), age, obesity in women (RR ×1.3), and a history of phlebitis or venous thrombosis.

ON DIAGNOSIS -

- Diagnosis is primarily based on thorough clinical history, detailed physical examination (➥I), and appropriate use of invasive and noninvasive investigations.
- Duplex scanning— (B- mode USS combined with wave Doppler scan) is the investigation of choice for CVI (➥I).
  - » Use the following cut off values in diagnosing venous insufficiency: retrograde flow lasting
    - ▷ more than 0.5s in superficial venous system, deep femoral vein, and calf veins
    - ▷ more than 1s in the common femoral vein, femoral vein, and popliteal vein
    - ▷ more than 0.35s in perforating veins.
- Consider phlebography, CTV or MRV in cases where other diagnostic tools are inconclusive (such as in the diagnosis of abdominal/pelvic vein diseases) (➥IIa).
- Disease severity is assessed using one of the following (➥IIa):
  - » CEAP classification: widely accepted as the best available (and most widely used) classification system. This system is most widely used and should be used by investigators reporting on CVD.
  - » Venous Clinical Severity Score (VCSS): A total of 10 clinical characteristics are evaluated and graded from absent (score 0) to severe (score 3), with a total of 30 points attributable.
  - » Venous Segmental Disease Score (VSDS): takes into account the anatomical and pathophysiological mechanisms involved. It provides a measure of severity.
  - » Venous Disability Score (VDS) provides a simple measure of the functional impact of CVD, using a 4-point scale.

» Villalta-Prandoni Scale - classifies the severity of post-thrombotic syndrome (PTS).
• Consider using a disease specific tool. For example, the Aberdeen Varicose Veins Questionnaire, Chronic Venous Insufficiency Questionnaire, or Venous Insufficiency Epidemiological and Economic study questionnaire (➠IIa).
• Do NOT use the traditional diagnostic tests (Trendelenburg, Perthes, etc.) in the workup of patients (➠III).
• Consider intravascular ultrasound scan where needed in iliocaval obstruction management (➠IIb).

ON NON-SURGICAL TREATMENT -

• Venous ulcers -
  » Consider zinc dressings and cadexomer iodine iodine (in this order) to promoter healing , in this order (➠IIb).
  » Consider compression bandages (at high pressure of 40 mmHg ➠IIs), elastic or non elastic, and walking exercises as the initial treatment modality (➠I).
  » Consider intermittent pneumatic compression after a 6-month treatment course when standard methods have failed (➠IIa).
  » Consider leg elevation when compression cannot be tolerated because of acute inflammation or as an adjunct to compression during resting periods (➠IIb).
  » Consider leg massage as an adjunct to compression to reduce oedema (➠IIb).
  » Consider Sulodexide and micronized purified flavonoi fraction as adjuvants to compression treatment (➠IIa).
  » Do not ROUTINELY use zinc, antibiotics, horse chestnut extracts for venous ulcerations.
  » Do NOT use acetylsalicylic acid to promote ulcer healing (III).
• Chronic venous disease without ulceration -
  » Consider elastic stockings as an effectivetreatment modality for improving symptoms and signs (➠I).This treatment should be temporary while awaiting investigations results, or in patients who are not managed by invasive methods (➠IIb).

» Consider intermittent pneumatic compression to provide symptomatic relief in patients with chronic venous disease (C3-C6) if standard methods are not indicated or if they have failed (➡I).

» Consider leg massage as an adjunct to reduce oedema (➡IIb).

» Consider venotonic drugs as a treatment option for swelling and pain (➡IIa). These include micronized purified flavonoid fraction (MPFF), horse chestnut extract (HCSE), Sulodexide, and pentoxifylline.

ON SURGICAL AND ENDOVASCULAR TREATMENT -

• Surgical treatment is recommended over conservative management to improve symptoms, cosmetics, and quality of life (➡I).

• Foam sclerotherapy -
  » recommended as a second choice treatment of varicose veins (C2)
  » Consider in more advanced stages of chronic venous disease (C3-C6) in patients who are not eligible for surgery or endovenous ablation (➡I).
  » Consider as primary treatment in patients with recurrent varicose veins (➡IIa).
  » Consider as primary treatment in elderly and frail patients with venous ulcers (➡IIa).
  » Consider liquid sclerotherapy as primary treatment for treating telangiectasias and reticular veins (C1) (➡IIa).

• Endothermal ablation (laser, radiofrequency ablation) -
  » recommended as a first choice treatment over surgery and foam sclerotherapy for treating great saphenous vein reflux (➡I).
  » recommended with caution for treating small saphenous vein reflux ➡IIa). Do not puncture below the mid-calf.

• Phlebectomy -
  » Consider adding ambulatory phlebectomy to treat tributary varicose veins (➡IIa).
  » Consider isolated phlebectomy (with preservation of the saphenous trunk) in less evolved varicose veins (➡IIa).

- » Consider transilluminated powered phlebectomy as an alternative to phlebectomy (➡️IIb). This method uses a low oscillation speed with a large volume of surrounding tumescence.
- Cure Conservatrice et Hemodymalique de l'Insuffisance Veineuse en Ambulatoire (CHIVA) -
  - » Can be consider as a treatment option, if performed by physicians exclusively performing CHIVA (➡️IIb).

On Follow up and Outcome -
- Always consider using compression after venous surgery, endovenous ablation, and sclerotherapy (➡️I).

Deep Venous Obstruction and Insufficiency Disease:

On Surgical and Endovascular Treatment -
- Consider percutaneous transluminal angioplasty and stent placement using large self expanding stents for patients with clinically relevant chronic ilio-caval or ilio-femoral obstruction. This may also be used in patients with symptomatic non-thrombotic iliac vein lesions (➡️IIa). Do NOT use angioplasty only (➡️III).
- Surgical correction of deep venous axial reflux may be considered in patients with severe and persistent symptoms and signs of chronic venous disease (➡️IIb).Do NOT consider treating reflux in asymptomatic patients ➡️III).

VARICOSE VEINS

Outcome of Foam Sclerotherapy

SYS REVIEW & META-ANALYSIS 2007

AT A GLANCE

- 69 studies included.

MAIN RESULTS

- Complete occlusion of treated veins achieved in 87%.
- Recurrence or development of new veins: 8%.
- Serious adverse events, including pulmonary embolism and deep vein thrombosis, were less than 1%.
- Other complications include visual disturbance (1.5%), headache (4%), thrombophlebitis (5%), matting/skin staining/pigmentation (18%), and pain at site of injection (26%).
- Meta-analysis for complete occlusion suggests that foam sclerotherapy is less effective than surgery (relative risk (RR) 0.86), but more effective than liquid sclerotherapy (RR 1.39).

REFERENCES:

- Br J Surg. 2007 Aug;94(8):925-36. PMID: 17636511

Outcome of Endovenous Ablation - LSV?

COCHRANE SYS REVIEW 2014

AT A GLANCE

- 13 studies (3081 patients) included.
- Comparison made between foam sclerotherapy (UGFS), laser (EVLT), radiofrequency ablation (RFA) and surgery.

MAIN RESULTS

- UGFS vs. surgery: no difference in rate of recurrences or symptomatic recurrence. Recanalisation at < 4 months occurred less in UGFS (OR 0.66), but less in surgery > 4 months (OR 5.05). No difference in technical failure rate was found.
- EVLT vs. surgery: no differences in recurrence. No difference in both early and late recanalization. Neovascularisation and technical failure were less in laser treatment (OR 0.05). Long-term (five-year) outcomes were maintained and simila .
- RFA vs. surgery: no differences in recurrence, recanalisation (early or late), or technical failure.
- Quality of life generally increased similarly in all treatment groups and complications were generally low, especially major complications. Pain was similar between the treatment groups.

REFERENCES:

- Cochrane Database Syst Rev. 2014 Jul 30. PMID: 25075589

Outcome of Endovenous Ablation - SSV?

COCHRANE SYS REVIEW 2016

AT A GLANCE

- 3 studies (343 patients) included.
- Comparison made between foam sclerotherapy (UGFS), laser (EVLT), and surgery.
- No trials were found for radiofrequency ablation (RFA). Studies has issues on imprecision and indirectness.

MAIN RESULTS

- EVLA vs. surgery: recanalisation or persistence of reflux at 6 weeks occurred less frequently in EVLA (OR 0.07).
  - » Recurrence of reflux at one year is less (OR 0.24), but clinical recurrence was not different.
  - » Disease-specific quality of life (QoL) was not di ferent.
  - » Main complications reported at 6 weeks were sural nerve injury, wound infection and deep venous thrombosis (DVT) (one DVT case in each treatment group; EVLA: 0.6%; vs. surgery 1%).
- UGFS vs. surgery: insuffici nt data to detect clear differences between treatment groups.

REFERENCES:

- Cochrane Database Syst Rev. 2016 Nov 29. PMID: 27898181

Outcome of Treatment for Venous Leg Ulcers

SYS REVIEW & META-ANALYSIS 2014

AT A GLANCE

- 11 studies included.
- Comparison made between surgical intervention (open or endovascular) vs. compression alone with respect to ulcer healing, ulcer recurrence, and time to ulcer healing.

MAIN RESULTS

- Open surgical vs. compression: healing rate increased (pooled risk ratio [RR], 1.06), and recurrence reduced (RR, 0.54).
- Endovenous vs. compression: no difference in time to ulcer healing and no significant di ference in ulcer healing.
- Open surgical venous ligation and stripping vs. endovenous laser: no significant di ference in ulcer recurrence.

REFERENCES:

- J Vasc Surg. 2014 Aug;60(2 Suppl):60S-70S. PMID: 24835693

Outcome of Compression for Venous Leg Ulcers

SYS REVIEW & META-ANALYSIS 2014

AT A GLANCE

- 36 studies included.
- Comparison made between different compression methods with respect to ulcer healing, ulcer recurrence, and time to ulcer healingg.

MAIN RESULTS

- Compression stockings vs compression bandages: no difference in ulcer healing, time to ulcer healing, or ulcer recurrence outcomes.
- Stockings vs short stretch bandages: stockings were superior with respect to ulcer healing.
- Stockings vs four-layer systems: no difference in ulcer healing.
- Four-layer systems vs less-than-four layers: no significa t difference in ulcer healing.
- Short stretch vs long stretch bandages: no difference in respect to ulcer healing, time to ulcer healing, or ulcer recurrence.
- Better wound healing was found for: compression compared vs no compression; multicomponent vs single component systems; compression systems with elastic vs no elastic component.
- Compression in patients with healed ulcers reduced recurrence.

REFERENCES:

- J Vasc Surg. 2014 Aug;60(2 Suppl):71S-90S.e1-2. PMID: 24877851

Venaseal for Chronic Venous Insufficiency

Sys Review 2020

AT A GLANCE

- 20 RCTs (4570 patients) included.
- VenaSeal closure system compared with endovenous laser ablation (EVLA), radiofrequency ablation (RFA), mechanochemical ablation, sclerotherapy, and surgery.

MAIN RESULTS

- Anatomic success: VenaSeal had the highest probability of being ranked first (P = .980); RFA was ranked 2nd, EVLA 3rd, surgery 4th, mechanochemical ablation 5th, and sclerotherapy 6th.
- VenaSeal system ranked 3rd for VCSS, 5th for EuroQol-5 Dimension, and 3rd for Aberdeen Varicose Vein Questionnaire.
- VenaSeal system was slightly inferior to some of the other interventions for health-related quality of life (HRQoL).
- VenaSeal system ranked 1st in reduction of postoperative pain score from baseline, and in occurrence of adverse events
- Odds of occurrence of adverse events was 3.3 times in the sclerotherapy arm, 2.7 times in the EVLA arm, 1.6 times with surgery, and 1.1 times with RFA vs VenaSeal system arm.

REFERENCES:

- J Vasc Surg Venous Lymphat Disord. 2020 May;8(3):472-481.e3. PMID: 32063522

DEEP VEIN DISEASES

Thrombolysis for Proximal Acute DVT

COCHRANE SYS REVIEW 2016

AT A GLANCE

- 17 RCTs (1103 patients with acute DVT within 21d of onset of symptoms).
- Comparison made between thrombolysis or anticoagulation only.

MAIN RESULTS

- Venous patency (blood flow in affected vein) was better maintained in thrombolysis patients vs. anticoagulation only.
- Postthrombotic syndrome (PTS) in 6mo: better for thrombolysis (45% vs 66% in standard anticoagulation treatment).
- Postthrombotic syndrome (PTS) in 5yrs: fewer people developed PTS when treated with thrombolysis.
- Complications - more bleeding complications in thrombolysis group (10% vs 8% with standard anticoagulation); mostly in older studies but improved when strict eligibility criteria was used and thrombolysis delivered directly to the clot by catheter or via bloodstream from another vein.

REFERENCES:

- Cochrane Database Syst Rev. 2016 Nov 10;11(11):CD002783. PMID: 27830895

Thrombolysis for Proximal Acute DVT

Sys Review & Meta-Analysis 2020

At a glance
- 45 studies (4740 participants) included.

Main Results
- Pooled estimates of PE studies indicate:
  - » Probable reduction in mortality with thrombolysis (risk ratio [RR], 0.61) (moderate certainty).
  - » Possible reduction in nonfatal PE recurrence (RR, 0.56) (low certainty).
- Pooled estimates of DVT studies indicate:
  - » Possible absence of effects on mortality (RR, 0.77) (low certainty).
  - » Possible absence of effects on Recurrent DVT (RR, 0.99) (low certainty)
  - » Possible reduction in postthrombotic syndrome (PTS) with thrombolytics (RR, 0.70) (low certainty).
- Pooled estimates of the complete body of evidence indicate increases in major bleeding (RR, 1.89) (high certainty) and a probable increase in intracranial bleeding (RR, 3.17) (moderate certainty) with thrombolytics.

References:
- Blood Adv. 2020 Apr 14;4(7):1539-1553. PMID: 32289164

Safety of Thrombolysis in Proximal Acute DVT

SYS REVIEW 2017

AT A GLANCE

- 24 studies included.
- Review focus is on safety factors in delivering thrombolsyis.

MAIN RESULTS

- Safety improved on using:
  - » strict patient selection criteria
  - » types of fibrinolytic drug
  - » mode of fibrinolytic drug injectio
  - » biochemical markers monitoring (fibrinogen, D-dimer, activated partial thromboplastin time, plasminogen activator inhibitor-1)
  - » timing of intervention
  - » usage of intermittent pneumatic calf
  - » ward monitoring
  - » thrombolysis imaging assessment (intravascular ultrasound).

REFERENCES:

- Vasc Specialist Int. 2017 Dec;33(4):121-134. PMID: 29354622

Thrombolysis in DVT in Upper Limb

SYS REVIEW 2017

AT A GLANCE

- No suitable trial was found in the past or ongoing to address this question.

REFERENCES:

- Cochrane Database Syst Rev. 2017 Dec 11;12(12):CD012175. PMID: 29226949

Surgery for Deep Venous Incompetency

COCHRANE SYS REVIEW 2015

AT A GLANCE

- 4 RCTs (273 patients).
- Trials involved performing ligation and valvuloplasty in study participants with primary valvular incompetence, compared with ligation only. No trials investigated surgical treatment of participants with DVI due to secondary valvular incompetence or the obstructive form of DVI.
- No trials compared results of surgical procedures vs. those of high compression therapy in participants with venous ulcers secondary to DVI.

MAIN RESULTS

- The included trials were of small scale. Participants suffered from mild to moderate DVI, and none was reported to have a past or present history of venous ulcers.
- All trials reported better long-term results with surgery. Nevertheless, no evidence can be solidly concluded for benefit or harm of valvuloplasty in the treatment of patients with DVI secondary to primary valvular incompetence.

REFERENCES:

- Cochrane Database Syst Rev. 2015 Feb 23;2015(2):CD001097. PMID: 25702915

Treatment for Distal DVT

COCHRANE SYS REVIEW 2020

AT A GLANCE
- Treatment of distal (below the knee) DVT.
- 8 RCTs reporting on 1239 participants.
- Primary outcomes of interest were recurrence of venous thromboembolism (VTE), DVT and major bleeding and follow up ranged from three months to two years.

MAIN RESULTS
- Anticoagulant compared to no intervention or placebo:
  » reduced risk of recurrent VTE during follow-up compared with participants receiving no anticoagulation (RR 0.34), and reduced risk of recurrence of DVT (RR 0.25).
  » There was no clear effect on risk of pulmonary embolism (PE) (RR 0.81).
  » There was little to no difference in major bleeding with anticoagulation compared to placebo (RR 0.76).
  » There was an increase in clinically relevant non-major bleeding events in the group treated with anticoagulants (RR 3.34).
  » There was one death, not related to PE or major bleeding, in the anticoagulation group.
- Anticoagulation for three months or more compared to anticoagulation for six weeks:
  » Anticoagulation with a VKA for three months or more reduced the incidence of recurrent VTE to 5.8% compared with 13.9% in participants treated for six weeks (RR 0.42)
  » Risk for recurrence of DVT was also reduced (RR 0.32).
  » There was probably little or no difference in PE (RR 1.05)
  » There was no clear difference in major bleeding events (RR 3.42), or clinically relevant non-major bleeding events (RR 1.76) between three months or more of treatment and six weeks of treatment.
  » There were no reports for overall mortality or PE and major bleeding-related deaths.

REFERENCES:
- Cochrane Database Syst Rev. 2020 Apr 9;4(4):CD013422. PMID: 32271939

Oral Direct Anticoagulants for DVT

COCHRANE SYS REVIEW & META-ANALYSIS 2015

AT A GLANCE

- 11 randomised controlled trials of 27,945 participants.
- Three studies tested oral Direct Thrombin Inhibitors - DTIs (two dabigatran and one ximelagatran), while eight tested oral factor Xa inhibitors (four rivaroxaban, two apixaban and two edoxaban).

MAIN RESULTS

- Oral DTIs vs. standard anticoagulation: no difference in the rate of recurrent VTE (OR 1.09), recurrent DVT (OR 1.08), fatal PE (OR 1.00), non-fatal PE (OR 1.12), or all-cause mortality (OR 0.82). Oral DTIs were associated with reduced bleeding (OR 0.68).
- Oral factor Xa inhibitors vs. standard anticoagulation:
  » similar rate of recurrent VTE.
  » Oral factor Xa inhibitors were associated with a lower rate of recurrent DVT (OR 0.75 - weak association).
  » Rate of fatal (OR 1.20), non-fatal PE (OR 0.94) and all-cause mortality (OR 0.90) was similar.
  » Oral factor Xa inhibitors were associated with reduced bleeding (OR 0.57).
- None of the included studies measured post-thrombotic syndrome or health-related quality of life.

REFERENCES:

- Cochrane Database Syst Rev. 2015 Jun 30;(6):CD010956. PMID: 26123214

Pentasaccharides for the Prevention for VTE?

COCHRANE SYS REVIEW 2016

AT A GLANCE

- Pentasaccharide are another type of anticoagulant, an indirect factor Xa inhibitor. Three types of pentasaccharides are available: short-acting fondaparinux, long-acting idraparinux and idrabiotaparinux.
- 25 randomised controlled trials of 21,004 participants.
- All investigated fondaparinux

MAIN RESULTS

- Fondaparinux vs. placebo: fondaparinux had less total VTE (risk ratio (RR) 0.24), less symptomatic VTE (RR 0.15), less total DVT (RR 0.25), less proximal DVT (RR 0.12), and less total pulmonary embolism (PE) (RR 0.16).
- Fondaparinux vs. LMWH: fondaparinux reduced total VTE and DVT (RR 0.55 & RR 0.54),and showed a trend toward reduced proximal DVT (RR 0.58). Symptomatic VTE and total PE showed no differenc.
- Fondaparinux increased major bleeding compared with both placebo and LWMH (RR 2.56)
- All-cause mortality was not different between fondaparinux and placebo or LMWH.
- Conclusion - fondaparinux is effective for short-term prevention of VTE when compared with placebo. Fondaparinux is more effective for short-term VTE prevention when compared with LMWH.

REFERENCES:

- Cochrane Database Syst Rev. 2016 Oct 31;10(10):CD005134. PMID: 27797404

Graduated Compression Stockings for prevention of DVT?

Cochrane Sys Review & Meta-Analysis 2015

At a glance
- 120 RCTs involving a total of 1681 individual participants and 1172 individual legs (2853 analytic units).
- Graduated compression stockings were applied on the day before surgery or on the day of surgery and were worn up until discharge or until the participants were fully mobile.
- Duration of follow-up ranged from seven to 14 days

Main Results
- In the GCS group, 9% developed DVT in comparison to 21% in the control group (without GCS) .
- The incidence of proximal DVT was 1% in the GCS group and 5% in the control group.
- The incidence of PE was 2% in the GCS group and 5% in the control group.
- Focusing on surgical patients, 9.8% developed DVT in the GCS group compared to 21.2% in the control group.
- The incidence of proximal DVT was 1.6% in the GCS group and 6.4% in the control group.
- Focusing on medical patients admitted following acute myocardial infarction, 0% developed DVT in the GCS group and 10% in the control group. None of the medical patients in either group developed a proximal DVT, and the incidence of PE was not reported.

References:
- Cochrane Database Syst Rev. 2015 Jun 30;(6):CD010956. PMID: 26123214

CHAPTER 7
LYMPHOEDEMA

Complete Decongestive Therapy (CDT)

Sys Review 2012

At a glance

- Literature review of published article. Included are randomized controlled trials with control groups, well-controlled interventions, with precise measurements of volume, mobility and/or function, and quality of life.
- 42 studies reviewed and included.
- Levels of evidence - moderately strong

Main Results

- Treatment interventions were often bundled, therefore difficult to determine the contribution of each individual component of treatment to the outcomes achieved.
- Manual lymph drainage and compression bandage are seen to be effective in reducing lymphoedema.

References:

- PM R. 2012 Aug;4(8):580-601. PMID: 22920313

Noncomplete Decongestive Therapy, complementary & alternative therapy

SYS REVIEW 2014

AT A GLANCE
- 16 articles on botanicals and pharmaceuticals and 22 articles for physical agent modality and/or modalities of contemporary value.
- Levels of evidence – limited high level
- Modalities reviewed included ultrasound (US), electrically stimulated lymphatic drainage (ESD), high-voltage electrical stimulation (HVES), diathermy, low-level laser therapy (LLLT), hyperbaric oxygen therapy (HBOT), and elastic taping.

MAIN RESULTS
- US - Although the outcomes of the study showed limited limb volume reduction, the benefits associated with the reduction of pain, the improvement of tissue pliability, and joint mobility suggest that US may provide an indirect therapeutic contribution to support the return of limb function. This treatment is ranked as "effectiveness not yet established".
- Electrically Stimulated Lymphatic Drainage - using a monophasic twin-peak wave form with an output greater than 150 V. Larger numbers are needed to show effectiveness. This treatment is ranked as "effectiveness not yet established".
- Electromagnetic short wave diathermy (SWD), generates a deep heating tissue response through the use of high-frequency electrical current. This treatment is ranked as "effectiveness not yet established".
- Low-Level Laser Therapy (LLLT) - LLLT uses energy within the spectrum of light to create biochemical changes to modulate the tissue, which causes physiochemical effects after controlled exposure. "Likely to be effective" was the quality assessment assigned to LLLT.
- Acupuncture - The term APS was used to represent various methods of acupuncture, including manual needling, needling combined with electric stimulation, and wrist band, magnet, laser, or heat applications. Studies presented with a small sample size, lack of controls, and lack of reported long-term outcomes. This treatment is ranked as "effectiveness not yet established".
- Some other modalities were also strudies, including elastic taping, endermoligie system (to reduce cellulite), Lymphease massaging units, and deep oscilitation therapy.

REFERENCES:
- PMR. 2014 Mar;6(3):250-74. PMID: 24056160

Outcome from Surgical Treatment

Sys Review 2012

At a glance

- 20 articles included: excisional procedures (n = 8), lymphatic reconstruction (n = 8), and tissue transfer (n = 4).

Main Results

- Reported incidence of volume reduction of lymphedema: 118% reduction to 13% increase over the follow-up intervals ranging from 6 months to 15 years.
- The largest reported reductions were noted after excisional procedures (91%), lymphatic reconstruction (55%), and tissue transfer procedures (478%).
- Procedure complications were rarely reported.

References:

- Ann Surg Oncol. 2012 Feb;19(2):642-51. PMID: 21863361

Reducing Seroma following axillary surgery using sealing agents

RANDOMIZED CONTROLLED TRIAL 2016

AT A GLANCE

- 91 axillary lymphadenectomies distributed into a control group (n = 47) and a test group in which a collagen sponge coated with human coagulation factors was used (n = 44).

MAIN RESULTS

- Seroma occurred in 31%.
- A significant direct relationship (P = 0.002) was only noted between use of the hemostatic and sealing agent and nonoccurrence of seroma.
- In the multivariate study, the only variable found to be significantly related to seroma occurrence was use of the above agent (P = 0.046; odds ratio: 3.36).

REFERENCES:

- J Surg Oncol. 2016 Sep;114(4):423-7. PMID: 27338717

Reducing arm lymphoedema by reducing weight

RANDOMIZED CONTROLLED TRIAL 2007

AT A GLANCE
- Some 20 women with breast cancer-related lymphedema were randomized to receive either dietary advice for weight reduction or a booklet on general healthy eating.
- The primary outcome measure was arm volume at 12 weeks

MAIN RESULTS
- Arm volume reduced signific ntly at the end of the 12-week period (P = .003) in the intervention group.
- Body weight and BMI also reduced (P = .02).

REFERENCES:
- Cancer. 2007 Oct 15;110(8):1868-74.. PMID: 17823909

Safety of supervised exercises and weight lifting

A Pilot and Feasibility Study 2010

At a glance

- Cancer survivors with a known diagnosis of lower-limb lymphedema (N=10) recruited into a twice weekly slowly progressive weight lifting,
- Patients supervised for 2 months, & unsupervised for 3 months.

Main Results

- Interlimb volume differences were 44.4% and 45.3% at baseline and 5 months, respectively (pre-post comparison, P=.70).
- Two unexpected cellulitis incidences occurred within 2 months and resolved.
- Bench and leg press strength increased by 47% and 27% over 5 months (P=.001 and P=.07, respectively).
- Distance walked in 6 minutes increased by 7% in 5 months (P=.01).
- No improvement was noted in self-reported quality of life.

References:

- Arch Phys Med Rehabil. 2010 Jul;91(7):1070-6. PMID: 20599045

Effects of weight-lifting or resistance exercise

Sys Review 2019

At a glance

- 15 papers met the inclusion criteria: 13 trials evaluated weight-lifting or resistance exercise alone and two trials evaluated weight-lifting or resistance exercise plus aerobic exercise.

Main Results

- No arm volume change was observed for either exercise modality.
- Weight-lifting or resistance exercise did not cause lymphedema or adverse events in patients at risk of breast cancer-related lymphedema.
- Change of swelling outcome measures were not significa tly different between the weight-lifting or resistance exercise group and the control group.
- However, three included studies reported that volume of arm was significantly more reduced in the weight-lifting or resistance exercise group than those in the control group.
- The findings suggest that supervised resistance exercise may be safe, feasible, and beneficial in patients with breast cancer-related lymphedema or at risk for breast cancer-related lymphedema.

References:

- Int J Nurs Sci. 2019 Jan 10; 6(1): 92–98. PMID: 31406873

Manual lymphatic drainage for lymphedema

SYS REVIEW 2015

AT A GLANCE

- Six trials included, totaling 208 participants

MAIN RESULTS

- MLD + standard physiotherapy vs. standard physiotherapy: significant improvements in both groups from baseline but no significant between groups differences.
- MLD + compression bandaging vs. compression bandaging: significant per cent reductions of 30% to 38.6% for compression bandaging alone, and an additional 7.11% reduction for MLD. Volume reduction was borderline significant (= 0.06).
- MLD + compression therapy vs. non-MLD treatment + compression therapy: too varied to pool.
  - » compression sleeve plus MLD vs. compression sleeve plus pneumatic pump. Volume reduction was statistically significant favoring MLD, but per cent reduction was borderline significant (P=0.07)
  - » compression sleeve plus MLD vs. compression sleeve plus self-administered simple lymphatic drainage (SLD): significant for MLD for LE volume but not for volume reduction or per cent reduction.
  - » MLD + compression bandaging vs. SLD + compression bandaging: not significant for per cent reduction.

REFERENCES:

- Cochrane Database Syst Rev. 2015; (5): CD003475. PMID: 25994425

Effect of Resistance training on arm lymphoedema

COCHRANE SYS REVIEW 2015

AT A GLANCE

- Ten trials involving 1205 participants included.
- Patient follow-up ranged from 2 days to 2 years after intervention

MAIN RESULTS

- Resistance training did not increase risk of developing lymphoedema (RR 0.5. two studies, 358 participants) provided that symptoms are monitored and treated immediately if they occur.
- Pain reported more often at 3 months and 6 months compared to control group (one study).
- Qol was not difference

REFERENCES:

- Lymphology, 2015, 48(4), 184-196. PMID: 27164764

Chapter 8
Intermittent
Claudication

Summary of Current Surgical Guidelines on Chronic Limb Ischaemia

►NICE GUIDELINES **2018 (UK)**
➡ESVS VASCULAR GUIDELINES **2018**
→SVS VASCULAR GUIDELINES **2015**

ON PREVENTION AND RISK FACTORS -

- Do NOT screen routinely for PAD in the absence of risk factors or symptoms (→2). However, certain patients such as those >70, diabetics, or smokers can be considered for screening for PAD (→2).
- Consider single antiplatelet therapy (SAPT) for:
  » All symptomatic PADs (➡I)
  » All patients who have had revascularisation (➡I).
  » Preferably use clopidogrel rather than Aspirin (➡IIb);
- Consider dual antiplatelet therapy (DAPT) for:
  » Infra-inguinal stenting - use for min of 1 month (➡IIa).
  » Below knee bypasses using prosthetic graft (➡IIb);
- Do NOT routinely use antiplatelet therapy for asymptomatic, incidental, isolated disease (without any other clinical cardiovascular condition requiring antiplatelet therapy) (➡III).
- Consider oral anticoagulation (OAC) :
  » In addition to SAPT (for at least 1 month) - in endovascular revascularisation cases, where the risk of thrombosis is considered high, and the risk of bleeding is considered acceptable (➡IIa). Do not add SAPT if the bleeding risk is high (➡IIa).
  » In patients with PAD and AF - where other risk factors indicate the use of OACs (such as congestive heart failure, Diabetes mellitus, Stroke or TIA, etc.) (➡I).
  » In patients already on OAC for another indication (AF, etc.), do NOT add antiplatelets (➡IIa).
  » In patients already on OAC for another indication (AF, etc.), but with clear indication for SAPT, use both for long term (➡IIb).

ON DIAGNOSIS -

- Beside thorough clinical history and physical examination including the use of handheld doppler, measurement of ABI is indicated as a first-line non-invasive test for screening and diagnosis (➡I, →1, ►R).

   » Alternatively, use toe-brachial index, Doppler waveform analysis or pulse volume recording if ABI is unrecordable or exceptionally high (➡I, ►R).

• Where confirmation of a vascular origin is required, or where an intervention is considered, the patient can be further investigated. (➡I, →1, ►R).

   » Treadmill test - is performed using a standard protocol of walking at a speed of 3 km/h and 10% slope. A post-exercise ankle SBP decrease >30 mmHg or a post-exercise ABI decrease >20% are diagnostic for PAD (➡R).

   » Ultrasound scan - is the gold standard (➡I), with 85-90% sensitivity and >95% specificity to detect stenosis >50% (➡R). DUS is operator dependent and good training is mandatory.

   » CTA - is able to detect aorto-iliac stenoses >50% with sensitivity and specificity of 96% and 98%, respectively. CTA provides sensitivity (97%) and specificity (94%) for the femoro-popliteal region (➡→R).

   » MRA - has ~95% for diagnosing segmental stenosis and occlusion. However, MRA tends to overestimate the degree of stenosis (➡→R). In the first instance, offer contrast-enhanced magnetic resonance angiography (where quality is assured) first where feasible (►R)

   » Diagnostic Digital subtraction angiography (DSA) - might be required for guidance of percutaneous peripheral interventional procedures or for the identification of patent arteries for distal bypass (➡R).

ON NON-SURGICAL TREATMENT -

• Exercise - supervised exercise training is highly recommended (➡I, →1, ►R). Non-supervised training is also recommended where supervision is not possible (➡I, →1). Exercise can improve maximal walking distance by 5 min, and pain-free and maximal walking distance by 82 and 109 m, respectively. Improvements have been observed for up to 2 years.

Exercise also improves QOL as well.

» Most studies use programmes of at least 3 months, with a minimum of 3 h/week, with walking to the maximal or submaximal distance (➽R, ►R).

• Pharmacotherapy -

» On top of general prevention, statins are indicated to improve walking distance (➽I, →1).

» The beneficial effects of most studied drugs (cilostazol, naftidrofuryl, pentoxifylline, buflomedil, carnitine and propionyl-L-carnitine), if any, are generally mild to moderate, with large variability (➽R). Nevertheless, a 3-months trial with Cilastozol (100 mg twice daily) or pentoxifylline (400 mg thrice daily) can be recommended (→2, ►R).

ON SURGICAL INDICATIONS -

• When daily life activities and quality of life are compromised despite exercise therapy, revascularisation should be considered when there is a reasonable likelihood of symptomatic improvement with treatment (➽IIa, →1, ►R). Revascularisation options have limited durability and may be associated with mortality and morbidity. Hence restricting them to debilitating symptoms that substantially alter daily life activities is advisable.

• The general condition of the patient should be evaluated. Revascularisation should only be considerd for reasonably fit patients.

ON TECHNIQUES -

• Aorto-iliac occlusive disease:

» Short (<5cm) lesions (➽I, →1), or long occlusive lesions in high risk patients (➽IIa), should be considered for `endovascular-firs ` strategy.

• Primary (selective →1) stenting should be always considered in treating occlusive (but not stenotic ►R) lesions (➽IIa).

• Consider bare metal stents for occlusive disease, and covered stents for severely calcified or aneurysmal disease (→1, ►R).

» Long occlusive aorto-iliac lesions in fit and young patients should be considered for `open surgery firs` strategy (➡️IIa, ▶️R). A full discussion and shared decision with the patient are recommended (→1).
» Occlusive aorto-iliac lesions extending to CFA, in fit patients, should be considered for a <u>hybrid approach </u>first (➡️IIa, →1).
» Consider <u>extra-anatomical bypass</u> where no other alternatives exist (➡️IIb).
» Where experience exists, and the procedure does not compromise future options, an endovascular approach can be considered for occlusive aorti-iliac disease (➡️IIb).
• Femoro-popliteal occlusive disease:
» Short (<25cm) lesions (➡️I, →1), or long occlusive lesions in high risk patients or lack of veins (➡️IIb), not involving the origin of SAF (→1) should be considered for `<u>endovascular-firs</u>` strategy.
  • Consider primary (selective) stenting for short lesions (➡️IIa) with unsatisfactory technical results (→1). Drug eluting balloons (➡️IIb) or stents (➡️IIb) may be considered.
  • Consider drug-eluting balloons for the treatment of in-stent restenosis (➡️IIb).
» Long occlusive lesions in fit patients with life expectancy >2yrs, should be considered for `<u>open/bypass surgery firs</u>` strategy , where an autologous vein is available (➡️I, →1). Consider prosthetic conduit where a suitable vein is not available (➡️IIa, →2).
  • Where endovascular approach is used, consider using self-expanding nitinol stents to improve patency (→1).
» CFA disease should be considered for a <u>hybrid approach</u> first (open endarterectomy and angioplasty of SFA/POP) (➡️IIa).

ON OUTCOME AND FOLLOW UP -
• Most patients with IC present increased 5-year cumulative CV-related morbidity of 13% vs. 5% in reference-control population.

- Regarding the limb risk, at 5 years, 21% progress to CLTI, of whom 4-27% have amputations (➡R →R).
- Consider following up patients with IC on annual basis (➡I).
  - » This allows for proper assessment of compliance with lifestyle measures (e.g. smoking cessation, exercise) and medical therapies. This also aids in determining whether there is evidence of progression in symptoms or signs of PAD (→1).
  - » A follow up programme should consist of clinical history and examination (including ABI), checking compliance with medical therapy, and record of subjective functional improvements (→2).
  - » Duplex scan surveillance is recommended where a vein bypass was used (→2). Lesions detected in duplex should be treated with an endovascular or open approach (→1).

Supervised Exercise for Claudication

COCHRANE SYS REVIEW & META-ANALYSIS 2018

AT A GLANCE

- Supervised exercise therapy (SET) versus home-Based exercise therapy (HBET) versus walking advice (WA) for intermittent claudication.
- 21 studies (1400 participants) included.
- SET and HBET programs consisted of three exercise sessions per week. Follow-up ranged from six weeks to two years.

MAIN RESULTS

- SET groups showed clear improvement in maximal treadmill walking distance or time (MWD/T) compared with HBET and WA groups, with overall standardized mean difference (SMD) at three months of 0.37 and 0.80, respectively.
- This translates to differences in increased MWD of approximately 120 and 210 meters in favor of SET groups.
- The HBET group did not show improvement in MWD/T compared with the WA group (SMD 0.30).
- Compared with HBET, SET was more beneficial for pain-free treadmill walking distance or time (PFWD/T) but had no effect on quality of life parameters nor on self-reported functional impairment.

REFERENCES:

- Cochrane Database Syst Rev. 2018 Apr 6;4(4):CD005263. PMID: 29627967

Perceived Benefits from Exercise in Claudication

Sys Review & Meta-Analysis 2015

At a glance
- 15 RCTs (1257 patients) with PAD.
- RCTs selected where exercise training vs. usual medical care is used.
- Outcome measured used walking Impairment Questionnaire (WIQ) and Short-Form Health Survey component summary scores.

Main Results
- Completing any form of exercise training significantly improves WIQ speed (mean difference (MD) 9.60,) WIQ distance (MD 7.41), and WIQ stair-climbing (MD 5.07)
- Walking significantly improved Short-Form Physical Component Summary (SF-PCS) score when compared to controls (MD 1.24), but not the Mental Component Summary score (MD -0.55).

References:
- Vasc Med. 2015 Feb;20(1):30-40. PMID: 25432991

Side Effects of Exercise in Claudication?

SYS REVIEW 2015

AT A GLANCE
- 74 studies (82,725 traing hours in 2876 IC patients).

MAIN RESULTS
- Eight adverse events were reported, six of cardiac and two of noncardiac origin, resulting in an all-cause complication rate of one event per 10,340 patient-hours.

REFERENCES:
- J Vasc Surg. 2015 Feb;61(2):512-518.e2. PMID: 25441008

Further Studies of Effect of Exercise in Claudication

Study	Treatment	Outcome
Gardner 2012	RCT 142 patients SET vs. usualk care	In SET: claudication onset time and peak walking time improved significantly within 2mo only.
Spafford 2014	RCT 52 patients. Nordic Pole Walking (NPW**) vs. standard home exercise	NPW improved immediately claudication and max walking distance beyond 12 weeks, with excellent compliance
Saxtonr 2011	RCT 104 patients. Effect of upper (UL) and lower limb (LL) aerobic exercise on IC	UL and LL improved severity of IC and other outcome measures beyond 72 weeks

*SET: Structured Excercise Training
**NPW: Nordic Pole Walking

Angioplasty vs. stenting for iliac artery lesions

COCHRANE SYS REVIEW 2015

AT A GLANCE
- Two RCTs (397 participants).
- One study included mostly stenotic lesions (95%), whereas the second study included only iliac artery occlusions

MAIN RESULTS
- Percutaneous transluminal angioplasty (PTA) with selective stenting and primary stenting (PS) resulted in similar improvement in the stage of peripheral arterial occlusive disease according to Rutherford's criteria, resolution of symptoms and signs, improvement of quality of life, technical success of the procedure and patency of the treated vessel.
- In one trial, PTA of iliac artery occlusions resulted in a significantly higher rate of major complications, especially distal embolisation.

REFERENCES:
- Cochrane Database Syst Rev. 2015 May 29;(5):CD007561. PMID: 26023746

Outcome of Iliac Angioplasty

BRITISH ILIAC ANGIOPLASTY STUDY (BIAS IV REGISTRY) 2019

AT A GLANCE
- 8,294 procedures were submitted during the study period.
- 12,253 iliac segments were treated in 10,311 legs.

MAIN RESULTS
- 65% of procedures done for claudication.
- 81% performed electively and 45% as a day-case.
- Stents used in 54% of the lesions.
- Successful endovascular intervention (residual stenosis ≤49%) was achieved in 97% of treated segments. 1.5% of lesions could not be crossed with a wire.
- Limb complications occured in 3.5% in the limbs, and systemic complications in 2.2%.
- 141 patients had an unplanned intervention.
- Deaths occured in 84%, 15% were procedure-related.
- Both systemic and limb complication rates were higher in patients undergoing treatment for critical ischaemia.

REFERENCES:
- Clin Radiol. 2019 Jun;74(6):429-434. PMID: 30846190

Covered vs. uncovered stents for aortoiliac and femoropopliteal disease

Sys Review & Meta-Analysis 2016

At a Glance
- 2 RCTS and 4 retrospective cohort studies (744 patients).

Main Results
- For aortoiliac disease: covered stent showed no significant improvement in primary patency, but higher ankle-brachial index (ABI) (MD 0.08) and lower reintervention rate (OR 0.19).
- For femoropopliteal disease: covered stents showed increased primary patency (OR 1.84), higher ABI (MD 0.08), and lower reintervention rate (OR 0.51).
- No significant differences in technical success, complications, limb salvage, or survival between groups.

References:
- J Endovasc Ther. 2016 Jun;23(3):442-52. PMID: 27099281

Drug-Coated Balloon (DCB) and Drug-eluting stent (DES) vs. angioplasty/bare-metal stent (PTA/BMS) for infrapopliteal disease

SYS REVIEW & META-ANALYSIS 2017

AT A GLANCE
- 9 studies (707 DCB/DES patients, 606 PTA).
- FU range from 1 to 50 months.

MAIN RESULTS
- DES resulted in significantly reduced risk of target lesion revascularization (TLR; OR 0.38), reduced restenosis rate (OR = 0.30), and reduced amputation rate (OR = 0.49).
- DCB vs PTA/BMS – similar overall survival (OR = 0.86), TLR (OR = 0.59), restenosis rate (OR = 0.49), amputation rate (OR = 1.32), and overall survival (OR = 1.40).

REFERENCES:
- Vasc Endovascular Surg. 2017 Feb;51(2):72-83. PMID: 28103754

Drug-coated balloon vs. uncoated balloon for PAD lesions

COCHRANE SYS REVIEW & META-ANALYSIS 2016

AT A GLANCE
- 11 studies (1838 patients).
- FU 1-5yrs.
- Including intermittent claudication (IC) or critical limb ischemia (CLI).
- 7 trials included femoropopliteal arterial lesions, 3 included tibial arterial lesions, and 1 included both.

MAIN RESULTS
- DCBs have better primary vessel patency (OR1.5 at 6 months; OR 1.9 at 12 months; OR 3.5 at two years), late lumen loss (mean difference (MD) -0.64 mm at 6mo ; MD -0.80 mm at 2 years), and remained superior for up to five years in target lesion and binary restenosis rate.
- No significant difference in amputation, death, change in ABI, change in Rutherford category and quality of life (QoL) scores, or functional walking ability, but none of the trials were powered to detect a significant di ference in these clinical endpoints.
- No advantage for DCBs in tibial vessels at 6 and 12 months compared with uncoated balloon angioplasty.
- No advantage for DCBs in CLI compared with uncoated balloon angioplasty at 12 months.

REFERENCES:
- J Endovasc Ther. 2016 Jun;23(3):442-52. PMID: 27099281

Paclitaxel-Coated Balloon Angioplasty for the Treatment of Femoropopliteal Artery Disease

SYS REVIEW & META-ANALYSIS 2019

AT A GLANCE

- 14 studies including 2504 patients included.
- Paclitaxel-coated balloons (DCB) compared to plain old balloon angioplasty (POBA).
- Random-effects meta-analysis was conducted to assess the main outcomes of freedom from target lesion revascularisation (FfTLR) and all-cause mortality.

MAIN RESULTS

- DCB significa tly increased the rate of FfTLR (favours DCB) with substantial heterogeneity (12-month: risk ratio [RR] 1·24; 24-month RR 1·39).
- The risk of 24-month all-cause mortality was increased after DCB (random-effects model: RR 1·53).
- Efficacy of DCB differed substantially across studies. Effect size depended on the type of DCB, treatment strategy, and lesion complexity.
- The risk of 2-year all-cause mortality at 2 years was increased, but without evidence of causation

REFERENCES:

- EClinicalMedicine. 2019 Oct 17;16:42-50. PMID: 31832619

Drug-eluting Balloon Angioplasty vs. Uncoated Balloon Angioplasty for the Treatment of In-Stent Restenosis

COCHRANE SYS REVIEW 2019

AT A GLANCE

- 3 trials (263 participants) included.
- All three trials examined the treatment of symptomatic in-stent restenosis within the femoropopliteal arteries.
- The certainty of evidence presented was very low for the outcomes of amputation, target lesion revascularization, binary restenosis, death, and improvement of one or more Rutherford categories.
- Most participants were followed up to 12 months, but one trial followed participants for up to 24 months.

MAIN RESULTS

- DEBs showed better outcomes for up to 24 months for target lesion revascularization (odds ratio (OR) 0.05 at six months; OR 0.24 at 24 months) and at six and 12 months for binary restenosis (OR 0.28 at six months; OR 0.34 at 12 months).
- DEBs correlated with improvement of one or more Rutherford categories at six and 12 months
- There was no difference in the incidence of amputation between DEBs and uncoated balloon angioplasty.
- There was no clear differences in death between DEBs and uncoated balloon angioplasty.

REFERENCES:

- Cochrane Database Syst Rev. 2019 Jan 26;1(1):CD012510. PMID: 30684445

Angioplasty vs. bare-metal stenting for SFA lesions

COCHRANE SYS REVIEW 2014

AT A GLANCE
- 11 studies (1387 patients).
- FU for 2yrs.
- Antiplatelet therapy protocols and inclusion criteria regarding affected arteries between trials showed marked heterogeneity.

MAIN RESULTS
- PTA plus stent – achieved more improvement in primary duplex patency at 6 and 12 months over lesions treated with PTA alone (odds ratio (OR) 2.90). This was lost by 24 months (P = 0.06).
- PTA plus stent – achieved significant angiographic patency benefit at 6 months (OR 2.49), but was lost by 12 months (OR 1.30).
- Ankle brachial index (ABI) and treadmill walking distance: no improvement at 12 months.
- Quality of life- no significant di ference between participants.

REFERENCES:
- Cochrane Database Syst Rev. 2014 Jun 24;(6):CD006767. PMID: 24959692

Angioplasty vs. stenting for Infrapopliteal lesions

COCHRANE SYS REVIEW & META-ANALYSIS 2018

AT A GLANCE

- 7 trials(542 participants) included.
- All procedures performed for critically ischaemic legs.
- all types of stents included irrespective of design (e.g. bare-metal, drug-eluting, bio-absorbable).
- Heterogeneity between studies was high for the outcomes procedure complications and primary patency.

MAIN RESULTS

- Technical success rate was greater in stent group vs. angioplasty group (odds ratio (OR) 3.00).
- No clear difference shown in short-term (within 6 months) patency between infrapopliteal arterial lesions treated with PTA and those treated with PTA and stenting (OR 0.88).
- No clear differences shown between treatment groups in procedure complication rate, rate of major amputations at 12 months, and rate of mortality at 12 months.

REFERENCES:

- Cochrane Database Syst Rev. 2018 Dec 8;12:CD009195. PMID: 30536919

Adjunct Procedures to Standard Angioplasty

Sys Review 2014

At a glance
- 40 studies (varying and small sample sizes).
- FU for at least 1mo.
- Trials compared modification or adjunct to standard P A.

Main Results
- Significantly reduced restenosis rates were shown in self-expanding stents (SES) {RR 0.67) and endovascular brachytherapy (EVBT) (RR 0.63) at 12mo.
- Significantly reduced restenosis rates were shown in drug-coated balloons (DCBs) at 6 months (RR 0.40).
- A single study of stent-graft and drug-eluting stent (DES), compared with PTA showed improvements with DES versus bare-metal stents (BMSs).
- Compared with PTA, walking capacity was not significantly affected by cutting balloon, balloon-expandable stents or EVBT;
- in SES, there was evidence of improvement in walking capacity after up to 12 months.
- These results were seen for both patient populations (IC and CLI).
- Sensitivity analyses showed that the results were robust to different assumptions about the clinical benefits attributable to the interventions.

References:
- Health Technol Assess. 2014 Feb;18(10):1-252. PMID: 24524731

Stent Type vs. Angioplasty Outcome

Sys Review and Bayesian Network Meta-analysis 2016

At a glance

- 16 studies (2532 patients – 4227 person-yr follow up).
- Trials compared bare nitinol stents, covered nitinol stents, paclita-xel- or sirolimus-eluting stents (PES or SES), and paclitaxel-coated balloons (PCB) with plain balloon angioplasty.

Main Results

- Technical success was highest with covered stents (pooled OR, 13.6) followed by uncovered stents (pooled OR, 7.0) when compared with balloon angioplasty.
- Vascular restenosis was lowest with PES (RR, 0.43) followed by PCB (RR, 0.43).
- Target lesion revascularization was lowest with PCB (RR, 0.36) followed by PES (RR, 0.42)
- Major amputations were rare in all treatment and control groups (pooled amputation rate of 0.7 events per 100 person-years).

References:

- J Endovasc Ther. 2016 Dec;23(6):851-863. PMID: 27708143

Atherectomy for PAD

COCHRANE SYS REVIEW 2014

AT A GLANCE
- 4 RCTs (220 patients).
- Trials compared atherectomy with angioplasty.
- No study was properly powered, or assessors blinded to the procedures.
- There was a high risk of selection, attrition, detection and reporting biases.

MAIN RESULTS
- The estimated risk of success was similar between treatment modalities for initial procedural success rate, patency at 6 months, and patency at 12 months.
- Cardiovascular events were not reported in any study.
- There was a reduction in rate of bailout stenting following atherectomy, and balloon inflatio pressures were lower following atherectomy.
- Complications such as embolisation and vessel dissection with more embolisations were higher in atherectomy group and more vessel dissections in angioplasty group, but data could not be pooled.
- There was no clear evidence of different rates of adverse events between atherectomy and balloon angioplasty groups for target vessel revascularisation and above-knee amputation.

REFERENCES:
- Cochrane Database Syst Rev. 2014 Mar 17;(3):CD006680. PMID: 24638972

Subintimal Angioplasty for Total Occlusion

COCHRANE SYS REVIEW 2016

AT A GLANCE
- 2 studies (147 participants) included.
- Treatment techniques and control groups of the 2 studies differed, precluding the combining of study results.
- subintimal angioplasty (SIA) vs. other treatment for people with lower limb arterial chronic total occlusions, looking at the effects on clinical improvement, technical success rate, patency rate, limb salvage rate, and morbidity rates.
- Patients were randomized to receive either SIA with stenting of the superficial femoral artery or remote endarterectomy (RE) with stenting of the superficial femoral arter .

MAIN RESULTS
- 3-year follow-up results showed improvement of 64% (Rutherford classification) in the SIA group compared to 80% in the RE group (risk ratio (RR) 0.79). Postexercise ABI improved in 70% of SIA group vs. 82% in RE group (RR 0.86).
- Technical success rate was 93% for SIA group vs. 96% for RE group.
- Primary patency at 12 months was 59% in SIA group vs. 79% in RE group. Primary patency at 24 months was 57% in SIA group vs. 77% in RE group. Primary patency at at 36 months was 48% in SIA group vs. 63% in RE group. Assisted primary patency was 53% in SIA group vs. 71% in RE group at 36 months. Secondary patency was better for RE group (P = 0.03) at 36 months.
- Limb salvage at 3 years was 95% in SIA group and 98% in RE group.
- No perioperative deaths reported. Complications in 2 SIA participants occured: femoral pseudoaneurysm and pulmonary edema. Complications in 3 RE participants occured: seroma, femoral pseudoaneurysm, and superficial femoral artery acute occlusion
- See reference below for further analysis of the 2nd study.

REFERENCES:
- Cochrane Database Syst Rev. 2016 Nov 18;11(11):CD009418. PMID: 27858952

Intravascular Brachytherapy (IVBT) for PAD

COCHRANE SYS REVIEW 2014

AT A GLANCE

- Eight trials with a combined total of 1090 participants included in this review.
- All included studies used the femoropopliteal artery.
- All studies compared PTA with or without stenting plus IVBT vs. PTA with or without stenting alone.
- Follow-up ranged from 6 months to 5 years.

MAIN RESULTS

- For brachytherapy, cumulative patency was higher at 24 months (odds ratio (OR) 2.36). Restenosis after IVBT was significantly less at 6, 12 and 24 months.
- Need for re-interventions was significantly reduced in IVBT vs. angioplasty alone (OR 0.51) at 6 month, but not at 12 and 24 months.
- Lower number of occlusions were reported in the control group at more than 3 months (OR 11.46) but no differences found at less than one month nor at 12 months after the procedures.
- ABI was better for IVBT at 12 month follow-up (mean difference 0.08) but no significantly di ferenct at 24 hours or at six months.
- Quality of life, complications, limb loss, cardiovascular deaths, death from all causes, pain free walking distance and maximum walking distance on a treadmill were similar.

REFERENCES:

- Cochrane Database Syst Rev. 2014 Jan 8;2014(1):CD003504. PMID: 24399686

Key Studies on Peripheral Angioplasty and Stenting

DRUG COATED BALLOONS (DCBs)

STUDY	COATING METHODS	COMMENTS
In.Pact Admiral	Paclitaxel+ Urea	
Elutax	Paclitaxel	TLR: PEB+BMS 25%
Moxy	Paclitaxel+ Hydro-philic carrier	
Pantera Lux	Paclitaxel+Butyryl-tri-hexyl Citrate	LLL ;0.03 ± 0.35 TLR: 2.6%
DIOR – I	Paclitaxel + Crystalline	LLL;PEB+BMS Proximal:0.58±0.65 Distal: 0.41±0.60 TLR: PEB+BMS 15%
DIOR – II	Paclitaxel+ Shellac	LLL 0.32 ± 0.73 PEB+BMS 14.3%
Sequent Please	Paclitaxel+ Paccocath (Iopromide)	TLR 4.2% LLL; PEB 0.28

* BMS: Bare metal stent; FU: Follow-up; LLL: Late lumen loss; MACE: Major adverse cardiac events; PEB: Paclitaxel eluting balloon; TLR: Targeted lesion revascularization

Key Studies on Peripheral Angioplasty and Stenting

DRUG ELUTING STENTS (DESs)

STUDY	COATING METHODS	COMMENTS
ACHILLES	Sirolimus-eluting stent versus PTA	
BELOW	Sirolimus-eluting stent versus PTA	
DESTINY	Sirolimus-eluting stent versus PTA	
YUKON-BTK	Everolimus- eluting stent versus BMS	
PADI	Paclitaxel-eluting stent versus BMS	
IN.PACT DEEP	Paclitaxel-eluting balloon versus. PTA	
DEBATE-BTX	Paclitaxel-eluting balloon versus PTA	
BIOLUX P-II	Paclitaxel-eluting balloon versus PTA	

Key Studies on Peripheral Angioplasty and Stenting

COVERED VS. UNCOVERED STENTS

STUDY	COATING METHODS	COMMENTS
LaMMER 2013 (VIASTAR)	Fempops	
MWIPATAYI 2011	Aortoiliac	

Antiplatelet following endovascular treatment

A META-ANALYSIS 2014

AT A GLANCE

- 3 randomized controlled trials with zotarolimus- or everolimus-eluting stents (6679 patients).
- Testing optimal duration of dual antiplatelet therapy (DAPT) after drug-eluting stent (DES).

MAIN RESULTS

- No significant differences between short-term DAPT and standard-term DAPT in the comparison of incidences of cardiac death, myocardial infarction, stent thrombosis, and target vessel revascularization.
- Short-term DAPT did not increase the risk of all-cause death, cerebrovascular accidents, and major bleeding events.

REFERENCES:

- J Cardiovasc Pharmacol. 2014 Jul;64(1):41-6. PMID: 24566464

Antiplatelet following endovascular treatment

A META-ANALYSIS 2016

AT A GLANCE

- 9 RCTs (.. patients). Studies comparing Dual antiplatelet therapy (DAPT) with mono antiplatelet therapy (MAPT) for stents throughout the arterial system (coronary, carotid, peripheral).
- Outcome included restenosis or stent thrombosis, major adverse cardiac events (MACE), target lesion revascularisation, cerebrovascular accident or transient ischemic attack, bleeding, and death.

MAIN RESULTS

- Coronary stents: The risk ratio on using DAPT vs. MAPT is 0.60 for restenosis, and 0.49 for myocardial infarction.
- Carotid artery stents: The risk ratio on using DAPT vs. MAPT is 0.22.
- Peripheral arterial stents: The risk ratio on using DAPT vs. MAPT is 1.02
- Bleeding risk of all the included trials showed a RR of 1.06 with DAPT.
- This analysis demonstrated no significant evidence for superiority of DAPT compared with MAPT, but also no evidence of increased bleeding risk with DAPT over MAPT.

REFERENCES:

- Eur J Vasc Endovasc Surg. 2016 Aug;52(2):253-62. PMID: 27241270

High-Pressure Intermittent Limb Compression for IC

SYS REVIEW AND META-ANALYSIS 2018

AT A GLANCE
- High-pressure intermittent limb compression (HPILC) are tested on IC patients.
- HPILC signific ntly increases flow rate in the popliteal artery by decreasing venous pressure as well as by promoting the release of angiogenic growth factors and nitric oxide, a potent vasodilator. These physiologic effects are postulated to improve symptoms in patients with claudication.
- 8 studies (290 subjects) included. 172 of whom were randomized to HPILC.

MAIN RESULTS
- There is persistent increase in walking distance for subjects receiving compression therapy.
- On meta-analysis, the mean difference of absolute claudication distance (ACD) from baseline to follow-up among subjects receiving compression compared with controls was 125 m.

REFERENCES:
- J Vasc Surg. 2018 Feb;67(2):620-628.e2. PMID: 29389425

CHAPTER 9
CRITICAL LIMB-THREATENING ISCHAEMIA

Summary of Current Surgical Guidelines for Critical Limb-Threatening Ischaemia (CLTI)

▶ NICE GUIDELINES 2018 (UK)
⇒ GLOBAL (ESVS, SVS, WFVS) VASCULAR GUIDELINES 2020

ON DEFINITIONS -

- CLI (outdated) - The presence of:
  - » Ischaemic <u>rest pain</u> with an ankle pressure (AP) <40 mm Hg
  - » or <u>tissue necrosis</u> (ulcer or gangrene) with an AP <60 mm Hg.
- CLTI (Preferable) - the presence of:
  - » <u>Ischaemic rest pain</u> with inadequate perfusion (measured using haemodynamic tests) sufficient enough to cause pain, to impair wound healing, and to increase amputation risk.
  - » <u>Ischaemic ulcer</u>, graded 0-3, based on depth, location, size and magnitude of ablative/wound coverage procedure required to achieve healing.
  - » <u>Ischaemic gangrene</u> - graded 0-3, based on depth, location, size and magnitude of ablative/wound coverage procedure required to achieve healing.
  - » <u>Regional ischaemia</u> - of any type (grade 0-3). Relatively normal hemodynamics when the limb or foot is considered as a whole but, nevertheless, suffers ulceration (or gangrene) as a result of diminished local perfusion (i.e. angiosomal or regional ischemia without adequate collateral flow), which can threaten the limb
  - » <u>Infection</u> - which is severe enough (grade 0-3) to require amputation despite apparent adequate perfusion.
- Abbreviations - **ABI**: Ankle-brachial index; **AP**: ankle pressure; **CLI**: critical limb ischemia; **DFU**: diabetic foot ulcer; **CLTI**: chronic limb-threatening ischemia; IDSA: Infectious Diseases Society of America; **PAD**: peripheral artery disease; **PEDIS**: perfusion, extent, depth, infection, and sensation; **PVR**: pulse volume recording; **TBI**: toe- brachial index; **TcPO2**: transcutaneous oximetry; **TP**: toe pressure; **WIfI**: Wound, Ischemia, foot Infection.

- **EBR** - Evidence-based revascularisation. For optimal management, all plans should include three independent axes: Patient risk, Limb severity, and ANatomic complexity (PLAN).
  - » *Average-risk and high-risk patients* are defined by the estimated procedural and 2-year all-cause mortality.
  - » *Limb severity* - as defined by WiFI classification system (see below)
  - » *ANatomic complexity* - as defined by the GLASS system and the preferred target artery path (TAP), which would then allow for estimating limb-based patency (LBP).

ON SCREENING AND PREVENTION -

- Optimise risk factors in all patients with CLTI (➡I):
  - » All CLTI patients should be on antiplatelets (unless clearly contra-indicated) (➡I). Clopidogrel, or Aspirin with low dose Rivaroxaban (2.5 mg bd) is recommended (➡II). Do not use warfarin for treating CLTI (➡I).
  - » All CLTI patients should be on moderate- or high-intensity statin therapy (unless clearly contra-indicated) (➡I).
  - » All CLTI patients should have their systolic (<140) and diastolic (<90) blood pressure controlled (➡I).
  - » All CLTI patients should have their diabetes well controlled, with HbA1c <7% (➡II).
  - » All CLTI patients should have their life style improved, including stopping smoking cessation, implementing a healthy diet (low-fat or Mediterranean type), weight control and exercise (➡I).
  - » All CLTI patients should have their pain managed well in preparation for revascularisation (➡G ▶R). Paracetamol +- Opioid are suitable.

ON ASSESSMENT AND DIAGNOSIS -

- A complete cardiovascular physical assessment, in addition to the peripheral arterial disease assessment, is essential in all patients with CLTI (➡G).
- Perform neuropathy test and a probe-to-bone test on all CLTI pts (➡G).
- Measure ABI, AP and doppler wave form in all patients with

suspected CLTI; If abnormal, proceed to TP and TBI especially in patients with tissue loss (➡️I).

» Consider obtaining DUS as a first line if the patient is a
candidate for revascularisation (➡️2).

» Use CTA/MRA if invasive angiography become required
(➡️2).

- Perform appropriate <u>clinical severity</u> staging in all CLTI patients:

  » Use a suitable lower extremity threatened limb classific -
  tion staging system (e.g. SVS's WIfI classification system
  - Wound, Ischemia, and foot Infection (WIfI)) in all CLTI
  patients (➡️I). In summary:

    - Wound (W) -
      ▷ 0: No ulcer. No gangrene
      ▷ 1: Small shallow ulcer. No bone exposed. No gang-
      rene
      ▷ 2: Deeper ulcer with exposed bone or tendon or shal-
      low heel ulcer. Digital gangrene
      ▷ 3: Extensive ulcer involving forefoot or midfoot or full
      thickness heel. Extensive gangrene

    - Ischaemia (I) -
      ▷ 0: ABI ≥0.80. AP ≥100. TP/TcPO$_2$ ≥60
      ▷ 1: ABI ≥0.60. AP ≥70. TP/TcPO$_2$ ≥40
      ▷ 2: ABI ≥0.40. AP ≥50. TP/TcPO$_2$ ≥30
      ▷ 3: ABI <0.40. AP <50. TP/TcPO$_2$ <30

    - Foot Infection (fI) -
      ▷ 0: No clinical infection
      ▷ 1: Localised infection. Localised signs. erythema
      <2cm around ulcer.
      ▷ 2: Regional infection. Erythema > 2cm. Infection in-
      volving deep structures such as bone or fasciitis.
      ▷ 3: Systematic infection.

- Perform appropriate <u>anatomical</u> staging in all CLTI patients:

  » Use the Global Limb Anatomic Staging System (GLASS):

    ▷ <u>Aorto-iliac (inflow) disease stagin</u> :

      AI 1: Any of: stenosis in infrarenal aorta; occlusion of
      CIA only; occlusion of EIA only; or stenosis of CIA

and/or EIA.

AI **2**: Aortic chronic occlusion; CIA+EIA total occlusion; severe diffuse disease/small-caliber (<6 mm) in CIA+EIA; severe diffuse in-stent restenosis in aorto and iliac system; concomitant aneurysm disease.

A: no significant C A disease.

B: significant (>50% stenosis) C A disease.

▷ Femoropopliteal (FP) disease grading:

FP 0: Mild or no significant disease.

FP 1: SFA disease < 1/3 of total length (<10cm); or focal single occlusion (<5cm) - POPLITEAL: normal or mildly diseased.

FP 2: SFA disease < 2/3 of total length (<20cm); or SFA occlusion <1/3 (<10cm - not flush occlusion); POPLITEAL: focal stenosis (<2cm - not in trifurcation).

FP 3: SFA disease > 2/3 of total length (>20cm); or non-flush occlusion (<20cm - or flush occlusion 10-20cm); POPLITEAL: short occlusion (<5cm - not in trifurcation).

FP 4: SFA occlusion - total length (>20cm); POPLITEAL: any occlusion; or disease > 5cm or involving trifurcation

▷ Infrapopliteal (IP) disease grade:

IP 0: Mild or no significant disease in the primary target tibial artery (TTA) path.

IP 1: Focal stenosis of TTA < 3cm.

IP 2: TTA stenosis <1/3 of total length; or TTA occlusion <3 cm. Not including TTA origin or TP trunk .

IP 3: TTA stenosis <2/3 of total length; or TTA occlusion up to 1/3. May include TTA origin but not TP trunk.

IP 4: TTA stenosis >2/3 of total length; or TTA occlusion >1/3. May include TTA origin. any occlusion of TP trunk (unless AT is the TTA).

▷ Pedal (infra-malleolar) disease grade:

P 0: TTA crosses ankle into foot, with intact pedal arch.

P 1: TAA crosses ankle into foot; absent or severely

diseased pedal arch
P 2: No TTA crossing ankle into foot

▷ Calcification grad :
Severe calcification is define as calcification >50% of circumference; diffuse, bulky, or coral reef plaques likely within the FP and IP segments of the target artery path (TAP).
If present, increase the segment grade by one.

▷ Estimate the Global Limb Anatomic Staging System (GLASS) stage:
Stage 0: FP: 0 & IP: 0
Stage 1: FP: 0 & IP <3 or IP: 0 & FP <3 or IP:1 & FP:1
Stage 2: everything else
Stage 3: FP or IP of grade 4; or FP 3 & IP 3

ON DECISION MAKING -

- Ensure all CLTI patients are discussed by a vascular multidisciplinary team prior to treatment decisions (▶R).
- Estimate periprocedural risk and life expectancy in all patients with CLTI where revascularisation is deemed suitable (➡I).
  » An anticipated mortality of < 5% and an estimated 2-year survival of >50% defines an `average` surgical risk (➡II). Any higher mortality or lower 2-yr survival defines a `high` surgical risk (➡II).
- Combine patient's risk, clinical severity (WIfI), and anatomic complexity (GLASS) to formulate an intergrated PLAN (Patient risk estimation, Limb staging, ANatomic pattern of disease) as follows:
  » Patients with limited life expectancy, poor functional status, or an unsalvageable limb should be offered a palliation or primary amputation after joint discussion and decision making (➡G).
  » Patient presenting with deep space foot infection or wet gangrene:
    ▷ Perform urgent surgical drainage, debridement, and/or

minor amputation. Commence antibiotic. Consider correcting inflow disease (if likely to be urgently essential) (➥G).

▷ Repeat staging before next major treatment decision (➥G).

» Patient presenting with significant limb disease (infection or wet gangrene):

▷ Mild limb disease (WIfI stage 1) + mild ischaemic grade (WIfI ischaemia grade 0 or 1): do NOT offer revascularisation. Optimise BMT first. If the wound fails to reduce in size by ≥50% within 4 weeks despite appropriate care, consider revascularisation (➥II). Consider improving circulation to an isolated ischaemic area if required (➥II).

▷ Intermediate or advanced limb disease (WIfI stage ≥1) + moderate ischaemic grade (WIfI ischaemia grade 1-2): Consider revascularisation where possible (➥II).

▷ Advanced limb disease (WIfI stage ≥2) + moderate or severe ischaemic grade (WIfI ischaemia grade ≥1): Consider revascularisation where possible (➥II).

▷ Advanced limb disease (WIfI stage ≥2) + severe ischaemic grade (WIfI ischaemia grade ≥1): Consider revascularisation where possible (➥I).

ON TREATMENT TECHNIQUES AND CHOICES -

• Successful revascularization in CLTI nearly always requires restoration of pulsatile in-line flo   to the affected part, particularly in patients with tissue loss. This does not apply to patients with rest pain only, in which case improving the inflow alone might be sufficient.

• Usie a high-quality imaging to chooses and define a TAP that is most likely to achieve that in-line flo .

• **The Conduit:**

» Map the ipsilateral GSV and small saphenous vein (➥I ►R).

» Map veins in the contralateral leg and both arms if ipsilateral vein is insufficient or inadequate ➥G).

» Consider arm/spliced vein bypass conduits based on the operator's experience.
» Where no veins are available, consider endovascular option first (even if anatomy is complex).
» Prosthetic or biologic conduits (e.g. cryopreserved vein allografts) may be reasonable in highly selected cases, such as in patients with failed endovascular intervention, with acceptable runoff, and in patients who are able to tolerate aggressive antithrombotic therapy.

- **Inflow treatment:**
  » Always correct the inflow first ➡️G).
  » Correct inflow ONLY without outflow correction (where both exist) for patients with:
    ◊ Low-grade ischemia grade.
    ◊ Limited tissue loss.
    ◊ Risk-benefit of additional outflow reconstruction is high or initially unclear (➡️I).
  » Re-stage the level of ischaemia AFTER correcting the inflow ➡️I).
  » AI disease -
    ◊ use endovascular-first approach for moderate to severe disease (➡️I).
    ◊ Use open surgical reconstruction for failed endovascular, extensive AI disease in an average risk patient (➡️II).
  » Femoral artery disease -
    ◊ Use open CFA endarterectomy with patch, with or without extension into the PFA, in patients with hemodynamically significant (>50% stenosis) disease of the common and deep femoral arteries (➡️I).
    ◊ Use open CFA endarterectomy and endovascular treatment to AI disease where needed (➡️II).
    ◊ Correct hemodynamically significant (>50% stenosis) PFA proximal disease where possible (➡️G).
    ◊ Very high-risk patients/hostile groin: consider angioplasty of CFA (but not stent) (➡️II).

- **Outflow treatment:**
  - » Correct the outflow either as staged or a combined procedure wherever needed, based on the three PLAN factors (➡I) as follows:
  - » In average-risk patients (with suitable autologous vein):
    - ▷ Mild disease severity (WIfI stage 1) - revascularisation (endo or open) is rarely required regardless of anatomical complexity (➡I).
    - ▷ Advanced disease severity (WIfI 2,3,4) - preferably offer endovascular for low anatomical complexity cases (Stage 1 +- 2), and open surgery preferably for high anatomical complexity cases (stage 3).
  - » In high-risk patients:
    - ▷ Intermediate disease severity (WIfI stage 2 or 3) with mild ischaemic derangement (WIfI ischaemic grade 1) - consider endovascular revascularisation if wound fails to reduce in size within 4 weeks despite appropriate infection control, wound care, and offloading ➡II).
    - ▷ Intermediate disease severity (WIfI stage 2) with significant ischaemic derangement (WIfI ischaemic grade 2 & 3) - consider endovascular revascularisation if at all possible (➡II).
    - ▷ Advanced disease severity (WIfI stage 3 or 4) with moderate ischaemic derangement (WIfI ischaemic grade 1) - consider endovascular revascularisation if wound fails to reduce in size within 4 weeks despite appropriate infection control, wound care, and offloading ➡II)
    - ▷ Advanced disease severity (WIfI stage 3 or 4) with significant ischaemic derangement (WIfI ischaemic grade 2 & 3) - consider endovascular revascularisation if at all possible (➡II).
    - ▷ Advanced disease severity (WIfI stage 3 or 4) with significant ischaemic derangement (WIfI ischaemic grade 2 & 3) and advanced complex anatomy (Glass III) - consider open surgery revascularisation primarily or after failed endovascular procedure (➡II).
  - » Endovascular technique choice:
    - ▷ Consider adjuncts to balloon angioplasty (e.g. stents,

covered stents, or drug-eluting technologies) when there is a technically inadequate result (residual stenosis or flow limiting dissection) or in the setting of advanced lesion complexity (e.g., GLASS FP grade 2-4) (➡️II).

• **Infra-malleolar disease:**
  » Endovascular interventions in the pedal arch have been reported. However, their durability and hemodynamic and clinical effectiveness remain unknown.
  » Open bypass surgery has also been successfully employed to tarsal and plantar arteries. However, techniques and outcomes are not established. The impact of IM disease on the success of proximal revascularization, whether open or endovascular, is also unknown.

• **Angiosome-guided revascularisation:**
  » Consider angiosome-guided revascularisation in patients with significant wounds (e.g. WIfI wound grades 3 and 4), particularly those involving the midfoot or hindfoot, and when the appropriate TAP is available (➡️II).

• **Interventional nonrevascularization treatments:**
  » Consider spinal cord stimulation (see page 75) to reduce risk of amputation and to decrease pain in carefully selected patients where revascularisation is not suitable (➡️II).
  » Do not use lumbar sympathectomy (page 76) for limb salvage in patients for whom revascularisation is not suitable (➡️II).
  » Consider Intermittent pneumatic compression therapy in carefully selected patients for whom revascularisation is not suitable (➡️II).

ON FOLLOW UP AND OUTCOME -
  • Emphasise on best medical therapy for all patients (➡️I).
  • Infra-inguinal vein bypass -
    » Single antiplatelet therapy, recommended as standard for long-term PAD management, should be continued in the-

se patients.

» Treatment with warfarin may be considered in patients with high-risk vein grafts (e.g. spliced vein conduit, or poor runoff) who are not at increased risk for bleeding.

» Consider regular follow up for at least 2 years with a clinical surveillance program consisting of interval history, pulse examination, and measurement of resting APs and TPs. Consider DUS scanning where available (➡️II).

» Consider intervention for DUS-detected vein graft lesions with PSV of >300 cm/s, PSV ratio >3.5 or grafts with significant low velocity (midgraft PSV <45 cm/s) ➡️I).

» Maintain long term surveillance to detect any recurrent in new lesions (➡️I).

• Infra-inguinal prosthetic bypass -

» Consider DAPT (aspirin plus clopidogrel) for 6-24 months (➡️II).

» Consider regular follow up for at least 2 years with interval history, pulse examination, and measurement of resting APs and TPs (➡️II).

• infrainguinal endovascular interventions -

» Consider DAPT for 12 months (➡️II).

» Consider follow up in a surveillance program that includes clinical visits, pulse examination, and noninvasive testing (resting APs and TPs) (➡️II).

» For repeated catheter-based interventions - consider DAPT for 1-6 months (➡️II).

» Consider reintervention for patients with DUS-detected restenosis lesions >70% (PSV ratio >3.5, PSV >300 cm/s) especially where symptoms are unresolved.

» Patients after catheter-based interventions

Axillo-Bifem Byass Trial

EPRMAT TRIAL

AT A GLANCE

- In 19 centres, 117 patients were randomised, 59 receiving a prosthesis with a flow splitter, and 58 a prosthesis with a 90° bifurcation.

MAIN RESULTS

- Analysis at 3 years with mean follow-up of 12 months showed that prosthesis with a flow-sp itter had significantly better patency rate after 2 years of 84% vs. patency rate of the prosthesis with a 90°-angled bifurcation of 38% (log-rank test, p < 0.0001).
- Death and graft infection did not differ significantl .

REFERENCES:

- Eur J Vasc Surg. 1992 Mar;6(2):115-23. PMID: 1572450

Ilio-Fem vs. Fem-fem bypass Trial

PROSPECTIVE MULTICENTRE RCT 2008

AT A GLANCE
- 143 patients with unilateral iliac artery occlusive disease and disabling claudication were randomized into two surgical treatment groups, ie, crossover bypass (n = 74) or direct bypass (n = 69).
- Median follow-up was 7.4 years.

MAIN RESULTS
- Primary patency at 5 years - higher in direct bypass group (92.7 vs 73.2, P = .001).
- Assisted primary patency and secondary patency at 5 years - higher after direct bypass (92.7 vs 84.3. P = .04 and 97.0 vs 89.8, P = .03, respectively).
- For crossover bypass, Patency at 5 years after significantly higher with no or low-grade SFA stenosis vs those with high-grade (≥50%) stenosis or occlusion (74.0 ± 12% vs 62.5, P = .04).
- Patency was comparable using polytetrafluoroethylene (PTFE) and polyester grafts.
- Overall survival was 59.5 ± 12% at 10 years.

REFERENCES:
- J Vasc Surg 2008;47:45-54. PMID: 17997269

Crossover Bypass for Iliac Atherosclerotic Lesions

RE-ACTION STUDY - LONG TERM RESULTS 2018

AT A GLANCE

- The long-term results of crossover bypass (CB) for iliac athero-sclerotic lesions in the era of endovascular treatment (EVT).
- 242 patients at multiple medical centers in Japan.

MAIN RESULTS

- Perioperative mortality was 1.7%.
- Primary patency rates were 86% at 5 years and 82% at 8 years.
- Univariate analysis showed that critical limb ischemia, vein graft, and superficial femoral artery occlusion were significantly associated with low primary patency.
- In multivariate analysis, only critical limb ischemia influenced primary patency.
- Secondary patency rate was 87% at both 5 and 8 years.
- Limb salvage rate was 98% at both 5 and 8 years.
- Overall survival rates were 71% at 5 years and 49% at 8 years.

REFERENCES:

- Ann Vasc Dis. 2018 Jun 25;11(2):217-222. PMID: 30116414

Dacron vs. PTFE in Fem-fem bypass graft

RCT 2006

AT A GLANCE
- 198 patients randomised to PTFE (n = 107) or fluoropolym r-coated Dacron grafts (n = 91).
- Median follow-up: 24 months.

MAIN RESULTS
- Primary patency rate of the two grafts was similar (log rank test: p = 0.35): Dacron 92% vs. PTFE grafts 94% at 12 months, and 87% vs. 93% at 24 months, respectively.

REFERENCES:
- Eur J Vasc Endovasc Surg. 2006 Oct;32(4):431-8. PMID: 16807001

Dacron vs. PTFE in AK Fem-Pop bypass graft

Sys Review & Meta-Analysis 2014

At a glance
- 8 RCTs included (1192 pts) - 601 Dacron and 591 PTFE (5-8mm) above-knee lower limb arterial bypasses.
- Only above-knee femoropopliteal arterial bypass included, involving adult patients older than 18 years, and presenting with disabling claudication, rest pain or tissue loss, occlusion of the superficial femoral artery, and reconstitution of the above-knee popliteal artery.

Main Results
- Primary and secondary patency rates at 12 months were not significantly di ferent.
- Primary patency at 24-, 36-, and 60-month primary patency rates were significantly better with Dacron compared with PTFE grafts (RR, 0.79; P = .003; RR, 0.80; P = .03; RR, 0.85; P = .02).
- Secondary patency rates for Dacron at 24 months (RR, 0.75; P = .02) and 60 months (RR, 0.76-0.77; P = .03-.27) were better than PTFE.
- At 10 yrs, Dacron had the best primary patency (49% vs. 28% for PTFE).
- No difference noticed in amputation, overall morbidity, or mortality rates between the two surgical graft populations.

References:
- J Vasc Surg. 2014 Aug;60(2):506-15. PMID: 24973288

Bypass vs Angioplasty for Severe Ischaemia of the Leg

BASIL TRIAL 2010

AT A GLANCE
- RCT
- Of 452 enrolled patients in 27 United Kingdom hospitals, 228 were randomized to a bypass-first and 224 to a balloon angioplasty-first revascularization strateg .
- All patients were monitored for 3 years and more than half for >5 years.

MAIN RESULTS
- At the end of follow-up, 56% of patients were dead, 38% alive without amputation, and 7% alive with amputation.
- Amputation-free survival (AFS) and overall survival (OS) did not differ between randomized treatments during the follow-up.
- Surgery had higher morbidity and longer hospital stay, while angioplasty had higher failure and intervention rate.

REFERENCES:
- J Vasc Surg. 2010 May;51(5 Suppl):52S-68S. PMID: 20435262

Outcome of Femoro-Popliteal Bypass Graft

A META-ANALYSIS 2006

AT A GLANCE
- 73 articles contributed 1 or more series that used survival analysis, assessed femoropopliteal bypasses in one of the foregoing configurations, reported a 1-year graft patency rate, and included at least 30 bypasses.
- Meta-analysis C: included claudicants. Meta-analysis CI: included critical limb ischaemia.

MAIN RESULTS
- In meta-analysis C:
  - » Primary graft patency at 5 years was 58% for above-knee PTFE, 77% for above-knee vein, and 65% for below-knee vein.
  - » Secondary graft patency was 73%, 80%, and 80%, respectively (P > .05).
- In meta-analysis CI:
  - » Primary graft patency at 5 years was 49% for above-knee PTFE, 70% for above-knee vein, and 70% for below-knee vein
  - » Secondary graft patency was 54%, 72%, and 79%, respectively.

REFERENCES:
- J Vasc Surg. 2006 Sep;44(3):510-517. PMID: 16950427

AK & BK Fem-Pop bypass graft Outcome

Cochrane Sys Review & Meta-Analysis 2018

At a glance

- 19 RCTs: 3123 patients. 2547 above-knee, 576 below-knee by-pass surgery.
- 9 graft types compared:
  - » autologous vein
  - » polytetrafluoroethylene (PTFE) with and without vein cu f
  - » human umbilical vein (HUV)
  - » polyurethane (PUR)
  - » Dacron and heparin bonded Dacron (HBD)
  - » FUSION BIOLINE and Dacron with external support.
- Follow-up ranged from six months to 10 years.

Main Results

- Above-knee bypass.
  - » Autologous vein grafts improve primary patency compared to prosthetic grafts by 60 months (Peto odds ratio (OR) 0.47). This benefit translated to improved secondary patency by 60 months.
  - » No clear difference between Dacron and PTFE graft types for primary patency by 60 months
  - » Dacron grafts improved secondary patency over PTFE by 24 months (Peto OR 1.54), an effect which continued to 60 months.
  - » Externally supported prosthetic grafts had inferior primary patency at 24 months when compared to unsupported prosthetic grafts (Peto OR 2.08). Secondary patency was similarly affected
  - » HUV showed benefits in primary patency over PTFE at 24 months (Peto OR 4.80). This benefit was still seen at 60 months. Results were similar for secondary patency at 24 months and at 60 months.
  - » HBD showed superior results to PTFE for primary patency at 60 months
  - » No difference in primary patency between HBD and HUV.
  - » PUR showed very poor primary and secondary patency rates

- Below-knee bypass
  - » No graft type showed to be superior to any other in terms of primary patency.
  - » PTFE alone compared to PTFE with vein cuff: very low-quality evidence indicates no effect to either primary or secondary patency at 24 months
  - » Limited data were available for limb survival, and those studies reporting on this outcome showed no clear difference between graft types for this outcome.
- Antiplatelet and anticoagulant protocols varied extensively between trials, and in some cases within trials.

REFERENCES:
- Cochrane Database Syst Rev. 2018 Feb 11;2:CD0014875. PMID: 29429146

Biological prosthesis (BP) vs. PTFE vs. autologous veins graft (VG) for bypass

A META-ANALYSIS 2017

AT A GLANCE
- 11 studies (4 randomized controlled trials (RCT) and 7 cohorts) comprising 2627 patients included.

MAIN RESULTS
- BP vs PTFE, pooled RR of graft patency is 1.54, indicating 54% higher graft patency.
- BP vs VG - pooled RR of graft patency was 0.74, indicating 26% lower graft patency in BP than VG.

REFERENCES:
- Ann Med Surg (Lond). 2017 Jan 25;15:26-33. PMID: 28224036

Interposition vein cuff for infragenicular pros-thetic bypass graft

COCHRANE SYS REVIEW & META-ANALYSIS 2012

AT A GLANCE
• Six trials (885 patients) included.

MAIN RESULTS
- **FEM–BK POP GRAFTS**
  » Vein cuff -
    » Primary patency rate statistically significantly higher in vein cuff group (80% versus 65% at 12 months and 52% versus 29% at 24 months, P = 0.03).
    » Secondary patency was not statistically significantly different at 12 and 24mo (82.9% versus 72.5% and 58.6% versus 34.9%, P = 0.14).
    » Limb salvage rates was no statistically significant difference (86.3% versus 71.8% and 82.6% versus 62.2%, P = 0.08) at 12 and 24 months respectively.
  » Vein collar -
    » no statistically significant difference between the groups at three years in the below knee femoro-popliteal bypasses (primary patency rate 26% vs. 43%, secondary patency rate 32% vs. 42% and limb salvage rate 64% vs. 61%
- **FEM – DISTAL BYPASS GRAFTS**
  » Vein cuff - no statistically significant difference at 12 and 24mo in primary patency (62% vs. 52% and 49% vs. 44%), secondary patency (66% vs. 53%, and 55% vs. 50%, P = 0.30) or limb salvage rate (75% vs 72%, and 62% vs. 65%).
  » Vein collar - primary patency, secondary patency and limb salvage rates were not statistically significant at 3 years (20% vs. 17%, 22% vs. 20%, and 59% vs. 44%).
  » Spliced vein vs. vein cuffed PTFE grafts., Secondary patency rate was statistically significantly higher at 24 months in spliced vein group (86% vs. 52%). No difference in primary patency rate (44% vs. 50%) or limb salvage rate.
  » Using Arterio-venous fistula in cuffed PTFE grafts - no significant difference at 24 months in primary patency rate (29% vs. 36%), secondary patency rate (40% vs. 40%) or limb salvage rate (65% vs. 70).

REFERENCES:
• Cochrane Database Syst Rev. 2012 Sep 12;(9):CD007921. PMID: 22972115

Smoking and the patency of lower extremity bypass grafts

A SYST REVIEW & META-ANALYSIS 2005

AT A GLANCE
- 29 eligible studies included 4 randomized clinical trials, 12 prospective studies, and 13 retrospective studies.

MAIN RESULTS
- The effect of smoking on graft patency in the randomized clinical trials and other prospective studies was 3.09-fold increase in graft failure.
- A comparison of patency rates among all studies that used autogenous or polyester grafts showed no difference.
- A clear dose-response relationship was present, with a decreased patency in heavy smokers compared with moderate smokers.
- Smoking cessation restores patency rates toward the never smokers group.

REFERENCES:
- J Vasc Surg. 2005 Jul;42(1):67-74. PMID: 16012454

Vein Graft duplex ultrasound (DUS) Surveillance

SYS REVIEW & META-ANALYSIS 2017

AT A GLANCE
- 15 studies included.
- ABI and clinical examination compared to Surveillance DUS fi - dings.

MAIN RESULTS
- DUS surveillance was not associated with a significant change in primary, secondary, or assisted primary patency or mortality.
- DUS surveillance was associated with a nonstatistically signifi- cant reduction in amputation rate (odds ratio, 0.70).
- The quality of evidence was low.

REFERENCES:
- J Vasc Surg. 2017 Dec;66(6):1885-1891. PMID: 29169544

Vein Graft duplex ultrasound (DUS) Surveillance

CASE-CONTROL SERIES 2007

AT A GLANCE
- Patients who had infrainguinal vein grafts were enrolled in a duplex surveillance program.
- All patients recieved first scan at 6 weeks after surger .
- Graft DUS outcme classified into four groups: (a) low risk grafts, (b) mild flow disturbance, (c) intermediate stenosis and (d) critical stenosis.
- 364 grafts followed-up for a median of 23 months.

MAIN RESULTS
- 65% had no flow abnormality at 6-weeks, and had a 40-month cumulative patency rate of 82%.
- 35% grafts had a flow disturbance.
- Grafts with untreated critical stenoses were associated with lower patency (p < 0.001).

REFERENCES:
- Eur J Vasc Endovasc Surg. 2007 Sep;34(3):327-32. PMID: 17521931

Autologous cells for 'no-option' CLI

COCHRANE SYS REVIEW 2018

AT A GLANCE

- To compare the efficacy and safety of autologous cells derived from different sources, prepared using different protocols, administered at different doses, and delivered via different routes for the treatment of 'no-option' CLI patients.
- 7 RCTs (359 participants).
- Quality of evidence was most often low to very low
- Comparing between:
  - » Bone marrow-mononuclear cells (BM-MNCs) vs. mobilised peripheral blood stem cells (mPBSCs)
  - » BM-MNCs vs. bone marrow-mesenchymal stem cells (BM-MSCs)
  - » High cell dose vs. low cell dose
  - » Intramuscular (IM) versus intra-arterial (IA) routes of cell implantation

MAIN RESULTS

- No clear difference in amputation rates between IM and IA routes.
- No clear difference in amputation rates between BM-MNC- and mPBSC-treated groups, between high and low cell dose
- Ulcer healing - similar numbers of participants reported between BM-MNCs and mPBSCs, and between IM and IA routes
- More participants appeared to have healing ulcers in BM-MSC group vs. BM-MNC group (RR 2.00).
- Reduction in rest pain between BM-MNCs vs. mPBSCs were similar.
- Reduction in rest pain between IM and IA routes were similar.
- Increase in ankle-brachial index (ABI; increase of > 0.1 from pre-treatment), not seen between BM-MNCs vs. mPBSCs, and between IM vs. IA routes
- ABI scores appeared higher in BM-MSC vs. BM-MNC groups.
- Improved transcutaneous oxygen tension (TcO) with IM vs. IA routes was similiar (RR 1.22). Higher TcO reading in BM-MSC vs. BM-MNC groups and in mPBSC- vs. BM-MNC-treated groups
- Study authors reported no significant short-term adverse effects attributed to autologous cell implantation.

REFERENCES:
- Cochrane Database Syst Rev. 2018 Aug 29;8:CD010747. PMID: 30155883

Lumbar sympathectomy vs. prostanoids

COCHRANE SYS REVIEW 2018

AT A GLANCE

- Randomised controlled trials (RCTs), with parallel treatment groups, that compared lumbar sympathectomy (surgical or chemical) with prostanoids (any type and dosage) in people with CLI due to non-reconstructable PAD.
- 1 RCT included (200 patients) with Burger's disease.
- Compared open surgical technique for lumbar sympathectomy with the prostanoid, iloprost, and followed participants for 24 weeks.
- Quality of evidence considered low.

MAIN RESULTS

- Participants received prostaglandins had complete ulcer healing without rest pain or major amputation when compared with those who received lumbar sympathectomy (RR 1.63).
- More participants who received prostaglandins reported adverse effects, such as headache, flushing, nausea and abdominal discomfort.
- Five participants who underwent lumbar sympathectomy reported minor wound infection.
- There was no reported mortality in either of the treatment groups.

REFERENCES:

- Cochrane Database Syst Rev. 2018 Apr 16;4:CD009366. PMID: 29658630

Gene Therapy for Ischaemic Legs

COCHRANE SYS REVIEW & META-ANALYSIS 2018

AT A GLANCE
- Randomised and quasi-randomised studies that evaluated gene therapy versus no gene therapy in people with PAD.
- 17 studies (1988 participants). (evidence current until November 2017). Studies included patients with intermittent claudication, varying levels of critical limb ischaemia, and two studies included people with either condition.
- Most studies evaluated growth factor-encoding gene therapy: vascular endothelial growth factor (VEGF)-encoding genes, hepatocyte growth factor (HGF)-encoding genes, fibroblast growth factor (FGF)-encoded genes, hypoxia-inducible factor 1-alpha (HIF-1α) gene therapy, endothelial locus-1 gene therapy, and a stromal cell-derived factor-1 (SDF-1) gene therapy.
- Most studies reported outcomes after 12 months of follow-up.
- Overall risk of bias varied between studies.
- Moderate or low quality evidence.

MAIN RESULTS
- No clear differences in amputation-free survival, major amputation, and all-cause mortality for gene therapy treated patients vs. no gene treatment.
- Low-quality evidence suggests improvement in complete ulcer healing with gene therapy (odds ratio (OR) 2.16).
- Ankle brachial index showed no clear differences between treatments.
- Pain symptom scores had no clear differences between treatment groups.

REFERENCES:
- Cochrane Database Syst Rev. 2018 Oct 31;10:CD012058. PMID: 30380135

CHAPTER 10
ACUTE LIMB
ISCHAEMIA (ALI)

Current Surgical Guidelines
on Acute Limb Ischaemia

ESVS 2020 CLINICAL PRACTICE GUIDELINES SUMMARY ⟹

IN ASSESSMENT -

⟹ Consider active revascularisation in selected patients with cancer; the immediate outcome is comparable to non-cancer patients [IIa]. Use Rutherford classification (viable, marginally threatened, immediately threatened, non-viable) when evaluating ALI [I].

⟹ Diagnostic imaging is always essential, providing this does not delay treatment significantl , and a primary amputation is not clearly indicated[I]. Consider using CTA as a first line imaging [I].

⟹ Do NOT use myoglobin or CK assessment to decide on what surgical option is available (revascularisation, primary amputation, etc.) [III].

⟹ Investigate the source of embolism, if present, [I] after revascularisation has taken place.

IN TREATMENT -

⟹ Start Heparin immediately (if not contraindicated and a spinal anaesthesia is not planned) [I] and administer oxygen [I]. Control the pain adequately [I].

⟹ Consider starting prostacyclin analogues perioperatively if an open surgery is decided [IIb].

⟹ Treat patients with ALI in appropriate fully equipped hybrid theatre.

⟹ If open thrombo-embolectomy is chosen:

⟹ Consider local or regional anaesthesia, but ONLY with anaesthetist involvement [IIB].

⟹ Always consider using over the wire embolectomy catheter under fluoroscopy guidance [IIa]

⟹ Use vein graft for a bypass (when indicated) if at all possible [IIa].

⟹ Always use completion angiography when done [I]. If a residual thrombus is found, consider using intraoperative local thrombolysis [IIc].

➥ For graft occlusion, always correct the mechanical cause of the graft occlusion if at all possible [I].

➥ When open surgery is conducted, consider using endo-vascular options for inflow and outflow corrections [IIa]

➥ Consider using preoperative or intraoperative thrombolysis as adjuvant [IIa].

➥   If open surgery is not chosen:

➥ Do NOT use intravenous thrombolysis [III].

➥ Do NOT use thrombolysis if ALI is very mild (Rutherford class I) [III].

➥ Always consider percutaneous catheter-directed thrombolysis as an alternative to surgery for Rutherford class IIa [I].

➥ Consider using suction thrombectomy or aspiration as an adjuvant [IIb].

➥ Use tPA or Urokinase as preferable agents [I].

➥ Do not routinely monitor plasma fibrinogen levels [III].

➥ Do NOT continue using heparin during thrombolysis [III].

➥ If a bleeding occured, continue treatment if minor, and stop if major [IIa and I].

➥   If ALI is caused by thrombosed popliteal artery aneurysm, repair the aneurysm, and use vein graft if at all possible [IIa]. Do NOT use stent grafting [III].

➥   Use four compartment fasciotomy if compartment syndrome is evident or suspected clinically [IIb], or if the ischaemia was profond or prolonged [IIa]. Do not use fasciotomy routinely [III].

➥   Perform emergency fasciotomy withinno more than 2 hours of diagnosing compartment syndrome [IIa].

IN FOLLOW UP -

➥   Keep patients on anticoagulation if the cause of ALI was an embolism [I]. Also consider anticoagulation for thrombosed prosthetic graft [IIB].

➥   Always consider antiplatelet or anticoagulation + statin for long term patients [I].

REFERENCES:

• Eur J Vasc Endovasc Surg (2020) 59, 173e218. PMID: 31899099

Thrombolysis vs. Surgery for ALI

COCHRANE SYS REVIEW 2018

AT A GLANCE

- 5 trials (1292 participants).
- Agents used for thrombolysis were recombinant tissue plasminogen activator and urokinase.
- Quality of evidence according to GRADE was generally low.

MAIN RESULTS

- There is icreased risk of major haemorrhage (OR 3.22) and distal embolisation (OR 31.68) with thrombolysis treatment at 30 days.
- There was no clear difference in stroke (OR 5.33).
- No clear differences in limb salvage, amputation, or death at 30 days (odds ratio (OR) 1.02), six months or one year between initial surgery and initial thrombolysis.
- No overall association with vessel patency.
- Initial thrombolysis had associated greater reduction in level of intervention required, compared with a pre-intervention prediction, at 30 days.
- None of the included studies evaluated time to thrombolysis as an outcome.

REFERENCES:

- Cochrane Database Syst Rev. 2018 Aug 10;8:CD002784. PMID: 30095170

Thrombolysis vs. Surgery Key Trials

REVIEW OF TRIALS 1994-2010

STUDY	TREATMENT	COMMENTS
Rochester 1994		114 pts
TOPAS 1996	Thrombolysis or Peripheral Arterial Sur- gery.	213 pts
STILE 1994	Surgery vs Thrombolysis for Ischemia of the Lower Extremity	393 pts
Alfimeprase HA004 and HA007 2010		402 pts

Thrombolysis Outcome

SYS REVIEW 2018

AT A GLANCE
- 10 articles included (1,249 patients and 1,361 lower extremities treats).
- Most cases were acute thrombosis of a limb artery or bypass graft.

MAIN RESULTS
- Overall technical success rate of the applied method reached 80%.
- Complications of any type occurred in 29% of patients: 20% of them experienced minor complications; 80% had a major life-threatening complication.
- Need for secondary interventions is 78%.
- Patients who suffered amputation because of a failed thrombolysis during the same period is 12%.
- Survival rate without amputation within 30 days is 89%Death rate during first month is 4%.

REFERENCES:
- Ann Vasc Surg. 2018 Oct;52:255-262. PMID: 29772326

Outcome of Acute Limb Ischaemia

CASE SERIES FROM NATIONAL DATABASE 2013

AT A GLANCE
- Case series from national database (USA)
- 20-year study duration (1.76 million cases of thromboembolism).

MAIN RESULTS
- In-hospital mortality decreased significantly from 8.3% between 1988 and 1997 to 6.4% between 1998 and 2007
- Treatments showed decreasing use of surgical bypass and amputation and increasing rates of catheter-based thrombolysis.

REFERENCES:
- Circulation. 2013 Jul 9;128(2):115-21. PMID: 23741056

Trends in Management of Acute Limb Ischaemia

CASE SERIES FROM NATIONAL DATABASE 2015

AT A GLANCE
- 11-year study duration (1.76 million cases of thromboembolism).

MAIN RESULTS
- Hospital admissions did rise significantly from 60 to 94 per 100,000 of the population - average annual increase is 6% since 2003 (p<0.001).
- The rise was greater in older age group.
- Procedures for ALI show significant decrease since 2000 - from 14 to 12.5 per 100,000 (p=0.013), independent of age and sex.
- Most common procedure is open embolectomy of the femoral artery
- Proportion of endovascular interventions showed a small increase.
- Only few deaths were attributed to ALI - range: 95–150 deaths per year.

REFERENCES:
- Ann R Coll Surg Engl. 2015 Jan;97(1):59-62. PMID: 25519269

Controlled reperfusion vs. conventional treatment

CRAIL Trial 2013
Randomized, Open-label, Multicenter Trial

At a glance
- Immediate reperfusion following thromboembolectomy is commonly assocaitaed with local and even systemic reperfusion injury. Controlled reperfusion is designed to mitigate this effect by reducing the reperfusion pressure (to about 60 mmHg), reperfusion timing, and by introducing additional crystalloid reperfusion solution to limit the damage by reactive oxidative species and to restore cellular energy and substrate metabolism.
- 174 patients from 14 centers randomised for thromboembolectomy and normal blood reperfusion (CT) vs thromboembolectomy followed by controlled reperfusion (CR) (see details in reference below).

Main Results
- Amputation-free survival (AFS) after 4 weeks : CT, 83%; CR, 83%.
- Secondary end points were AFS after 1 year: CT, 63%; CR, 63%.
- Overall survival after 1 year: CT, 72%; CR, 77%.
- Age >80 years and central localization of the occlusion had independent negative prognostic effects on AFS.
- No differences between treatment groups CT and CR were found, neither overall nor in the per-protocol population.

References:
- Circ Cardiovasc Interv. 2013 Aug;6(4):417-27. PMID: 23881815

Ultrasound-Accelerated Thrombolysis

DUET STUDY 2015
RANDOMIZED, PLACEBO-CONTROLLED, TRIAL

AT A GLANCE
- 60 patients with recently (7-49 days) thrombosed infrainguinal native arteries or bypass grafts causing acute limb ischemia were randomised.
- Comparing standard catheter-directed vs. ultrasound-accelerated thrombolysis (UST).

MAIN RESULTS
- Thrombolysis was significan ly faster in the UST group (17.7 ± 2.0 hours) than in the ST group (29.5 ± 3.2 hours) and required significantly fewer units of urokinase for uninterrupted fl   .
- Technical success was achieved in 84% patients in the ST group vs. 75% patients in the UST group.
- 30-day death and severe adverse event rate was 19% in the ST group and 29% in the UST group.
- 30-day patency rate was 82% in the ST group as compared with 71% in the UST group.

REFERENCES:
- J Endovasc Ther. 2015 Feb;22(1):87-95. PMID: 25775686

CHAPTER 11
DIABETIC FOOT DISEASE

Effectiveness of revascularization for ulcer healing

Sys Review 2016

At a glance
- 56 articles included.
- No randomized controlled trials found; four nonrandomized studies with a control group included.

Main Results
- Major outcomes following endovascular or open bypass surgery were broadly similar among the studies.
- For open surgery: 1-year limb salvage rates is 85%
- For endovascular revascularization:, 1-year limb salvage rates is 78%
- At 1-year follow-up, 60% or more of ulcers had healed following revascularization with either open bypass surgery or endovascular techniques.
- Studies appeared to demonstrate improved rates of limb salvage associated with revascularization compared with results of conservative treatment only.

References:
- Diabetes Metab Res Rev. 2016 Jan;32 Suppl 1:136-44. PMID: 26342204

Examining the Angiosome Model

A CASE CONTROL STUDY 2013

AT A GLANCE

- 201 patients treated with Direct revascularisation (DR) compared to indirect (IR) technique.
- Factors included rates and values of partial and complete ulcer healing, restenosis, major and minor amputation, limb salvage, and percutaneous oximetry (TcPO2).

MAIN RESULTS

- At a mean follow-up of 17.5 months: mortality rate was 3.5 %, major amputation rate 9.4 %, limb salvage rate 87 %, with a statistically significa t increase of TcPO2 values at follow-up compared to baseline (p < 0.05).
- In both DR and IR in both groups, there was a statistically significant increase of TcPO2 values at follow-up compared to baseline (p < 0.05), without statistically significant di ferences in therapeutic efficac .
- DR and IR appears of comparable results.

REFERENCES:

- Cardiovasc Intervent Radiol. 2013 Jun;36(3):637-44. PMID: 23358605

Prognostic markers for ulcer healing

SYS REVIEW 2016

AT A GLANCE
- 11 articles included. No randomized controlled trials found; four nonrandomized studies with a control group included.

MAIN RESULTS
- In 10 studies, skin perfusion pressure $\geq$ 40 mmHg, toe pressure $\geq$ 30 mmHg and transcutaneous pressure of oxygen (TcPO2) $\geq$ 25 mmHg were associated with at least a 25% higher chance of healing.
- In 4 studies, ankle pressure < 70 mmHg and fluorescein toe slope < 18 units each increased the likelihood of major amputation by around 25%.
- Combined test of ankle pressure < 50 mmHg or ankle brachial index (ABI) < 0.5 increased the likelihood of major amputation by approximately 40%.

REFERENCES:
- Diabetes Metab Res Rev. 2016 Jan;32 Suppl 1:128-35. PMID: 26342129

Effect of interventions for ulcer healing

Sys Review 2016

At a glance
- 30 articles (out of 2161 papers) included.

Main Results
- Interventions studied: sharp debridement and wound bed preparation with larvae or hydrotherapy; wound bed preparation using antiseptics, applications and dressing products; resection of the chronic wound; oxygen and other gases, compression or negative pressure therapy; products designed to correct aspects of wound biochemistry and cell biology associated with impaired wound healing; application of cells, including platelets and stem cells; bioengineered skin and skin grafts; electrical, electromagnetic, lasers, shockwaves and ultrasound and other systemic therapies
- With the possible exception of negative pressure wound therapy in post-operative wounds, there seems to be little published evidence to support the use of newer therapies with high level confidence

References:
- Diabetes Metab Res Rev. 2016 Jan;32 Suppl 1:154-68. PMID: 26344936

Effect of debridement methods for ulcer healing

SYS REVIEW & META-ANALYSIS 2016

AT A GLANCE
- 11 RCTs and 3 non-randomised studies (800 patients) included.

MAIN RESULTS
- Autolytic debridement significantly increased the healing rate (relative risk 1.89).
- Larval debridement reduced amputation (RR, 0.43) but did not increase complete healing (RR, 1.27).
- Surgical debridement was associated with shorter healing time compared with conventional wound care.
- Insufficient evidence was found for comparisons between autolytic and larval debridement, between ultrasound-guided and surgical debridement, and between hydrosurgical and surgical débridement.

REFERENCES:
- J Vasc Surg. 2016 Feb;63(2 Suppl):37S-45S.e1-2. PMID: 26804366

Effect of Low-frequency Ultrasonic vs. Nonsurgical Debridement

Sys Review & Meta-Analysis 2018

At a glance
- Reviewing the effectiveness of nonsurgical sharp debridement (NSSD) versus low-frequency ultrasonic debridement (LFUD) for diabetes-related foot ulceration in adults.
- 4 RCTs met the inclusion criteria. Only 2 RCTs included. 173 patients.

Main Results
- Percentage of ulcers healed: no significant difference was found between the two methods of debridement (RR = 0.92).
- Risk of bias for both studies was low.

References:
- Ostomy Wound Manage. 2018 Sep;64(9):39-46. PMID: 30256750

Growth Factors for Treating Diabetic Foot Ulcers

COCHRANE SYS REVIEW & META-ANALYSIS 2015

AT A GLANCE
- 28 RCTs (2365 participants).
- Assessing 11 growth factors in 30 comparisons: platelet-derived wound healing formula, autologous growth factor, allogeneic platelet-derived growth factor, transforming growth factor β2, arginine-glycine-aspartic acid peptide matrix, recombinant human platelet-derived growth factor (becaplermin), recombinant human epidermal growth factor, recombinant human basic fibroblast growth factor, recombinant human vascular endothelial growth factor, recombinant human lactoferrin, and recombinant human acidic fibroblast growth facto .
- Topical intervention was the most frequent route.

MAIN RESULTS
- Any growth factor vs. placebo increased the incidence of reporting complete wound healing (53% vs. 35%; RR 1.51).
- Main growth factors reporting those results were platelet-derived wound healing formula (RR 2.45), and recombinant human platelet-derived growth factor (becaplermin) (RR 1.47).
- No clear evidence of a difference between any growth factor vs. placebo for lower limb amputation rate (13% vs. 18%).
- Growth factors showed a slight increased risk of overall adverse event rate compared with compared with placebo (RR 0.83).

REFERENCES:
- Cochrane Database Syst Rev. 2015 Oct 28;(10):CD008548. PMID: 26509249

Three Adjunctive Therapies for Diabetic Foot Ulcers

SYS REVIEW & META-ANALYSIS 2016

AT A GLANCE

- 18 interventional studies included (9 RCTs, 1526 patients).
- Risk of bias is moderate.
- Adjuvant therapies included: hyperbaric oxygen therapy (HBOT), arterial pump devices, and pharmacologic agents (pentoxifylline, cilostazol, and iloprost).

MAIN RESULTS

- The addition of HBOT to conventional therapy: healing rate significantly increased (Peto odds ratio, 14.25) and major amputation rate reduced (odds ratio, 0.30).
- Arterial pump devices (small trial) had a favorable effect on complete healing compared with HBOT or placebo.
- Neither iloprost nor pentoxifylline had a significant effect on amputation rate compared with conventional therapy.
- Cilostazol: No comparative studies were found.

REFERENCES:

- J Vasc Surg. 2016 Feb;63(2 Suppl):46S-58S.e1-2. PMID: 26804368

Hyperbaric Oxygen Therapy for Diabetic Foot Ulcers

SYS REVIEW 2014

AT A GLANCE
- 7 studies included (376 patients).
- Trials included ischaemic ulcers and non-ischaemic ulcers.

MAIN RESULTS
- Rates of complete healing at 1-year follow-up increased (number needed to treat (NNT) 1.8).
- No difference in amputation rates.
- Major amputation rates significantly reduced with HBOT (NNT 4.2).
- Non-ischaemic ulcers - no differences reported in wound healing or amputation rates.
- HBOT did not influence the need for additional interventions.

REFERENCES:
- Eur J Vasc Endovasc Surg. 2014 Jun;47(6):647-55. PMID: 24726143

Hyperbaric Oxygen Therapy for Diabetic Foot Ulcers

SYS REVIEW & META-ANALYSIS 2020

AT A GLANCE
- 11 studies (729 patients) included.
- Hyperbaric Oxygen Therapy for diabetic foot ulcers with arterial insufficienc .

MAIN RESULTS
- Meta-analysis showed a significantly fewer major amputations in the HBOT group (11% vs 26%; number needed to treat, 7).
- No difference found for minor amputations (risk difference, 8%).
- Complete wound healing results showed contrasting results.
- No significant difference was found for mortality or amputation-free survival.

REFERENCES:
- J Vasc Surg. 2020 Feb;71(2):682-692.e1. PMID: 32040434

Skin Grafting & Tissue Replacement for Diabetic Foot Ulcers

COCHRANE SYS REVIEW 2016

AT A GLANCE
- 17 studies (1655 patients).
- Comparing skin grafts or skin replacement vs. standard treatment.
- Skin substitutes consisted of bioengineered or artificial skin, autografts (taken from the patient), allografts (taken from another person) or xenografts (taken from animals).
- nearly all studies (15/17) reported industry involvement.

MAIN RESULTS
- Skin grafts and tissue replacement products used in the trials increased the healing rate of foot ulcers compared to standard care (risk ratio (RR) 1.55).
- No specific type of skin graft or tissue replacement showed superior effect on ulcer healing over another type of skin graft or tissue replacement.
- No extra adverse effects reported.
- Fewer amputation reported in experimental group vs. control (RR 0.43).

REFERENCES:
- Cochrane Database Syst Rev. 2016 Feb 11;2:CD011255. PMID: 26866804

Topical Antimicrobial Agents for Diabetic Foot Ulcers

COCHRANE SYS REVIEW 2017

AT A GLANCE

- 22 Trials (2310 participants).
- Most had small numbers of participants (from 4 to 317) and relatively short follow-up periods (4 to 24 weeks).
- Various topical antimicrobial treatments included: Antimicrobial dressings (e.g. silver, iodides), super-oxidised aqueous solutions, zinc hyaluronate, silver sulphadiazine, tretinoin, pexiganan cream, and chloramine.
- Topical antimicrobial therapy used either as a treatment or to prevent infection.

MAIN RESULTS

- Antimicrobial vs. non-antimicrobial dressings: More wounds may heal with antimicrobial dressings (risk ratio (RR) 1.28). This correspond to an additional 119 healing events in the antimicrobial-dressing arm per 1000 participants.
- Antimicrobial topical treatments (non dressings) vs. non-antimicrobial topical treatments (non dressings): proportion of wounds healed is slightly higher (RR 2.82|), achieving [almost similiar] resolution of infection RR 1.16.
- Topical antimicrobials vs. systemic antibiotics : there is probably little difference in the risk of adverse events.
- Topical antimicrobial agents vs. growth factor: data was uncertain.

REFERENCES:

- Cochrane Database Syst Rev. 2017 Jun 14;6:CD011038. PMID: 28613416

Phototherapy for Diabetic Foot Ulcers

COCHRANE SYS REVIEW 2017

AT A GLANCE
- 8 trials (316 participants) included.
- Most are single-centre studies with a sample size ranging from 14 to 84. Studies are of high risk of bias.

MAIN RESULTS
- Phototherapy reported greater proportion of wounds completely healed during follow-up vs.no phototherapy/placebo (65% vs. 37%; risk ratio 1.57).
- There were no device-related adverse events.
- After two to four weeks of treatment, phototherapy may result in a greater reduction in ulcer size.
- Change in quality of life: no clear difference between phototherapy group and no phototherapy/placebo group.

REFERENCES:
- Cochrane Database Syst Rev. 2017 Jun 28;6:CD011979. PMID: 28657134

Negative Pressure for Diabetic Foot Ulcers

SYS REVIEW & META-ANALYSIS 2017

AT A GLANCE
- 11 RCTs (1,044 patients).
- Testing the clinical efficac , safety, and cost-effectiveness of negative-pressure wound therapy (NPWT) compared to standard dressing.

MAIN RESULTS
- NPWT has:
  - » higher rate of complete healing of ulcers (relative risk, 1.48)
  - » shorter healing time (mean difference, -8.07)
  - » greater reduction in ulcer area (mean difference, 12.18)
  - » greater reduction in ulcer depth (mean difference, 40.82)
  - » fewer amputations (relative risk, 0.31)
  - » and no increased treatment-related adverse effects (relative risk, 1.12).
- NPWT is more cost-effective than standard dressing changes.

REFERENCES:
- Ther Clin Risk Manag. 2017 Apr 18;13:533-544. PMID: 28458556

Offloading for Diabetic Foot Ulcers

SYS REVIEW 2016

AT A GLANCE

- Studying the effect of footwear and offloading interventions to prevent heal foot ulcers and reduce plantar pressure in diabetes.
- 19 controlled studies (13 RCTs) – 1605 patients.

MAIN RESULTS

- Wound healing improved with total contact casting over removable cast walker, therapeutic shoes, and conventional therapy.
- No advantage of irremovable cast walkers over total contact casting.
- Healing improved with half-shoe compared with conventional wound care.
- Therapeutic shoes and insoles reduced relapse rate in comparison with regular footwear.

REFERENCES:

- J Vasc Surg. 2016 Feb;63(2 Suppl):59S-68S. PMID: 26804369

Therapeutic Footwear for Diabetic Foot Ulcers

SYS REVIEW 2019

AT A GLANCE
- Therapeutic footwear is one of the main strategies to prevent foot ulceration.
- 26 articles included.

MAIN RESULTS
- The use of therapeutic footwear is linked to the reduction of the risk of ulceration or its recurrence in people with diabetes who already have diabetic neuropathy as chronic complication of the disease.

REFERENCES:
- J Diabetes Metab Disord. 2019 Aug 14;18(2):613-624. PMID: 31890687

Gabapentin for Neuropathic Pain in diabetes

COCHRANE SYS REVIEW 2017

AT A GLANCE

- Current clinical guidelines for pain management in diabetes recommend the treatment of painful diabetic polyneuropathy (pDPN) through the use of amitriptyline (tricyclic antidepressant), duloxetine (serotonin norepinephrine reuptake inhibitor), gabapentin and pregabalin (α2-δ ligands), tramadol and tapentadol (μ receptor agonists and norepinephrine reuptake inhibitors) and topical agents such as capsaicin (transient receptor potential V1 receptor desensitizer), although the latter is known to cause degeneration of small nerve fibers.
- 37 studies (5914 participants).
- Most studies used oral gabapentin or gabapentin encarbil at doses of 1200 mg or more daily.
- Different neuropathic pain conditions, predominantly postherpetic neuralgia and painful diabetic neuropathy.
- Study duration was typically four to 12 weeks.
- High risk of bias occurred mainly due to small size and handling of data after study withdrawal.

MAIN RESULTS

- In painful diabetic neuropathy, more participants had substantial benefit (at least 50% pain relief) with gabapentin at 1200 mg daily or greater compared with placebo (RR 1.9. NNT 5.9).
- More participants had moderate benefit (at least 30% pain relief) with gabapentin compared to placebo
- Averse event withdrawals were more common with gabapentin (11%) than with placebo (8.2%) (RR 1.4).
- Serious adverse events were no more common with gabapentin (3.2%) than with placebo (2.8%)
- Participants taking gabapentin experienced dizziness (19%), somnolence (14%), peripheral oedema (7%), and gait disturbance (14%).

REFERENCES:

- Cochrane Database Syst Rev. 2017 Jun 9;6:CD007938. PMID: 28597471

Pregabalin for Neuropathic Pain in diabetes

COCHRANE SYS REVIEW 2019

AT A GLANCE
- 45 studies (11,906 participants).
- Oral pregabalin doses of 150 mg, 300 mg, and 600 mg daily were compared with placebo.
- Cases inlcuded postherpetic neuralgia, painful diabetic neuropathy, and mixed neuropathic pain predominated.
- High risk of bias occurred mainly due to small size.

MAIN RESULTS
- Painful diabetic neuropathy: More participants had at least 50% pain intensity reduction with pregabalin 300 and 600 mg compared to placebo
- Somnolence and dizziness were more common with pregabalin than with placebo: somnolence 300 mg 11% versus 3%, 600 mg 15% versus 5%; dizziness 300 mg 13% versus 4%, 600 mg 22% versus 5%.

REFERENCES:
- Cochrane Database Syst Rev. 2019 Jan 23;1:CD007076. PMID: 30673120

Effect of Neurolysis on Diabetic Patients with Compressed Nerves

Sys Review & Meta-Analysis 2013

At a glance
- Assessing efficiency of lower extremity (LE) nerve compression in diabetic patients.
- 10 clinical series (875 diabetic patients and 1053 LEs).

Main Results
- Pain relief >3 points on visual analog scale occurred in 91% of patients; sensibility improved in 69%.
- Postoperative ulceration/amputation incidence was significantly reduced compared to preoperative incidence (odds ratio = 0.066).

References:
- Plast Reconstr Surg Glob Open. 2013 Aug 7;1(4):e24. PMID: 25289218

Tendon Lengthening and Fascia Release for Ulcer Healing

SYS REVIEW & META-ANALYSIS 2015

AT A GLANCE
- 11 studies (614 participants) included.
- Comparing achilles tendon lengthening or gastrocnemius recession vs. total contact casting.

MAIN RESULTS
- No statistically significant difference for time to healing of diabetic foot ulcers, or rate of ulcers healed.
- Ulcer recurrence was significantly lower following Achilles tendon lengthening or gastrocnemius recession compared to total contact casting (RR, 0.45).

REFERENCES:
- J Foot Ankle Res. 2015 Jul 30;8:33. PMID: 26300980

CHAPTER 12
MINOR & MAJOR AMPUTATIONS

Summary of Current Surgical Guidelines for Lower Limb Amputation

▶VASCULAR SOCIETY'S BEST PRACTICE CLINICAL CARE PATHWAY FOR MAJOR AMPUTATION SURGERY 2016 (UK)
➡GLOBAL (ESVS, SVS, WFVS) VASCULAR GUIDELINES 2020

ON DEFINITIONS -

- Minor amputations - include digital and ray amputation of the toe, transmetatarsal amputation of the forefoot, and Lisfranc and Chopart amputations of the midfoot.
- Primary amputation - is amputation without an antecedent open or endovascular attempt at limb salvage. Indications are 1) relief of ischemic pain; (2) removal of all lower extremity diseased, necrotic, or grossly infected tissues; (3) achievement of primary healing; and (4) preservation of independent ambulatory ability for patients who are capable (➡R).
- Secondary amputation - is amputation performed where revascularisation has failed and the likelihood of a successful and durable redo procedure is limited. The goal is to allow for rehabilitation to independent ambulation.

ON INDICATIONS -

- Always consider revascularisation and clearly document the rationale behind proposing the amputation to patients (▶R).
- Consider primary amputation for CLTI patients with pre-existing dysfunctional or unsalvageable limb or a poor functional status (➡I).
- Consider amputation for CLTI patients with incapacitating pain, nonhealing wounds, or uncontrolled sepsis in the affected limb where revascularisation has failed or considered inappropriate (➡II).
- Consider amputation for non-CLTI patients to enhance the possibility of rehabilitation; such as in patients with flexio contracture, dense hemiplegia, or cancer (➡II).
- If pain can be managed differently and life cannot be saved, then consider quality of death first (▶R)

ON PREPARATION-

- Multidisciplinary team (MDT) discussion should always take place before proceeding to amputation (▶R).

- The MDT team should include vascular surgeons, Vascular Anaesthetists, Vascular Specialist Nurses, Interventional Radiology, Diabetes Medicine, Tissue Viability Nurses, Acute Pain specialists, Specialist Amputation Rehabilitation physiotherapy team, Occupational Therapists, Prosthetics Department, Rehabilitation Medicine and Complex Discharge Co-ordinator, Critical care, and other medical specialties as required (▶R).
- Councelling and proper discussion should always take place with patients, families and carers (▶R).
- A consultant vascular anaesthetist should be involved in the optimisation of the patient (▶R).

ON TYPES AND TECHNIQUES -

- Amputations should be done electively on a planned operating list and in normal working hours (▶R). Operations should NOT be deferred more than once (▶R).
- The Unit should always aim at having above to below knee amputation ratio below one (▶R).
- Consider improving inflow with a suitable revascularisation where the healing of the amputation at a more distal functional amputation level (eg, AKA to BKA) may be at risk (➤➤II).
- Consider transmetatarsal amputation if more than two digital ray amputations are required, especially when the hallux is involved (➤➤II).
- Diabetes, pain team, and rehabilitation teams should all review the patient within 12 hours of decision, and regularly thereafter (▶R).
- The author's recommended summary for a quality major amputation stump, based on St Mary's Hospital Standards for Stump Classification (PMID: 6856447):
  - » Above Knee Amputation:
    - ➤ Length of stump:
      - ▷ Suitable: l ongest possible length with clearance of 12-14cm above the contralateral knee joint line.
      - ▷ Acceptable: Without clearance of 12-14cm for prosthetic knee components.
      - ▷ Unsuitable: Shorter than 10cm from the crotch to end

of soft tissue.
- ➤ Shape of stump:
  - ▷ Suitable: When proximal circumference is more than 2cm greater than the distal measurement; the stump is considered tapered.
  - ▷ Acceptable: If the difference between the proximal and distal measurements is within 2cm, then the stump is considered cylindrical.
  - ▷ Unsuitable: If the distal measurement Is more than 2cm than the proxim measure, then the stump is considered bulbous.
- ➤ Bone end:
  - ▷ Suitable: Evidence of circumferential rounding of bone edge, no evidence of loose periosteum or bone spike.
  - ▷ Acceptable: Evidence of smooth anterior cortical border only, rest of the bone edges appearing sharp. Presence of asymptomatic bone spike.
  - ▷ Unsuitable: Sharp edges all around with no evidence of bone contouring. Sharp symptomatic spike.
- ➤ Muscle Cover:
  - ▷ Suitable: Evidence of both myodesls and myoplasty and with optimal shape.
  - ▷ Acceptable: Unable to confirm myodesis but sufficien cushioning and shape.
  - ▷ Unsuitable: Inadequate muscle cover likely abscence of myodesis.
- » Below Knee Amputation:
  - ➤ Length of stump:
    - ▷ Suitable: Between 13-18cm, taking into account patients height and 18cm clearance for components.
    - ▷ Acceptable: 5cm-13cm or less than 18cm from end of stump to contralateral foot.
    - ▷ Unsuitable: Shorter than 5cm.
  - ➤ Shape of stump:
    - ▷ Suitable: If the difference between the proximal and distal measurements is within 2cm; the stump is considered tapered.
    - ▷ Acceptable: If the proximal circumference Is more than 2cm than the distal measurements; the stump is consi-

dered cylindrical.

▷ Unsuitable: If the distal me.measurement is more than 2cm greater than the proximal measurement, the stump is considered bulbous.

➤ Bone end:

▷ Suitable: Anterior bevelling, edges made smooth all around, fibula trimmed 1-1.5 cm shorter than tibia and bevelled. See x·ray.

▷ Acceptable: Partial bevelling, insufficient rounding of edges, fibula not trimmed shorter or inadequately bevelled.

▷ Unsuitable: Clinically protuberant & tender tibial crest, no evidence of bevelling or edges being made smooth or flbula equal or longer than tibia on X-Ra .

➤ Muscle Cover:

▷ Suitable: Adequate calf muscle covering tibia and fibula ends.

▷ Acceptable: Thin and insufficient muscle flaps

▷ Unsuitable: Inadequate cushioning with prominent and tender bone ends.

ON OUTCOME -

• Continue to observe CLTI patients who have undergone amputation on a yearly basis (as a minimum) to monitor progression of disease in contralateral limb and to maintain optimal medical therapy . Up to 44% of patients are at risk of losing their contralateral limb (➡I).

• The primary healing rate, need for a revision to a higher level, perioperative mortality, and ambulation is up to 92%, 20%, 10%, and 80% for below knee amputation, compared to 95%, 12%, 20%, and 40% for above knee amputation; and 81%, 20%, 17%, and 70% for through knee amputation (➡R).

ON REHABILITATION -

• A discharge coordinator should be involved from the preoperatiove period (►R).

Epidemiology of Amputation

THE GLOBAL LOWER EXTREMITY AMPUTATION STUDY GROUP
2000

AT A GLANCE

- Epidemiology of lower extremity amputation in centres in Europe, North America and East Asia.
- Ten centres included, all with populations greater than 200 000, in Japan, Taiwan, Spain, Italy, North America and England.

MAIN RESULTS

- The lowest in Madrid, Spain (2.8 per 100 000 per year), and the highest amputation rates were in the Navajo population (43.9 per 100 000 population).
- The incidence rises steadily and steeply with age (most over 60 years).
- The incidence was higher in men than women in most centres
- The incidence of major amputations was greater than that of minor amputations.
- Diabetes was associated with between 25 and 90% of amputations.

REFERENCES:

- Br J Surg. 2000 Mar;87(3):328-37. PMID: 10718803

Selection of Amputation Level: a Review

SYS REVIEW 1991

AT A GLANCE

- Different tests were examined: Doppler indices, segmental pressures, skin blood flo , skin perfusion pressure, TcpO2, and thermography.

MAIN RESULTS

- Reducing the AK to BK ration requires increasing awareness among surgeons of the importance of this principle, as well as ensuring revascularisation is done appropriately.
- More specialiised tests need to more evidence.

REFERENCES:

- Eur J Vasc Surg. 1991 Dec;5(6):611-20. PMID: 1756874

Gritti-Stokes vs. through-knee amputations

CASE SERIES 1987

AT A GLANCE
- Twenty-two patients (median age – 79) had 24 amputations.

MAIN RESULTS
- Nine of 12 (75%) Gritti-Stokes amputations had uncomplicated primary healing vs. only 2 of 12 (17%) through-knee procedures had uneventful healing (P = 0.04).
- Two through-knee amputations required revision to above the knee (17%) vs. all Gritti-Stokes amputations healed.
- Three patients in each group became mobile on a prosthesis, the remainder being bilateral amputees or unable to manage an artificial lim
- .

REFERENCES:
- Ann R Coll Surg Engl. 1987 Jan; 69(1): 1–4. PMID: 3566109

Skewflap vs. long posterior flap in below-knee amputations

RCT 1991

AT A GLANCE

- Surgeons in 11 centres randomized 191 patients with end-stage vascular disease to two different methods of stump construction (Skewflap - 98 pts, long posterior flap – 93

MAIN RESULTS

- 30-day mortality rate: skew 11% vs. long posterior flap 17%; wound primary healing 60% - both groups; surgical revision at the same level 7% vs. 8%; revision to higher level 10% vs. 8%.
- Prosthetic limb fitted to 84% of skew flaps vs. 77% of long posterior flaps
- Walking, alone or with support, was achieved in 78% and 71%, respectively. None of these differences reached statistical significance
- Skew flap is found as effective as the long posterior flap and is an excellent option for below-knee amputation.

REFERENCES:

- J Vasc Surg. 1991 Mar;13(3):423-7. PMID: 1999863

Type of Incision for Below Knee Amputation

SYS REVIEW 2014

AT A GLANCE

- Three studies with a combined total of 309 participants
- One study compared two-stage versus one-stage BKA; one study compared skew flaps BKA versus long posterior flap BKA; and one study compared sagittal flaps BKA versus long posterior flap BKA.

MAIN RESULTS

- BKA using skew flaps or sagittal flaps conferred no advantage over the well established long posterior flap technique (primary stump healing - 60% for skew flaps and long posterior flap, 58% for sagittal flaps and 55% for long posterior fla
- Wet gangrene benefited more from a two-stage procedure with a guillotine amputation at the ankle followed by a definiti e long posterior flap amputation vs. one-stage procedure.
- Post-operative infection rate, wound necrosis, redo amputation, and mobility with a prosthetic limb were similar among all groups.

REFERENCES:

- Cochrane Database Syst Rev. 2014 Apr 8;(4):CD003749. PMID: 24715679

Pharmacologic interventions for treating phantom limb pain

Sys Review 2016

At a glance
• 14 studies included (269 participants).

Main Results
• Botulinum toxin A (BoNT/A) did not improve phantom limb pain intensity during 6mo follow-up compared to lidocaine/methylprednisolone.
• Morphine (PO and IV) is effective in decreasing pain intensity short term.
• N-methyl D-aspartate (NMDA) receptor antagonists ketamine (vs. placebo; vs. calcitonin) and dextromethorphan (vs. placebo), had analgesic effects. Adverse events of ketamine were more serious than placebo and calcitonin.
• Gabapentin results for pain relief were conflicting; combining results favoured treatment group (gabapentin) over control group (placebo) (mean difference -1.16). Gabapentin did not improve function or sleep quality.
• Amitriptyline was not effective for pain.
• Calcitonin (vs. placebo; vs. ketamine) and local anaesthetics (vs. placebo) were variable.
• Most of the studies were limited by their small sample sizes.

References:
• Cochrane Database Syst Rev. 2016 Oct 14;10:CD006380. PMID: 27737513

CHAPTER 13

REVISION

VASCULAR

SUREGRY

GRAFT FAILURE

Prevention of Graft thrombosis

COCHRANE SYS REVIEW 2015

AT A GLANCE
- 16 studies (5683 participants).
- Nine different treatment groups were evaluated:
  - » Aspirin (ASA) or aspirin and dipyridamole (ASA/DIP) vs. placebo or nothing (six studies)
  - » ASA or ASA/DIP vs. pentoxifylline (two studies)
  - » ASA/DIP vs. indobufen (one study)
  - » ASA or ASA/DIP vs. vitamin K antagonists (two studies)
  - » ASA/DIP vs. low molecular weight heparin (one study)
  - » ticlopidine vs. placebo (one study)
  - » ASA vs. prostaglandin E1 (one study)
  - » ASA vs. naftidrofuryl (one study)
  - » Clopidogrel and ASA vs. ASA alone (one study)

MAIN RESULTS
- Aspirin (ASA) or ASA and dipyridamole (ASA/DIP) vs. placebo or nothing: graft patency improved in the ASA or ASA/DIP treatment group, odds ratio (OR) 0.42).
  - » No difference noted for prosthetic grafts.
  - » Secondary patency shows no difference.
  - » No difference for any of the side effects: general, gastrointestinal, bleeding and wound/graft infection, amputations, cardiovascular events and mortality.
- ASA or ASA/DIP vs. vitamin K antagonists: no differences between treatment for primary graft patency at 3, 6, 12 or 24 months.
  - » No evidence of a difference for limb amputation, cardiovascular events or mortality.
- Clopidogrel and ASA vs. ASA alone: no evidence of a difference of primary patency at 24 months (all types of grafts).
  - » Total bleeding increased in the clopidogrel and ASA group.
  - » No difference in severe or fatal bleeding.
  - » No difference between the treatment groups for limb amputation or mortality.
- Not currently enough evidence to draw any robust conclusions about the efficacy or safety of the other treatments.

REFERENCES:
- Cochrane Database Syst Rev. 2015 Feb 19;(2):CD000535. PMID: 25695213

Vein Graft Surveillance Outcome

VEIN GRAFT SURVEILLANCE RANDOMISED TRIAL (VGST) 2005

AT A GLANCE
- 594 patients with a patent vein graft at 30 days after surgery randomized to either a clinical or duplex follow-up program at 6 weeks, then 3, 6, 9, 12, and 18 months postoperatively.

MAIN RESULTS
- Both groups had similar amputation rates (7%) and mortality rates (3% vs. 4%) over 18 months.
- Primary patency, primary assisted patency, and secondary patency rates, were similar in clinical (69%, 76%, and 80%) and duplex groups (67%, 76%, and 79%).
- More patients in the clinical group had vein graft stenosis at 18 months (19% vs. 12%, P=0.04).
- Duplex surveillance program cost £495 more.

REFERENCES:
- Circulation. 2005 Sep 27;112(13):1985-91. PMID: 16186435

Angioplasty and stenting for failing (stenotic) vein grafts

REVIEW OF STUDIES 1991-2015

STUDY	TREATMENT	PATENCY
J Vasc Surg. 1991	54 graft stenosis angioplasty	3-yr: 59% (drops to 6% if repeated) 5-yr: 18%
EJVES 2009	96 (of 411 grafts) developed stenosis. 76 had 99 angioplasties	78% technical success. 30-month patency: 73.2%(1st), 82.6% (1st assis) and 84.3% (2nd)
EJVES 2016	178 angioplasties in 114 bypass grafts	At 5yrs: patency 46%. Amputation-free survival 58%. Pt survival 65%.
J Vasc Surg. 2004	19 stenosis; 4mm cutting balloon Angioplasty	Technical success: 100% 11mo FU: 1 recurrent stenosis
J Vasc Surg. 2008	161 stenosis in 124 bypass. cutting balloon(CB), Balloon(B), and open surgery(OS) Angioplasty	At 48mo: patency 62%(CB), 34%(B), and 74%(OS)
J Vasc Surg. 2015	175 vein graft Balloon(B), and open surgery(OS)	At 12mo patency: Lesion favourable: 59%(B), 66%(OS). Lesion unfavourable: 34%(B), 62%(OS)
JVS 2016	RCT. 293pts with AV fistula. Balloon(B) vs. Viabahn(V)	At 6mo: Patency 52%(V) vs. 34% (B).
NEJM 2010	RCT. 190pts with AV fistula. Balloon(B) vs. Viabahn(V)	At 6mo: Patency 51%(V) vs. 23% (B).
J Vasc Interv Radiol. 2015	RCT. 14 pts with AV fistula. Balloon(B) vs. Viabahn(V)	At 6mo: Patency 67%(V) vs. 0% (B).

Technical factors affecting autogenous vein graft failure

OBSERVATIONS FROM PREVENT III MULTICENTER TRIAL 2007

AT A GLANCE
- Trial database includes 1404 North American patients with critical limb ischemia (CLI).

MAIN RESULTS
- Vein diameter <3.5 mm and composite graft type were significan - ly associated with early (30 day) graft failure.
- At 1 year, patency rates were negatively associated with diameter <3.5 mm, non-great saphenous vein (GSV) type, and graft lengths >50 cm.
- Limb salvage and survival at 1 year were not significantly impacted by technical variables.
- High-risk conduits (diameter <3mm or nonsingle segment GSV was associated with a 2.1-fold increased risk of 30 day graft failure (P < .05), and increased index length of stay (mean 9.37 vs 8.71 days, P = .03) and a greater number of reinterventions (mean 0.67 vs 0.42, P < .0001) over the ensuing year.

REFERENCES:
- J Vasc Surg. 2007 Dec;46(6):1180-90. PMID: 18154993

Prophylactic Mesh Reinforcement following AAA repair

SYS REVIEW AND META-ANALYSIS 2018

AT A GLANCE
- 4 RCTs (388 patients).

MAIN RESULTS
- Mesh reinforcement significantly reduced risk of incisional hernia after AAA repair compared with standard sutured closure (RR 0.27).
- Re-operations was not different between groups.
- Mesh reinforcement did not cause more intra-operative or post-operative complications than sutured closure.

REFERENCES:
- Eur J Vasc Endovasc Surg. 2018 Jul;56(1):120-128. PMID: 29685678

Surgical vs. Endovascular revision of vein graft stenosis

MID-TERM ANALYSIS OF RCT (PREVENT III TRIAL) 2007

AT A GLANCE
- 156 open surgical and 134 endovascular reinterventions performed. Mean follow-up after revision of 193 and 151 days, respectively.

MAIN RESULTS
- 12-month amputation-/revision-free survival - 75% for open surgical group; 56% for endovascular group (hazard ratio, 2.2; P = .043).
- Thrombosed grafts undergoing salvage benefited most from open surgery (P = .006).
- Stenotic grafts had similar early outcomes, with a trend favoring open surgical group developing beyond 6 months.
- At 12mo: 80% of open surgical and 64% of endovascular-revised grafts required no further intervention; endovascular revisions necessitated significantly more reinterventions to maintain patenc .

REFERENCES:
- J Vasc Surg. 2007 Dec;46(6):1173-1179. PMID: 17950564

Thrombolysis for Acute artery/graft Occlusions

REVIEW OF STUDIES 2017-2018

STUDY	TREATMENT	OUTCOME
EJVES 2017	689 Cases: grafts/Stents(G) 40%; thrombosis (T) 28%; embolus(E); 25%% pop aneurysm(A) 8%	*FU 60mo – success rate: G86%;T74%; E87%; A74% *Overall Adjuvant revasc 78% *Overall major bleeding 14% *Overall 30d Survival 96% *Amputation-free survival 86% *2nd Patency 1,5yr: 80%,75%
Cochrane Sys review 2018	5 trials (1283 Cases): grafts; / Stents/ thrombosis/etc. Initial thrombolysis vs. initial surgery Meta-analysis performed	No sig difference in death or limb salvage at 30d, 6mo, 12mo. Stroke rate 0.9% vs. 0%. Major bleeding 9% vs 4%. Distal embolis. 13% vs 0% Level of complexityx5 for surgery

GRAFT INFECTION

Summary of Current Surgical Guidelines for Vascular Graft and Endograft Infections (VGEI)

▶NICE GUIDELINES - NO SPECIFIC GUIDELINES (UK)
➡ESVS CLINICAL PRACTICE GUIDELINES 2020 (EU)

ON DEFINITIONS -

- **Superficial vs. deep surgical site infection (CDC criteria):**
  » Superficia :
  1. infection within 30 days of surgery
  2. Infection only in skin and subcutaneous tissue, and
  3. Presence of one of the following: purulent discharge; isolated organisms from aseptically obtained culture; clear signs or symptoms of infection; or clinical impression of infection by the surgeon.

  » Deep:
  1. infection within 30 days of surgery, or within 1yr of using an implant
  2. Infection in deep soft tissue, and
  3. Presence of one of the following: purulent discharge (or deep abscess); spontaneous dehiscence of deep incision, isolated organisms from the deep site with clear signs or symptoms of infection; or clinical impression of infection by the surgeon.

- **Szilagyi, Samson, and Bunt classification** See original guidelines.

- **The Management of Aortic Graft Infection (MAGIC) classificatio** :
  » Major criteria:
  1. **Clinical** - Graft exposed (direct or sinus); Pus around graft; Fistula with the graft; Graft inserted in infected site.
  2. **Radiological** - Perigraft gas (>7 wks) or fluid (>3 mo) after insertion; Increase in gas volume [< 7wks] on serial imaging.
  3. **Laboratorial** - organisms recovered from graft explanted, from intraoperative specimen, or from perigraft fluid aspiration.

  » Minor criteria:
  1. **Clinical** - Localised clinical features of infection in graft area; fever with graft infection the most likely cause.
  2. **Radiological** - suspicious perigraft gas; pseudoaneu-

rysm formation; focal bowel wall thickening; discitis/os-teomyelitis; suspicious metabolic activity on FDGPET/CT; radiolabelled leukocyte uptakeuptake.

3. **Laboratorial** - positive blood culture(s) and no apparent source except graft infection; markers with graft infection as most likely cause.

ON RISK FACTORS & PREVENTION -

- **Early VGEI** most likely results from a breach in sterility during surgery, or presence of bacteria in the field of surgery. **Late VGEI** results most likely from a bacteraemia (mostly arising from the urinary or respiratory tract), from bacterial transloca-tion, or due to iatrogenic contamination during catheterisation.
- **Post-implantation syndrome** - a transitory fever associated with elevated leukocytes and CRP. This should be distinguis-hing from an actual infection.
- **Risk factors include**: groin incision, lower limb infection or gangrene, re-intervention, emergency operation, infection in another site, prolonged operation, postoperative wound infec-tion, graft thrombosis, chemotherapy, malnutrition, diabetes mellitus, chronic kidney disease, liver disease, and immuno-suppression, among other things.
- **Preventing graft and endograft infection** -
  - » Staphylococcus nasal decontamination - despite some sup-porting evidence, this is not yet recommended (➡).
  - » Shower regimen and hair removal - no difference has been shown between use of antiseptics vs. normal shower (➡).
  - » Peri-operative systemic antimicrobial prophylaxis - should be used In every case where a vascular graft/endograft is implanted. Antimicrobials should cover the first 24 hours, by intravenous administration of a first/second generation cephalosporin or vancomycin in the event of penicillin al-lergy (➡I).
  - » Changing gloves before handling graft - there is no current evidence to support this practice (➡).
  - » Meticulous wound closure with monofilament absorbable suture has been shown consistently to reduce risk of infec-tion compared to using staples (➡R).
  - » Dental procedures - antimicrobial prophylaxis should be considered before any dental procedure involving the ma-nipulation of the gingival or peri-apical region of teeth (➡II).

On Diagnostic -
- Perform exhaustive of clinical status, signs of infection and patient comorbidities. Use preferably MAGIC criteria (➡I).
- Obtain microbiological specimens (preferably 3 deep) if at all possible (➡I).
- Common responsible pathogens are:
  » Gram positive bacteria (58%) including enterococci, staphylococcus aureus, and coagulase negative staphylococci
  » Gram negative bacteria (34%)
  » Anaerobes (8%).
- CTA is currently the recommended first line diagnostic modality (➡I). Use MRI as a second choice if CT is not possible.
- If CTA raises suspicion, obtain 18F-FDG-PET combined with low dose CT (➡I). If diagnostic enhanced accuracy is still required, consider WBCS with SPECT/CT as a second line after PET (or as alternative if the infection is in peripheral grafts) (➡I).

On Management -
- Perform exhaustive check of clinical status, signs of infection and patient comorbidities. Use preferably MAGIC criteria (➡I).

- Antibiotics -
  » Start with broad spectrum. Target the most likely pathogen. Consider adding antifungal esp. for visceral fistuals ➡).
  » Duration -
    ▷ Prosthetic material removed: give IV antibiotics for min two weeks, followed by 2-4 weeks of oral regime.
    ▷ Infected material replaced by a new graft: give IV antibiotics for 4-6 weeks, followed by oral antibiotics for 4-6 months (up to 12 months).
    ▷ Patients at particularly high risk and infection of low virulence: consider similar regime for 6-12months, or in some cases, life-long(➡).
  » Isolation - isolate patients infected multidrug resistant (MDR) bacteria (such as MRSA, extended spectrum beta lactamase producing Enterobacteriaceae, or glycopeptide resistant enterococi). They should remain so during their hospital stay.

- Principles of surgical management - historically, the gold standard of management includes excision of the infected graft, extensive debridement, and extra-anatomic bypass. Due to the complexity and duration of such procedures, it is now more acceptable to debride the infected graft and its bed, perform and in situ bypass using infection resistant material, and covering anastomosis site with appropriate material such as omentum, muscles or pericardium patch.

- Head and neck arteries VGEI:
  - » Those include carotid stent graft, subclavian stent graft, and brachiocephalic and subclavian bypasses or stents.
  - » Infection is rare.
  - » Carotid patches tend to occur in the first few months.
  - » S. aureus is most commonly encountered in acute setting, while S. epidermidis is predominantly more common in late infections.
  - » Management -
    - Total removal of infected material followed by reconstruction with autologous material is recommended (➡I).
    - Avoid conservative approach in fit patients.
    - A stent graft as a definitve management with long term antibiotics or as a bridging therapy (EndoVAC technqiue) should be considered, especially in emergency cases (➡IIb).
    - Muscle falps can also be considered.
    - Patients unfit for surgery can be treated with antibiotics only (➡IIb).

- Thoracic and thoraco-abdominal VGEI:
  - » Incidence is 6% and mortality rate reaches 75%.
  - » In summary:
    - Patients presenting with acute bleeding should be considered for a bridging stent graft (➡IIa), followed by a definitive treatment or palliation if unfit.
    - Patients unfit for surgery should be considered for palliative treatment, including antibiotics, drainage and irrigation (➡IIb).
    - Patients fit for surger :
      ▷ *VGEI with no evidence of a fistula*: should be considered for graft explantation (total (➡I) if possible, or

partial (➡llb) if well incorporated). Vascular reconstruction should be implanted with an in-situ graft (first choice
(➡l), using cryoprerved allografts, treated PET grafts or
biological xenografts, and covered with with autologous,
and ideally vascularised, tissue(➡l)) or extra-anatomical
bypass (➡lla).

▷ *VGEI with oesophageal fistula*: Do NOT treat conservatively (unless in a palliative setting)(➡lll). Do NOT use
aortic endograft and oesophageal endoprosthesis (with
antibiotics) alone (➡lll). Instead, aim at explantation of
the infected material, repair of the oesophagus, and coverage with viable tissue (➡l).

▷ *VGEI with airway fistula*: Do NOT treat conservatively
(unless in a palliative setting)(➡lll). Closure of the airway defect and explantation of the infected material with
in situ reconstruction (➡lla) is recommended. Preservation of the endograft should also be considered after
closure of the airway defect and coverage with viable
tissue (➡lla).

- Abdominal Aorta VGEI:
  » Incidence is generally low: 0.19% after open surgery vs.
  0.16% after EVAR and 0.2% in both elective and non-elec-
  tive patients in one series.
  » In summary:
    - Patients presenting with acute bleeding should be consi-
    dered for a bridging stent graft (➡lla), followed by a defi-
    nitive treatment or palliation if unfit.
    - Patients unfit for surgery should be considered for palliati-
    ve treatment, including antibiotics, drainage and irrigation
    (➡llb).
    - Patients fit for surger :
      ▷ *VGEI with no evidence of a fistula*: should be conside-
      red for complete excision of all graft material and infec-
      ted tissue (➡l). Vascular reconstruction should be done
      with an in-situ graft (first choice (➡lla), using preferably
      an autologous vein(➡l), cryopreserved allografts, silver
      coated grafts, rifampicin bonded polyester grafts, or bo-
      vine pericardium (➡lla). Patients with a large abscess or
      multiresistant microorganisms can be considered for an
      extra-anatomic reconstruction (➡llb).
      ▷ *VGEI with aorto-enteric fistula*: Do NOT use aortic

endograft (with antibiotics) alone unless in palliative treatment or in cases with very minimal signs of infection (➡III). Instead, aim at explantation of the infected material, repair of the bowel, and coverage with viable tissue (➡I). Omentoplasty or transfer of autologous vascularised tissue to cover the vascular reconstruction is recommended (➡IIa).

▷ *VGEI with arterio-ureteral fistula*: Consider complete explantation of the graft combined with urological treatment with or without in situ arterial reconstruction (➡IIa).

- Peripheral Arteries VGEI:
  » Incidence reported in up to 2.5% in fem-fem prosthetic bypasses and in up to 2.8% in fem-pop prosthetic bypasses.
  » In summary:
    - Palliative treatment is rarely an option as mortality reaches 45% in 5 years.
    - Infection involving full graft:
      ▷ Offer in situ reconstruction with autologous vein if removal of the infected graft is likely to lead to limb ischaemia (➡I).
      ▷ Cryopreserved allografts should be considered as an alternative after infected graft removal if it is likely to lead to limb ischaemia (➡IIa).
    - Infection involving part of the graft:
      ▷ Offer local irrigation and/or negative pressure wound therapy in selected (or unfit) patients ➡IIb).
    - Adjunct techniques:
      ▷ Muscle flap coverage - should bve considered to manage the complex wound. Sartorius muscle flap (SMF), rectus femoris flap (RFF), gracilis muscle flap (GMF), rectus abdominis flap (RAF), and musculocutaneous anterolateral thigh flap have all been used for this purpose.
      ▷ Antibiotic loaded beads - Different types of beads are available, including vancomycin, tobramycin, and gentamicin, or a combination of the aforementioned.
      ▷ Extra-anatomic reconstruction - using obturator bypass (OB), lateral retrosartorius bypass (LRSB), perigeniculate arteries (PGAs), and lateral approach to crural arteries (LACA).

Diagnosing Aortic Graft Infection (AGI) – Collaborative criteria

MANAGEMENT OF AORTIC GRAFT INFECTION COLLABORATION **[MAGIC] 2016**

AT A GLANCE
- AGI is suspected where 1 Major + >2 minor same-category criteria. Diagnosis is made with 1 Major + 1 minor different-category criteria.

MAIN RESULTS
- (i) Clinical/surgical – major: intraoperative peri-graft pus or direct communication with nonsterile site (fistulae, exposed grafts, mycotic aneurysm); minor - localized AGI features or fever where AGI is most likely.
- (ii) Radiological - major perigraft gas volume, perigraft gas (>7wk) or fluid ≥3 mo); minor - other CT features; or evidence from alternative imaging.
- (iii) Laboratory - major isolation of microorganisms from perigraft aspirates or explanted grafts; minor - +ve blood cultures or infla - matory indices with no alternative source.

REFERENCES:
- Eur J Vasc Endovasc Surg. 2016 Dec;52(6):758-763. PMID: 27771318

Aortic Stent-graft Infection

SYS REVIEW AND META-ANALYSIS **2018**

AT A GLANCE

- 11 studies (402 patients) included. met the inclusion criteria.
- Most endografts were implanted for EVAR (87%) or TEVAR.
- 10% patients presented with aortic rupture. 24% had aortoenteric fistula (AEF).

MAIN RESULTS

- 17% died in hospital or within 30 days after operation. 28% died during follow-up.
- 27% had negative culture, and multiple microorganisms were identified in 26%.
- Most frequently isolated microorganisms were Staphylcoccus species (30%), Streptococcus (15%), and fungus (9%).
- 10% received conservative treatment, whereas 90% underwent surgical treatment.
- Surgery included stent graft removal with in situ reconstruction or extra-anatomical bypass, and secondary endovascular procedure.
- Survival rate was higher in the surgical group compared with conservative group (58% vs. 33%, P = 0.002).
- Survival rate was higher in patients with infected EVAR than TEVAR (58% vs. 27%, P = 0.000).
- Patient with AEF had a worse prognosis (survival rate 72% vs. 33%, P = 0.002).

REFERENCES:

- Ann Vasc Surg. 2018 Aug;51:306-313. PMID: 29772328

Diagnostic Imaging in Vascular Graft Infection

SYS REVIEW AND META-ANALYSIS 2018

AT A GLANCE

- 14 articles included, containing eight prospective and six retrospective articles.

MAIN RESULTS

- Pooled sensitivity for CTA was 0.67, in contrast to FDG-PET of 0.94, FDG-PET/CT of 0.95, WBC scintigraphy of 0.90, and WBC scintigraphy with SPECT/CT of 0.99.
- Pooled specificities were for CTA 0.63, FDG-PET 0.70, FDG-PET/CT 0.80, WBC scintigraphy 0.88, and WBC scintigraphy SPECT/CT 0.82.
- Pre- and post-test results showed that WBC SPECT/CT favours FDG-PET/CT, with a positive post-test probability of 96% vs. 83%.

REFERENCES:

- Eur J Vasc Endovasc Surg. 2018 Nov;56(5):719-729. PMID: 30122333

Prevention of infection in peripheral arterial Surgery

SYS REVIEW AND META-ANALYSIS 2007

AT A GLANCE
- 34 RCTs included
- Followed up graft infection outcomes to 2 years in 2 trials.

MAIN RESULTS
- Prophylactic systemic antibiotics reduced the risk of wound infection (RR, 0.25) and early graft infection in a fixed-e fect model (RR, 0.31).
- Antibiotic prophylaxis for >24 hours appeared to be of no added benefit (RR, 1.28)
- Prophylactic rifampicin bonding to Dacron grafts - no evidence that it reduces graft infection at 1 month.
- Suction groin wound drainage - no evidence of significant benefit
- Preoperative bathing with antiseptic agents compared with unmedicated bathing - no evidence of any significant di ference.

REFERENCES:
- J Vasc Surg. 2007 Jul;46(1):148-55. PMID: 17606135

Endovascular treatment of carotid blowout syndrome

SYS REVIEW & META-ANALYSIS 2017

AT A GLANCE

- Carotid blowout syndrome (CBS) is a life-threatening complication of head and neck cancer and radiation therapy.
- Outcomes of CBS patients treated with coil embolisation and covered stents are analysed.
- 25 noncomparative studies (559 patients) included.

MAIN RESULTS

- Technical success rate was 100% in both coiling and covered stenting groups.
- Median survival time was 3 months for all CBS patients.
- Overall perioperative mortality was 11%.
- Postoperative rebleeding rate was 27%.
- Perioperative stroke and infection rates were 3% and 1% , respectively.
- At last follow-up, 39% of patients were alive .

REFERENCES:

- J Vasc Surg. 2017 Mar;65(3):883-888. PMID: 28236928

Post-operative Infection of Prosthetic Materials

Sys Review 2018

At a glance

- 49 articles included (140 cases of prosthetic material infections).
- Most were infected carotid patches.

Main Results

- Patch infection:
  » Surgical treatment was mostly based on complete removal of the infected material followed by in situ arterial reconstruction.
  » Peri-operative complications included cranial nerve injury (13%), stroke (7%), bleeding (3%), re-infection (4%), and cardiac failure (2.2%).
- Stent infections
  » Reported in 12 patients.
  » Treatment not described for 1 case, conservative in 1 case, stent removal with venous reconstruction in 6 cases, stent removal without reconstruction in 2 cases, and carotid embolisation in 2 cases.
  » Complications included intra-operative death (9%), stroke (18%), reinfection (9%), bleeding (9%), and cardiac failure (9%).

References:

- Eur J Vasc Endovasc Surg. 2018 Dec;56(6):885-900. PMID: 30121172

CHAPTER 14
CAROTID &
VERTEBRAL
ARTERIES
DISEASES

Summary of Current Surgical Guidelines for Carotid and Vertebral Arteries Disease

▶NICE - STROKE GUIDELINES 2019 (UK)
▶▶ESC VASCULAR GUIDELINES 2017 (EU)
→VSV CAROTID GUIDELINES 2011 (US) - NO UPDATES AVAILABLE

CAROTID ARTERY DISEASE GUIDELINES

ON DEFINITIONS -
- World Health Organization (WHO) clinical definitions
  » Stroke is a focal, occasionally global, loss of neurological function lasting >24 hours (or leading to death) and which has a vascular aetiology.
  » TIA a similar presentation, but the duration is <24 hours.
- American Heart Association (AHA) definitions (tissue-based) -
  » Stroke is an episode of neurologic dysfunction caused by focal cerebral or retinal infarction (defined here as cell death), attributable to ischaemia, based on neuropathologic, neuroimaging, and/or clinical evidence of permanent injury.
  » TIA is a brief episode of neurologic dysfunction resulting from focal temporary cerebral ischaemia, with no associated infarction.
- Carotid territory symptoms are those presenting in the last 6 months, and include:
  » Hemi-sensory impairment: numbness, paraesthesia of face, arm and/or leg.
  » Hemimotor deficits: weakness of face/arm/leg, or limb clumsiness.
  » Higher cortical dysfunction: dysphasia/ aphasia, visuospatial problems
  » "Crescendo TIAs" involve multiple TIAs within a short time period, for example 3 per week, with full recovery in between.
  » "Stroke-in-evolution" refers to a fluctuating deficit (never fully back to normal) or a progressively worsening deficit
  » Amaurosis Fugax, or transient monocular blindness, refers

to transient impairment or loss of vision in one eye.

On Diagnosis -

- Duplex ultrasound (as first-line), CTA and/or MRA are recommended for evaluating the extent and severity of the stenoses (➡I, ►R, →1).
  - » Where surgical approach is considered, a dual imaging modality (CTA, MRA, or a repeated duplex by a second operator) is indicated (➡I).
  - » Duplex scan is not enough on its own if a carotid stent is considered (➡I).
  - » Consider other imaging modalities if the duplex was inconclusive (→1).
- Duplex ultrasound (DUS) is low cost and accessible. B-mode imaging is combined with colour flowand Doppler flow velocity measurements to estimate the degree of stenosis.
- Diagnostic angiography is NOT indicated unless a signific nt discrepancy between non-invasive imaging modalities exists (➡III).
- NASCET (North American Symptomatic Carotid Endarterectomy Trial) method is currently the most widely used method for measuring stenosis (➡R,►R).
- In NACET, the stenosis is calculated by measuring the luminal diameter at the maximum stenosis area (N), and the diameter of the normal internal carotid artery distal to the lesion (D). The ratio between them (1-N/D)*100 gives the stenotic percentage.
- In ECST (European Carotid Surgery Trial) method, the stenosis is calculated by measuring the luminal diameter at the maximum stenosis area (N), and the diameter of the carotid artery at the lesion level (E) (out to out). The ratio between them (1-N/E)*100 gives the stenotic percentage.

On Medical Management -

- Best medical therapy (healthy diet, smoking cessation, and physical activity) are recommended for all patients with carotid artery disease (➡I, ►R).
- Asymptomatic carotid disease -

» Low dose Aspirin is indicated for prevention of late myo-cardial infarction and other cardiovascular events, *rather than* preventing the stroke itself (➡ I). Clopidogrel should be considered if Aspirin is not tolerated (➡IIa).

» Statin therapy is recommended for long-term prevention of stroke, myocardial infarction and other cardiovascular events (➡I, ▶R).

» Do NOT consider routine screening for asymptomatic ca-rotid disease in the population (➡III, →1). However, in SE-LECTED patients with multiple risk factors screening may be beneficial to help in optimising medical therapy and en-suring adherence to treatment (➡IIb). Bruit per se is not indication for screening (→1)

• Symptomatic carotid disease -

» All patients should be on low dose Aspirin (75mg) or Clopi-dogrel (75mg) PLUS modifie release dipyridamole 200 mg twice daily (➡ I).

• If the patient is having CEA:

☞ consider early usage of Aspirin and Clopidogrel after TIA or minor stroke in the perioperative period (➡IIb). Apply the same principle to patients receiving carotid stenting (➡I).

☞ do NOT stop antiplatelets (➡I).

☞ do NOT use high dose Aspirin (➡I).

☞ do NOT use long-term dual antiplatelets AFTER sur-gery (➡III), unless indicated for other reasons.

» Statin therapy is recommended for long-term prevention of stroke, myocardial infarction and other cardiovascular events (➡I).

• Start statin in the preoperative period and continue throug-hout and after surgery (➡I).

» Treat hypertension and diabetes mellitus appropriately.

» Do NOT offer redo CEA for patients with late ipsilateral stro-ke/TIA in the presence of an ipsilateral <50% restenosis (➡I).

• Concurrent coronary and carotid disease -

» Do NOT routinely screen for carotid disease in patients un-dergoing open heart surgery(➡ III). Only consider screening in selected high risk patients (→1).

» In symptomatic carotid patients - staged or synchronous carotid endarterectomy should be considered where symptoms have occurred in the preceding 6 months and a 50-99% carotid stenosis is found (➡ IIa).

» In asymptomatic carotid patients - consider a staged or synchronous carotid endarterectomy where 70-99% carotid stenosis is found (➡ IIa,→1). Similarly, consider intervention for asymptomatic bilateral carotid disease or where one artery is blocked (➡ IIa,→2).

» Asymptomatic - consider a staged or synchronous carotid endarterectomy where symptoms occurred in the preceding 6 months and a 50-99% carotid stenosis is found

ON SURGICAL INDICATIONS -

• Asymptomatic carotid disease -

» Carotid stenosis of < 60%: ensure BMT is in place. Do NOT offer any surgery (➡I,→1).

» Carotid stenosis 60-99%: consider surgery (➡IIa, →1) or stenting (➡IIb) for patients who are of "average surgical risk" in the presence of one or more imaging characteristics, where the centre/surgeon has a documented perioperative stroke/death rates are <3% and the patient's life expectancy exceeds 3-5 years.

» The following clinical and imaging characteristics have been associated with an increased risk of late ipsilateral stroke in asymptomatic patients:

• Silent infarction on CT scan (annual stroke rate 3.6% vs 1% - OR x3).

• stenosis progression (annual stroke rate 2% vs 1% - OR x1.92).

• High plaque area > 80 mm^2 on computerised plaque analysis (annual stroke rate 4.6% vs 1.4% - OR x5.8).

• existence of intra-plaque haemorrhage on MRI (annual stroke rate OR x 3.6).

• Predominantly echolucent plaque on Duplex (annual stroke rate 4.2% vs. 1.6% for echogenic. OR x 2.6).

• Presence of spontaneous embolisation on TCD (annual stroke OR x 7.46); Additional uniformly or echolucent plaque adds significantly to the risk (OR 10.6).

- Presence of contra-lateral TIA/Stroke (annual stroke rate 3.4% vs. 1.2% for echogenic. OR x 3).

» Surgery+ BMT vs. BMT alone: risk of stroke in 4-5 yrs in three major trials (VACS, CAS, ACST-1) is 10.4% vs. 12%, 12.4% vs. 17.8%, and 6.4% vs. 11.8%, respectively.

» Currently, there is NO indication to perform carotid intervention to improve cognitive impairment (➡III).

» Consider redo CEA for patients with asymptomatic restenos in the presence of an ipsilateral >70% restenosis (➡IIb).

- Symptomatic carotid disease -
  » WHICH PATIENTS?
    - Offer <u>carotid endarterectomy</u> to patients with carotid territory symptoms, within the preceding 6 months, who have a <u>70-99%</u> carotid stenosis, provided the centre/ surgeon documented procedural death/stroke rate is <6% (➡I).
      ◊ Surgery+ BMT vs. BMT alone: risk of stroke in 5 yrs in three major trials (ESCT, NASCET, and SVACS) is 17% vs. 32%, ARR of +16%, RRR of 48%, and NNT to prevent one stroke is 6.
      ◊ It is also possible to consider <u>stenting</u> as alternative to surgery where the patient is <70 yr-old and the centre documented procedural death/stroke rate is <6% (➡IIb).
      ◊ Do not consider stenting if the patient is >70 yr-old (➡I).
    - Symptomatic patients with <u>50-69%</u> stenosis should also be considered for CEA (➡IIa).
      ◊ Surgery+ BMT vs. BMT alone: risk of stroke in 5 yrs in three major trials (ESCT, NASCET, and SVACS) is 20% vs. 27%, ARR of +8%, RRR of 28%, and NNT to prevent one stroke is 13.
    - Do NOT offer surgery or stenting for patients with <u>stenosis <50%</u> unless they suffer recurrent symptoms despite best medical therapy and following multidiscipli-

nary team review (➡IIb, ▶R).

- Offer redo CEA for patients with late ipsilateral stroke/ TIA in the presence of an ipsilateral 50-99% restenosis (➡I).
- Do NOT offer symptomatic patients with <u>near occlusion</u> any surgery or stenting (➡III), unless they are suffering from recurrent ipsilateral symptoms (despite optimal medical therapy) and following multidisciplinary team review.
    - ◊ Neurologic symptoms may be secondary to embo- lisation from the distal aspect of the occluded ICA segmented other areas. These patients may be ma- naged by endarterectomy with transection and flush ligation of the ICA to remove the "stump" as a cause of the symptoms (→1).
    - ◊ Carotid dissection causing occlusion or stenosis should be managed with anticoagulation first (→1). Where symptoms are not responding to BMT, an intervention (possibly stenting) can be considered (→2).
- » Surgery+ BMT vs. BMT alone: risk of stroke in 5 yrs in three major trials (ESCT, NASCET, and SVACS) is 23% vs. 23%, ARR of -0.1%, RRR of none, and NNT to prevent one stroke is none (no benefit).

- » RISK FACTORS: The following clinical and imaging charac- teristics have been associated with an increased risk of late ipsilateral stroke in asymptomatic patients:
    - Increasing age (5 yr ARR conferred by CEA: 6% for <65yr vs. 19% for >75yr).
    - Recent symptoms (5 ry ARR conferred by CEA: 19% for <2w vs. 0.8% for >12w).
    - Gender (5 yr ARR conferred by CEA: 11% for malevs. 3% for female).
    - Extent of ischaemia (5 yr ARR conferred by CEA: 5% for occular vs. 15-18% for hemisphere).
    - Depth of ischaemia (3 yr ARR conferred by CEA: 9% for lacunar vs. 15% for non-lacunar).

- Comorbidities (2 y ARR conferred by CEA: 11% for 0-5comorbidities vs. 8% for >7comorbidities).
- Plaque features (5 yr ARR conferred by CEA: 8% for smooth vs. 17% for irregular).
- Contralateral occlusion (5 yr ARR conferred by CEA: 24% for presence of occlusion vs. 13% for no occlusion).

» TIMING?
- Offer urgent carotid endarterectomy (preferably <24h) for patients with 50-99% stenosis and stroke-in-evolution or crescendo transient ischaemic attacks (➡️IIa, →1).
- Otherwise, offer carotid endarterectomy otherwise as soon as possible, and preferably within 14 days of symptom onset (➡️I,→1).
  - The risk of a major stroke/death has been shown in three national audits (UK, Sweden, Germany) to be highest in tyhe first 48 hours (4%, 12%, 3% respectively), and drops as time passes (2.3%, 5.4% and 2.3%, respectively, after 15 days of index event).
- Do NOT consider stenting if the procedure is planned within 14 days of symptoms onset (➡️I).

» UNRESOLVED STROKE:
- Defer CEA in patients with 50-99% stenoses who suffer (➡️I):
  - A disabling stroke (modified Rankin score 3
  - The area of infarction exceeds one-third of the ipsilateral middle cerebral artery territory
  - With altered consciousness/ drowsiness
- This is to minimise the risks of postoperative parenchymal haemorrhage.
- • Patients with significant comorbidities that render them unsuitable for surgery can be considered for carotid stenting within appropriate discussion and governance framework (➡️IIa).

<u>ON SURGICAL TECHNIQUES -</u>

- Consent process should be thorough, including (➡R):
  - » indication for surgery
  - » any atypical symptoms require further investigation later
  - » degree of stenosis
  - » procedural risks
  - » if the patient is receiving optimal BMT
  - » carotid disease location (high, normal)
  - » any pre-existing cranial nerve injuries
  - » and operative side (marked clearly).
- Focus on four key preoperative questions (➡R):
  - » quoting your own operative risks (not a general trial-based risk)
  - » any previous carotid surgery (esp. if contralateral), parathyroid surgery or radical neck surgery - arrange indirect laryngoscopy if so, as vocal cord palsy can be fatal. Consider having ENT surgeon at the time of extubation.
  - » any missing antiplatelets, statins or hypertension (>180mmHg)
  - » and the liklihood of need to mobilise upper ICA - if so, double up or plan for more complicated exposure.
- Consider targeted monitoring and quality control strategies to reduce the risk of perioperative stroke (➡IIb).
- Consider general or local/regional anaesthesia (➡I), antegrade or retro-jugular approach (➡I), transverse or longitudinal incision (➡R), shunting selectively, routinely or never (➡I) based on and left to the discretion of the operating surgeon.
- Do NOT perform carotid sinus block routinely. There is no robust supportive evidence that this procedure positively affects hypertension postoperatively (➡III).
- Consider to patch more routinely than to primarily close more routinely. There is no evidence that the patch type influen es outcome (➡I).
- Consider using eversion CEA over routine primary arteriotomy closure (➡I). Nevertheless, The choice between eversion or patched endarterectomy should be left to the discretion of the operating surgeon (➡I). Other guidelines recommend patch or eversion technique more than primary closure (→1).

- Do NOT consider surgery routinely for isolated ICA coils/kinks (➡III). Symptomatic lesions can be considered for surgery after MDT discussion (➡IIb).
- Consider using protamine reversal of heparin to prevent neck haematomas requiring re-exploration (➡IIa).
- Consider creating a carotid bypass (interposition, etc.) in the following cases (➡R):
  » extensive atherosclerotic disease, carotid aneurysms, or excessive kinking.
  » previous radiotherapy with severe fibrosi
  » complicating large intimal flap on completion angi
  » treatment of carotid body tumour, patch infection, or restenosis.

ON SURGICAL COMPLICATIONS -

- <u>Intraoperative stroke:</u>
  » Suspect when a new neurologic deficit appears immediately following recovery from anaesthesia, and lasts >24h.
  » Common origin is a thrombus that has been dislodged during carotid dissection, while using the shunt, or upon restoration of flo . Less commonly is a hypoperfusion stroke due to inadequate contralateral perfusion or shunt malformation.
  » Prevention can likely be achieved by using targeted monitoring and quality control strategies (➡R).
  » Treatments include immediate re-exploration, to exclude accumulation of thrombus within the endarterectomy zone (➡R,→1). Where deemed safe, an urgent mechanical embolectomy (using dedicated neuro-interventional retrieval devices), thrombolysis (using 500k to 1m Units of Urokinase) and an intra-operative angiogram should be considered (➡I).
- <u>Postoperative stroke:</u>
  » Suspect when a new neurologic deficit appears following full recovery from anaesthesia, and lasts >24h.
  » Common reasons are thrombosis forming in the carotid (with the first 6 hours) or hyper perfusion syndrome (HPS) when onset is later.

» Prevention may be achieved by using using DAPT perioperatively (➨R), and by appropriate management of hypertension.
» Treatment include CTA/MRA, immediate re-exploration where needed, and the reduction of high intracranial pressure (➨R).
- Postoperative hypotension:
  » Mostly related to exposure of carotid sinus baroreceptors to the pulse pressure, without the dampening effect of the excised plaque (➨R).
  » There is conflicting evidence of the risk of hypotension on developing stroke postoperatively.
  » First-line treatment should be the administration of intravenous crystalloids together with volume expanders (➨IIb).
    - If this fails, titrated intravenous vasopressors (dobutamine, dopamine, noradrenaline, phenylephrine) should be considered
    - Maintain systolic blood pressure >90 mmHg.
- Postoperative hypertension:
  » Can affect up to two thirds of patients. . The condition is more common in patients with preoperative hypertension, GA cases, and emergency CEA>
  » Unknown cause, but can be related to denervation of the carotid bulb and increased cerebral norepinephrine and/or renin production by the central nervous system (➨R).
  » Postoperative hypertension increases the risk of TIA/stroke and neck haematoma postoperatively.
  » Treatment should be agreed and written as a protocol (➨R).
- Postoperative wound haematoma:
  » Not uncommon. The re-exploration for neck haematoma may be required in 1.2% of CEA patients on aspirin, 0.7% on clopidogrel, and 1.4% in patients taking aspirin and clopidogrel according to VSGNE report. (➨R).
  » Dual antiplatelets is NOT a risk facvtor Small drains do not reduce reexploration, while large ones do (➨R).
  » Any evidence of stridor or tracheal deviation mandates immediate evacuation (➨I).
- Cranial nerve injury:

> » Most common is the vagus nerve, followed by hypoglossal nerve. (➡R).
> » Risk increases in emergency cases and reexploration for haematoma (➡R).
> » To avoid injury, consider division of the sternocleidomastoid artery, apply a tie to the divided ansa cervicalis to retract the hypolossal, avoid jaw retraction by curving the skin incision posteriorly toward the mastoid process, , this ensures avoidance on the mandibular branch of the facial nerve (➡R). Some evidence suggest that administering dexamethasone perioperatively can reduce risk of CN injuries (➡R).

On Outcome and Follow-up -

- Admit all CEA and CAS patients to recovery area of theatre or angio suite for 3-6 hours for neurological and intra-arterial BP monitoring (➡I).
  - » Up to 40% of patients may require treatment for post-CEA hypertension in the early postoperative period.
    - Most patients require only a single bolus of intravenous labetalol to control their BP.
    - If no further spikes of hypertension exist, these patients can usually return to the vascular ward 2-3 hours later (➡I).
  - » Where BP and other parameters are stable, transfer the patient back to the vascular ward for ongoing surveillance (➡I). Obtain hourly non-invasive BP and neurological monitoring for the first 24 hours and 4-hourly thereafter until discharge.
  - » A written pathway and clear criteria are recommended (➡I).
- Arrange a DUS follow up within 30 days of surgery (→2). Where a patch or eversion technique are used, and no significant (>50%) stenosis is found, consider further DUS ONLY if other risk factors exist (→2). In patients with a normal DUS study result and primary closure of the endarterectomy site, ongoing imaging is recommended to identify recurrent stenosis (→2).
- Consider monitoring the contralateral asymptomatic disease where it has a significant (>50%) stenosis (→2).

VERTEBRAL ARTERY DISEASE GUIDELINES

- Over 20% of ischaemic cerebrovascular events involving the posterior circulation are related to vertebral artery disease (➡R).
- CTA/MRA have a higher sensitivity (94%) and specificit (95%) compared to than duplex scan (sensitivity 70%) (➡R). However, in patients with known vertebral artery stenoses, it is reasonable to use DUS to assess stenosis progression (➡R).
- In patients with symptomatic extracranial vertebral artery stenoses, consider revascularisation for lesions ≥ 50% where recurrent ischaemic events occur despite optimal medical management (➡IIb).
  » Surgery of extracranial vertebral stenoses include transposition to CCA, trans-subclavian vertebral endarterectomy, distal venous bypass. These can be performed with low stroke/death rates in experienced surgical teams.
  » Endovascular revascularisation has mostly replaced open surgery in many centres.
- Do NOT offer revascularisation for asymptomatic vertebral artery stenosis, irrespective of the degree of severity (➡III).

Treatment for Carotid Artery Aneurysm

REVIEW OF PRACTICE 2016

AT A GLANCE

- <4% of peripheral arterial aneurysms
- Caused by genetic predisposition, atherosclerosis, trauma, or infection.

MAIN RESULTS

- No trials identified
- Treatment include resection with primary anastomosis, interposition graft or endovascular stenting.

REFERENCES:

- Vascular. 2016 Oct;24(5):549-51. PMID: 26767605

Treatment for Carotid Dissection

REVIEW OF PRACTICE

AT A GLANCE

- Causes 2% of stokes; 20% of stroke in young patients; found in 20% of trauma with unexplained neuro defici
- Result from trauma, iatrogenic, central dissection, or spontaneous
- Three types: I-irregularity; II-stenosis; III-occlusion.

MAIN RESULTS

- No trials identified
- Treatment include conservative (I and III), or open/Endovascular (II).

Treatment for Carotid Body Tumour (CBT)

REVIEW OF PRACTICE

AT A GLANCE

- Uncommon. 5% is bilateral. 5% is metachronous. 5% is malignant.
- Originates from neural crest ectoderm (chemoreceptors).
- Classification – Chamblain.

MAIN RESULTS

- No trials identified.
- Treatment include:
  » Open surgical resection.
  » Consider ICA covered stent before resection (reduce bleeding).

Treatment for Carotid Kinks and coiling

RCT 2005

At a glance

- 92 patients randomly assigned for surgery and 90 for medical treatment.
- Some 37 patients (41.1%) randomly assigned to medical treatment crossed over to the surgical group within a mean of 16.8 months after randomization due to new hemispheric symptoms or worsening nonhemispheric complaints.

Main Results

- There were no perioperative strokes or deaths.
- The incidence of late hemispheric and retinal transient ischemic attacks was significantly lower in the surgical than in the medical group, respectively, 8% vs 21%, and 3% vs 12%.
- Late strokes, 2 (2.2%) of which were fatal, occurred only in the medical group.
- Late carotid occlusions also developed only in the medical group (5 of 90, 5.5%; P = .02).
- All surgically treated carotid elongations were analyzed histologically and 56%showed atypical and typical patterns of fibromusc - lar dysplasia.

References:

- J Vasc Surg. 2005 Nov;42(5):838-46; PMID: 16275432

Treatment for Carotid Artery Stenosis - guidelines

SYS REVIEW OF GUIDELINES 2015

AT A GLANCE

- 34 guidelines reviewed from 23 different regions/countries in 6 languages.

MAIN RESULTS

- **Asymptomatic carotid stenosis 50-99%** - 85% endorsed CEA (recommended it should or may be provided) for average-surgical-risk pts, 61% endorsed CAS, 29% opposed CAS, and 4% endorsed medical treatment alone.
- **Asymptomatic carotid stenosis in high risk pts** - 46% endorsed CAS.
- **Symptomatic carotid stenosis 50-99%** - 94% endorsed CEA in average-risk pts, 58% endorsed CAS and 27% opposed CAS.
- **Symptomatic carotid stenosis in high-risk pts** – 82% endorsed CAS
- Guideline recommendations were based on results of trials in which patients were randomized 12 to 34 years ago, rarely reflected medical treatment improvements but often understated potential CAS hazards

REFERENCES:

- Stroke. 2015 Nov;46(11):3288-301. PMID: 26451020

Carotid artery stenting vs. endarterectomy

COCHRANE SYS REVIEW & META-ANALYSIS 2020

AT A GLANCE

- 22 trials (9753 participants) included.

MAIN RESULTS

- Symptomatic carotid stenosis:
  - » Stenting has higher risk of periprocedural death or stroke (OR 1.7). Patients under 70 years old have OR of 1.11, while those over 70 yrs-old have OR of 2.23.
  - » Stenting has lower risks of myocardial infarction (OR 0.47), cranial nerve palsy (OR 0.09), and access site haematoma (OR 0.32).
  - » The combination of periprocedural death or stroke favoured endarterectomy (OR 1.51).
- Symptomatic carotid stenosis:
  - » Stenting caused a non-significant increase in periprocedural death or stroke (OR 1.72).
  - » Moderate or higher carotid artery restenosis (50% or greater) or occlusion during follow-up was more common after stenting (OR 2.00).

REFERENCES:

- Cochrane Database Syst Rev. 2020 Feb 25;2:CD000515. PMID: 32096559

Carotid artery stenting vs. endarterectomy

EVA-3S TRIAL 2014

AT A GLANCE
- 527 pts with symptomatic severe carotid stenosis in 30 centres in France Median follow-up- 7.1 yrs included.

MAIN RESULTS
- Cumulative probabilities of stroke was 11% in CAS vs. 6.3% in CEA at 5-year follow-up (hazard ratio, 1.85)
- At 10 yrs the probability was 11.5% in CAS vs.7.6% in CEA (hazard ratio, 1.70).
- No difference observed in ipsilateral stroke rate, severe carotid restenosis (≥70%) or occlusion, death, or myocardial infarction beyond the procedural period.

REFERENCES:
- Stroke. 2014 Sep;45(9):2750-6. PMID: 25082808

Restenosis and Risk of Stroke After Stenting or Endarterectomy

INTERNATIONAL CAROTID STENTING STUDY (ICSS) 2018

AT A GLANCE

- CSS is a parallel-group randomised trial at 50 tertiary care centres in Europe, Australia, New Zealand, and Canada. Patients aged 40 years or older with symptomatic carotid stenosis measuring 50% or more were randomly assigned either stenting or endarterectomy in a 1:1 ratio.
- 1713 patients were enrolled and randomly allocated treatment, of whom 1530 individuals were followed up with ultrasound for a median of 4·0 years.

MAIN RESULTS

- At least moderate restenosis (≥50%) occurred in 41% (cumulative 5-year risk) after stenting, and 30% after endarterectomy. The unadjusted hazard ratio [HR] is 1·43 (p<0·0001).
- Patients with at least moderate restenosis (≥50%) had a higher risk of ipsilateral stroke than did individuals without restenosis in the overall patient population (HR 3·18), and in the endarterectomy group alone but not in stenting.
- No difference was noted in the risk of severe restenosis (≥70%) or subsequent stroke between the two treatment groups.

REFERENCES:

- Lancet Neurol. 2018 Jul;17(7):587-596. PMID: 29861139

Carotid artery stenting vs. endarterectomy

CAROTID REVASCULARIZATION ENDARTERECTOMY VERSUS STENTING TRIAL (CREST) 2015

AT A GLANCE
• RCT – CEA vs CAS. 2502 pts followed up to 4 yrs.

MAIN RESULTS
• Collective stroke, MI, and death were not different between CAS and CEA (7.2% versus 6.8%; hazard ratio, 1.11).
• Outcomes were slightly better after CAS for patients aged <70 years and better after CEA for patients aged >70 years.
• There were differences in outcome components, CAS versus CEA (stroke 4.1% versus 2.3%, P=0.012; and myocardial infarction 1.1% versus 2.3%, P=0.032).

Restenosis rate from CREST (Stroke. 2015 Mar)
• Out of 1151 patients who underwent CEA, 65% had patch and 29% had primary closure.
• Significant reduction in 2-year risk of restenosis noted when patched is used (hazard ratio, 0.35)
• No significant differences found in periprocedural stroke or death rate or in 4-year risk of ipsilateral stroke.

10-yrs outcome from CREST (N Eng J Med. 2016 Mar)
• No significant difference in the rate of the primary composite end point between CAS (11.8%) and CEA (9.9%) over 10 years of follow-up (hazard ratio, 1.10).
• Ipsilateral stroke –6.9% in CAS vs. 5.6% in CEA (hazard ratio, 0.99).
• No significant di ferences for symptomatic vs. asymptomatic pts.
• Restenosis rate from CREST (Stroke. 2015 Mar)
• Out of 1151 patients who underwent CEA, 65% had patch and 29% had primary closure.
• Significant reduction in 2-year risk of restenosis noted when patched is used (hazard ratio, 0.35)
• No significant differences found in periprocedural stroke or death rate or in 4-year risk of ipsilateral stroke.

REFERENCES:
• Stroke. 2010 Oct;41(10 Suppl):S31-4. PMID: 20876500
• N Engl J Med. 2016 Mar 17;374(11):1021-31. PMID: 26890472
• Stroke. 2015 Mar;46(3):757-61. PMID: 25613307

CAS vs. CEA for carotid stenosis

META-ANALYSIS BY CAROTID STENTING TRIALISTS' COLLABORATION 2016

AT A GLANCE

- 4754 patients were randomly assigned to either CEA or CAS treatment in four studies.

MAIN RESULTS

- CAS pts - periprocedural hazard ratio (HR) for stroke and death in patients aged 65-69 years compared with patients younger than 60 years was 2·16. Patients >70 years has HR of 4.
- CEA pts –no evidence of increased periprocedural risk by age group
- CAS-versus CEA - periprocedural HR is 1·61 for patients aged 65-69 years, and HR is 2·09 for patients >70.
- Within-treatment stroke rate didn't differ with age.
- CEA remains the standard treatment in patients with recently symptomatic carotid stenosis; CAS is a safe and effective alternative option in patients younger than 70 and can be also considered when a contraindication to CEA exists.

REFERENCES:

- Lancet. 2016 Mar 26;387(10025):1305-11. PMID: 26880122

CEA vs. CAS in re-stenosis

SYS REVIEW AND META-ANALYSIS 2015

AT A GLANCE
- 50 articles involving 4,399 patients.

MAIN RESULTS
- No differences in 30-day perioperative mortality, stroke and transient ischemic attack rates.
- Patients undergoing redo CEA suffered more cranial nerve injuries (CNIs) than those undergoing CAS (P < .05). Most recovered within 3 months.
- Similar MI rate noted for CEA vs. CAS (rate was higher for CEA in non-comparative studies
- Non-significant difference noted in freedom from stroke at 36 months in comparative studies and at 12 months in non-comparative studies.
- Risk of restenosis was greater in CAS patients than in redo CEA patients.

REFERENCES:
- Surgery. 2015 Jun;157(6):1166-73. PMID: 25840718

Safety of Stenting and Endarterectomy for Asymptomatic Disease

Sys Review and Meta-Analysis 2018

At a glance

- 5 studies involving 3901 patients (1585 with CEA; 2316 with CAS) included.

Main Results

- Risk of any stroke is signific ntly lower in patients with CEA vs. CAS (OR 0.53).
- The difference could be driven by minor stroke (OR 0.50).
- Risk of death, major stroke, ipsilateral stroke, and MI were not significantly di ferent.
- No robust conclusion could be drawn regarding mid to long-term complications.

References:

- Eur J Vasc Endovasc Surg. 2018 May;55(5):614-624. PMID: 29559195

Eversion (EC) or Conventional (CC) Carotid Surgery

NATIONAL DATABASE (SOCIETY FOR VASCULAR SURGERY QUALITY INITIATIVE) 2015

AT A GLANCE
- 2365 EC and 17,155 CC compared.

MAIN RESULTS
- CC more often performed under GA (92% vs 80%) and with a shunt (59% vs 24%).
- Immediate perioperative ipsilateral neurologic events (EC, 1.3% vs CC, 1.2%) and ipsilateral stroke (EC, 0.8% vs CC, 0.9%) were uncommon and insignificantly di erent.
- EC tend to take less time (median 99 vs 114 minutes; P < .001), but required more return to theatre for bleeding (1.4% vs 0.8%; P = .002)
- Estimated survival at 1 year was similar (96.7% vs 95.9%).
- 1-year freedom from recurrent stenosis >50% was lower for EC (88.8% vs 94.3%, P < .001). Freedom from reoperation at 1 year was similar and very low (99.5% vs 99.6%).

REFERENCES:
- J Vasc Surg. 2015 May;61(5):1216-22. PMID: 25925539

Risk of stroke after TIA event

SYS REVIEW AND META-ANALYSIS 2007

AT A GLANCE
- 11 studies. random effects model.

MAIN RESULTS
- Pooled early risk of stroke was 3.5%, 8.0%, and 9.2% at 2, 30, and 90 days after TIA, respectively.
- When active ascertainment of stroke outcome is used, early risk of stroke was 9.9%, 13.4%, and 17.3% at 2, 30, and 90 days, respectively.

REFERENCES:
- Arch Intern Med. 2007 Dec 10;167(22):2417-22. PMID: 18071162

Risk of stroke after TIA event

SYS REVIEW AND META-ANALYSIS 2015

AT A GLANCE
- 10 studies (2634 pts) included.

MAIN RESULTS
- Pooled stroke risk in studies with active follow-up: 6% at 2-3 days, 11% at 7 days and 18% at 14 days.
- Pooled stroke risk in studies with uncensored populations: 6.4% at 2-3 days, 19.5% at 7 days and 26.1% at 14 days.
- Risk of recurrent cerebrovascular events in patients with symptomatic carotid stenosis: 6.4%, 19.5% and 26.1% after 2-3, 7 and 14 days respectively.

REFERENCES:
- J Cardiovasc Surg (Torino). 2015 Dec;56(6):845-52. PMID: 26399273

Risk of stroke after TIA event

SYS REVIEW AND META-ANALYSIS 2017

AT A GLANCE
- 15 papers that included 14,889 patients.

MAIN RESULTS
- Reported risk of stroke ranged from 0 to 1.5% 2 days after TIA , 0-2.6% 7 days after TIA, 1.9-2.9% 30 days after TIA, and 0.6-4.8% 90 days after TIA.
- Pooled stroke risk was 3.4% at 90 days, 2.8% at 30 days, 2% at 7 days and 1.4% at 2 days.

REFERENCES:
- Cerebrovasc Dis. 2017;43(1-2):90-98. PMID: 27992865

Early Intervention for Symptomatic Carotid Stenosis

NATIONWIDE INPATIENT SAMPLE DATABASE 2014

AT A GLANCE

- 72,797 admissions who had ultra-eraly (within 48h of admission) or deferred (up to 2w) procedure.

MAIN RESULTS

- Ultra-early intervention significantly decreased cost and length of stay
- Ultra-early procedure - in Pts without infarction - mortality and iatrogenic stroke rate are significantly lower compared to deferred ones. In Pts with infarction - mortality and iatrogenic stroke have increased odd compared to deferred group.
- Stenting in pts with infarction experienced increased odds of mortality (but not stroke) in comparison with those receiving endarterectomy.
- Recombinant tissue plasminogen activator (rtPA) administration on the day of revascularization greatly increased the odds of iatrogenic stroke and mortality.

REFERENCES:

- J Stroke Cerebrovasc Dis. 2014 Oct;23(9):2341-9. PMID: 25200243

Safety of Carotid Intervention Following Thrombolysis

NATIONWIDE INPATIENT SAMPLE DATABASE 2018

AT A GLANCE
- 310 257 patients included.

MAIN RESULTS
- Receiving tissue plasminogen activator (tPA) significantly increased risk of developing an intracerebral hemorrhage (ICH) or post-procedural stroke (PPS) than patients having CEA or CAS without tPA administration.
- The increased risk diminished with time, and became similar to patients who underwent carotid revascularization without tPA administration by 7 d after thrombolysis.
- Patients who received tPA and underwent CEA or CAS also had higher odds of poor outcome and in-hospital mortality.

REFERENCES:
- Neurosurgery. 2018 Nov 1;83(5):922-930. PMID: 29136204

Combined carotid and coronary bypass surgery

SYS REVIEW AND META-ANALYSIS 2014

AT A GLANCE

- 12 studies (17,469 and 7,552 patients in the combined and staged group, respectively).

MAIN RESULTS

- No difference found in early mortality (RR 1.36), post operative stroke (RR 1.14), combined early mortality or stroke (RR 1.08) and combined endpoint of MI or stroke (RR 0.75) between the 2 surgical approaches.

REFERENCES:

- Ann Thorac Surg. 2014 Jan;97(1):102-9. PMID: 24090581

Local vs. General Anaesthetic for carotid surgery

COCHRANE SYS REVIEW AND META-ANALYSIS 2013

AT A GLANCE
- 14 RCTs (4596 ops - 3526 were from GALA trial).

MAIN RESULTS
- No statistically significant difference in incidence of stroke within 30 days of surgery between local and general anaesthesia group.
- Incidence of strokes in local anaesthesia group: 3.2% vs. 3.5% in general group (Peto OR 0.92).
- LA patients - 3.6% of patients had a stroke or died; GA pts: 4.2% (Peto OR 0.85).
- Non-significant trend noticed towards lower operative mortality with local anaesthetic. However, neither the GALA trial nor the pooled analysis were adequately powered to reliably detect an effect on mortality.

REFERENCES:
- Cochrane Database Syst Rev. 2013 Dec 19;(12):CD000126. PMID: 24353155

Carotid surgery with contralateral carotid occlusion

SYS REVIEW 2013

AT A GLANCE

- 46 articles (3120 occluded contralateral carotid vs. 25,726 c/l carotid).

MAIN RESULTS

- Patients with occluded c/l carotid had increased incidence of stroke (OR 1.65), TIA (OR 1.57), stroke/TIA (OR 1.52), and death (OR, 1.76) ≤30 days of treatment.
- No difference in incidence of MI was noted.

REFERENCES:

- J Vasc Surg. 2013 Apr;57(4):1134-45. PMID: 23462196

Carotid surgery with contralateral carotid occlusion

SYS REVIEW AND META-ANALYSIS 2018

AT A GLANCE
- 35 articles included.

MAIN RESULTS
- Patients with C/L occlusion had:
  » higher rate of preoperative symptoms (Stroke + transient ischemic attack [TIA]) (odds ratio [OR] = 1.20).
  » increased risk of perioperative neurological complications (Stroke + TIA) (OR = 1.63).
- There is no significant difference in the perioperative mortality rate and stroke-free survival rate at 5 years.

REFERENCES:
- J Stroke Cerebrovasc Dis. 2018 Oct;27(10):2587-2595. PMID: 29941392

Routine or Selective Carotid Artery Shunting

COCHRANE SYS REVIEW AND META-ANALYSIS 2014

AT A GLANCE
- 1270 participants included.

MAIN RESULTS
- For routine vs. no shunting, there was no significant difference in the rate of all stroke, ipsilateral stroke or death up to 30 days.
- No significant di ference in postoperative neurological deficit.

REFERENCES:
- Cochrane Database Syst Rev. 2014 Jun 23;2014(6):CD000190. PMID: 24956204

Routine or Selective Carotid Artery Shunting

Vascular Quality Initiative database 2018

At a glance
- 28,457 endarterectomies included.

Main Results
- Unadjusted rates of in-hospital death and stroke were 0.30% and 0.78% for routine shunting vs. 0.22% and 0.91% for selective shunting, respectively.
- Unadjusted rate of in-hospital death was significantly lower in the awake monitoring group than in routine shunting group (0.05% vs 0.30%).
- After adjustment for patient risk factors, there was no difference in rates of any primary outcomes among the groups.
- There was a shorter postoperative length of stay for the awake monitoring group compared with the routine shunting group (1.55 days vs 2.00 days).

References:
- J Vasc Surg. 2018 Aug;68(2):416-425. PMID: 29571621

Role of Carotid Stump Pressure

SYS REVIEW AND META-ANALYSIS 2020

AT A GLANCE
- A total of 179 studies dating back to 1971 included.

MAIN RESULTS
- There is higher incidence of stroke in shunted CEAs solely based on CSP measurement alone (OR, 0.14).
- Similar patterns of stroke was found at 25 mmHg, 30 mmHg and 40 mmHg.
- This effect on end points of mortality and TIA demonstrated no benefit in either direction.
- carotid stump pressure, as a single criterion, is not a reliable parameter in reduction of TIA, mortality, and ischemic stroke at any given pressure range.

REFERENCES:
- Ann Vasc Dis. 2020 Mar 25;13(1):28-37. PMID: 32273919

Patching in CEA

RCT 2015

AT A GLANCE
- 753 patients had patch vs. 329 didn't (primary closure).

MAIN RESULTS
- Overall 52 patients had resetenosis (symptomatic in 52% of them).
- Restenosis significantly less in patch patients (HR 0.26)

REFERENCES:
- Stroke. 2015 Mar;46(3):757-61. PMID: 25613307

Patching in CEA

RCT 2019

AT A GLANCE

- 29 articles (9 randomized studies and 20 nonrandomized studies)
- Total of 12,696 patients and 13,219 CEAs.

MAIN RESULTS

- Overall 30-day stroke risk was higher in the patch closure (PAC) group (odds ratio [OR], 1.9). After exclusion of nonrandomized studies, this difference was not statistically significant anymore (OR, 1.8).
- Restenosis rate was higher after primary closure (PRC) group (OR, 2.2).
- No differences in bleeding complications.

REFERENCES:

- J Vasc Surg. 2019 Jun;69(6):1962-1974.e4 PMID: 30792057

Eversion vs. Conventional Carotid Endarterectomy

RCT 2000

AT A GLANCE
- 1353 patients randomly assigned to undergo eversion (n = 678) or standard CEA (n = 675; primary closure, 419; patch, 256).
- Mean follow-up interval was 33 months.

MAIN RESULTS
- Restenosis rates was 8% in primary closure vs. 1.5% in patched population.
- Cumulative restenosis risk at 4 years was significantly lower in eversion CEA vs. standard group (3.6% vs 9.2%; P =.01 - absolute risk reduction of 5.6%).
- Ilpsilateral stroke was 3.3% in eversion vs. 2.2% in standard group.
- No significant differences in cumulative risks of ipsilateral stroke and death
- Eversion CEA and patch CEA were negative independent predictors of restenosis.

REFERENCES:
- J Vasc Surg. 2000 Jan;31(1 Pt 1):19-30. PMID: 10642705

Protamin use in CEA

SYS REVIEW 2016

AT A GLANCE

- Protamine sulfate can be administered at the conclusion of carotid endarterectomy (CEA) to reverse the anticoagulant effects of heparin
- 7 studies included.
- 3,817 patients receiving protamine after CEA and 6,070 patients not receiving protamine for heparin reversal.
- Only one study was randomised.

MAIN RESULTS

- After heparin reversal with protamine - a statistically significant reduction in wound haematoma requiring re-operation was recorded (OR 0.42).
- No significant difference was observed in stroke rates between groups of patients that received and did not receive protamine
- Meta-regression analysis did not reveal any significant effect mediated by the modifiers examined.

REFERENCES:

- Eur J Vasc Endovasc Surg. 2016 Sep;52(3):296-307. PMID: 27389942

Protamin use in CEA

Sys Review & Meta-Analysis 2016

At a glance
- 12 observational studies (10,621 patients) included.

Main Results
- Event rates did not differ significantly between the two groups
  - » stroke - RR, 0.84
  - » myocardial infarction - RR, 0.89
  - » mortality - RR, 0.9
- The use of protamine was associated with a significant decrease in major bleeding complications requiring reoperation (RR, 0.57).

References:
- JAMA Surg. 2016 Mar;151(3):247-55. PMID: 26501944

Cranial Nerve Injury After Carotid Endarterectomy

SYS REVIEW & META-ANALYSIS 2017

AT A GLANCE
- 26 articles (20,860 CEAs) included.

MAIN RESULTS
- Vagus nerve is the most frequently injured cranial nerve (pooled injury rate 4%), followed by hypoglossal nerve (3.8%).
- Fewer than one seventh of these injuries are permanent .
- Injury rate decreased from about 8% to 2% and 1%, respectively, over the last 35 years.
- Urgent procedures (OR 1.59) and return to operating room for a neurological event or bleeding (OR 2.21) were associated with an increased risk of CNI.
- No statistically significant association found between CNIs and the type of anaesthesia, use of a patch, redo operation, and use of a shunt.

REFERENCES:
- Eur J Vasc Endovasc Surg. 2017 Mar;53(3):320-335. PMID: 28117240

Risk Prediction Models to Detect Asymptomatic Carotid Stenosis

Sys Review & Meta-Analysis 2020

At a glance

- 975 studies reviewed and 6 prediction models identified [3 for moderate and 3 for severe ACS]).
- Models validated using data from 596,469 individuals who attended commercial vascular screening clinics in the United States and United Kingdom.

Main Results

- The best model included age (defined as per year increase), sex (male), smoking (current), hypertension (, hypercholesterolemia, diabetes mellitus, vascular and cerebrovascular disease (defined as a medical history of either coronary heart disease or stroke), measured blood pressure (defined as per mmHg increase), and blood lipids (HDL, LDL, and TC/HDL ratio, per mmol/L increase).
- The area under the receiver operating characteristic curve for this model was 0.75 for ≥50% ACS and 0.78 for ≥70% ACS.
- The prevalence of ≥50% ACS in the highest decile of risk was 6.5% (number needed to scan (NNS) of 15), and 1.4% for ≥70% ACS (NNS of 70).
- Targeted screening of the 10% highest risk identified 35% of cases with ≥50% ACS (NNS of 21) and 42% of cases with ≥70% ACS (NNS of 102).

References:

- J Am Heart Assoc. 2020 Apr 21;9(8):e014766. PMID: 32310014

Stenting for Vertebral Artery Disease

SYS REVIEW & META-ANALYSIS 2011

AT A GLANCE

- 27 articles (993 patients) included.
- Majority (56%) had contralateral vertebral artery stenosis or occlusion
- 92% were symptomatic at the time of treatment.

MAIN RESULTS

- Only 1.3% of patients in this review experienced a vertebrobasilar territory infarct during a mean follow-period of 21 months, suggesting that stenting may confer secondary stroke protection.
- 8 (0.8%) experienced a transient ischemic attack within 30 days of the procedure.
- Drug-eluting stents were associated with lower restenosis rates (11%) compared to bare metal stents (30%) at a mean of 24 months of follow-up.

REFERENCES:

- Stroke. 2011 Aug;42(8):2212-6. PMID: 21700936

CHAPTER 15
ACUTE
MESENTERIC
ISCHAEMIA

ECT Guidelines Summary

GUIDELINES

AT A GLANCE

- Definition – sudden acute arterial or venous occlusion or drop in circulating pressure and inability to meet metabolic demands
- A normal lactate does not exclude AMI and should not be used for diagnosis (III)
- Multi-detector CT or IV contrast is the method of choice. In addition, oral contrast can be considered in addition. Meta-analysis of six primary studies: sensitivity 93.3% specificit 95.9%
- Angiography should NOT be used for diagnostic purposes. III
- Routine use for laparoscopy has insufficient supportive evidence (IV).
- Vasopressors should be avoided (IV)
- Antibiotics should always be given (IV)
- If immediate intervention is needed, then open surgery is indicated. If not, endo or open can be considered based on local experience.
- If an embolus is identified, there must be an attempt to remove it (IV).
- Arterial thrombosis – try endo first if there is no compromise for gut (III)
- Venous ischaemia – start systematic anticoagulation (III). Offer endo if patient continues to deteriorate. (IV).
- Non-occlusive mesenteric ischaemia – treat medically (III).
- Perforated gut and unsalvageable – consider for palliative treatment. (IV).
- Avoid bowel anastomosis in shocked patients (III).
- Plan a second evaluation within 48h (III). This practice is associated with improved mortality.

- Follow up vascular bypass with regular surveillance (IV). .

REFERENCES:

- Eur J Trauma Emerg Surg. 2016 Apr;42(2):253-70. PMID: 26820988

CHAPTER 16
MISCELLANEOUS

Endovasc Treatment for renal artery stenosis

COCHRANDE SYS REVIEW AND META-ANALYSIS 2014

AT A GLANCE
- Eight RCTs (2222 pts)
- Overall quality of evidence - moderate.

MAIN RESULTS
- Change in diastolic blood pressure (BP) - small improvement in diastolic BP in the angioplasty group (MD -2.00 mmHg)
- Change in systolic BP no significant improvement (MD -1.07 mmHg)
- Effect on renal function as measured by serum creatinine – no effect (MD -7.99 µmol/L)
- Number of antihypertensive drugs - small decrease in antihypertensive drug requirements for the angioplasty group (MD -0.18).
- Cardiovascular (OR 0.91) or renal adverse events (OR 1.02) – no difference between the angioplasty and medical treatment groups.
- Procedural complications of balloon angioplasty – small numbers reported
- No side effects of medical therapy were reported.

REFERENCES:
- Cochrane Database Syst Rev. 2014;2014(12):CD002944. PMID: 25478936

Endovascular Therapy for Vasculogenic Erectile Dysfunction

SYS REVIEW AND META-ANALYSIS 2019

AT A GLANCE

- 16 articles (total of 212 patients with VOD and 162 with AI).
- Treatment of the two most common etiologies of vasculogenic erectile dysfunction (ED): veno-occlusive dysfunction (VOD) and arterial insufficiency (AI)

MAIN RESULTS

- VOD cohort were treated either percutaneously (61%) or after surgical exposure of the deep dorsal vein (34%).
- ost common embolic used was n-butyl cyanoacrylate.
- Clinical success rate: 60% in VOD patients.
- Complications occurred in 5% of patients
- AI most commonly treated via stenting of the internal pudendal artery (40).
- Overall clinical success rate of 63%.
- Complications occurred in 5%.

REFERENCES:

- J Vasc Interv Radiol. 2019 Aug;30(8):1251-1258.e2. PMID: 31104902

Subclavian Artery Disease

➡️ESC Guidleines 2020

At a glance

- Upper body/Limb lesions are mostly situated at the level of the brachiocephalic trunk and the subclavian and axillary arteries.
- Duplex scans, CTA and MRA can all be used for diagnosis.
- When subclavian steal syndrome is suspected, flow reversal should be assessed in the ipsilateral extracranial vertebral artery by hyperaemia testing.
- Best medical therapy should be ensured for all patients.
- Clinical presentation includes TIA/stroke, coronary subclavian steal syndrome, ipsilateral haemodialysis access dysfunction or impaired quality of life (QOL) due to pain.
- Symptomatic patients - should be considered for revascularisation where appropriate (➡️IIa). Surgery or endovascular approaches can be considered, based on experience, lesion location and characteristics, as well as patient's risk factors (➡️IIa).
  - » Surgical options which include subclavian-carotid bypass (using prosthetic graft) have shown good long-term patency results (5-year patency 96%) (➡️R). Other options include extrathoracic extra-anatomic bypass procedures such as axillo-axillary, carotid-axillary or carotid-carotid bypass (➡️R).
- Asymptomatic patients - can be considered for revascularisation if the patient is undergoing CABG using the ipsilateral internal mammary artery. This may also be considered for patients who already have the ipsilateral internal mammary artery grafted to coronary arteries with evidence of myocardial ischaemia, and for patients with planned ipsilateral arteriovenous fistula for dialysis ➡️IIa).

CHAPTER 17
ATLAS OF
VASCULAR
ANATOMY AND
SURGICAL
TECHNIQUES
FACTS AND
FIGURES

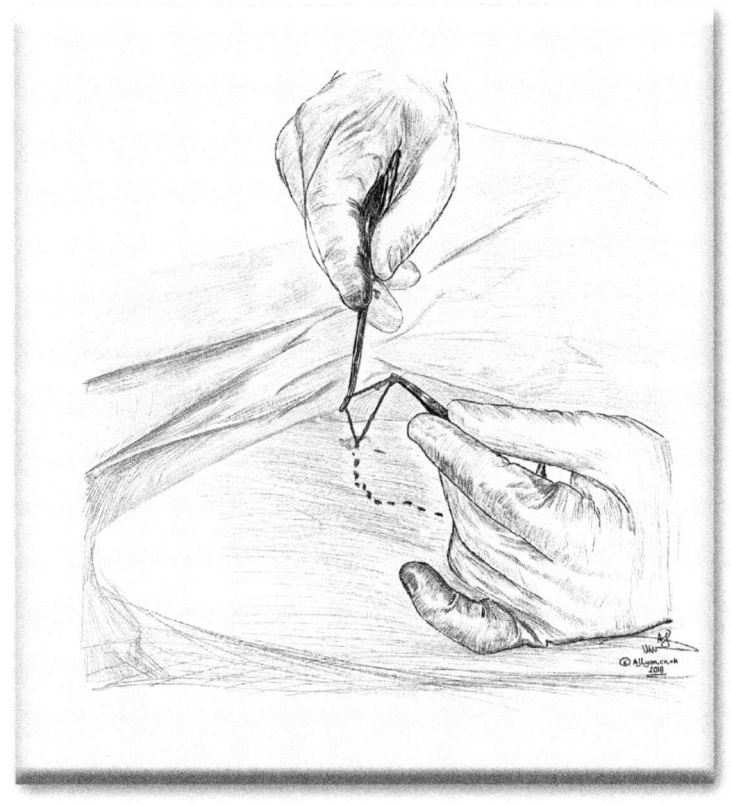

Anatomy of the Head and Neck

SUPERFICIAL MUSCLES

1. Sternocleidomastoid m.
2. Digastric m.
3. Omohyoid m.
4. Trapezius m.
5. Deltoid m.
6. Scalenus Anterior m.
7. Scalenus Medius m.
8. Levator Scapulae m.
9. Splenius Capitis m.
10. Temporalis m.

Anatomy of the Head and Neck - Superficial Muscles

SUPERFICIAL MUSCLES

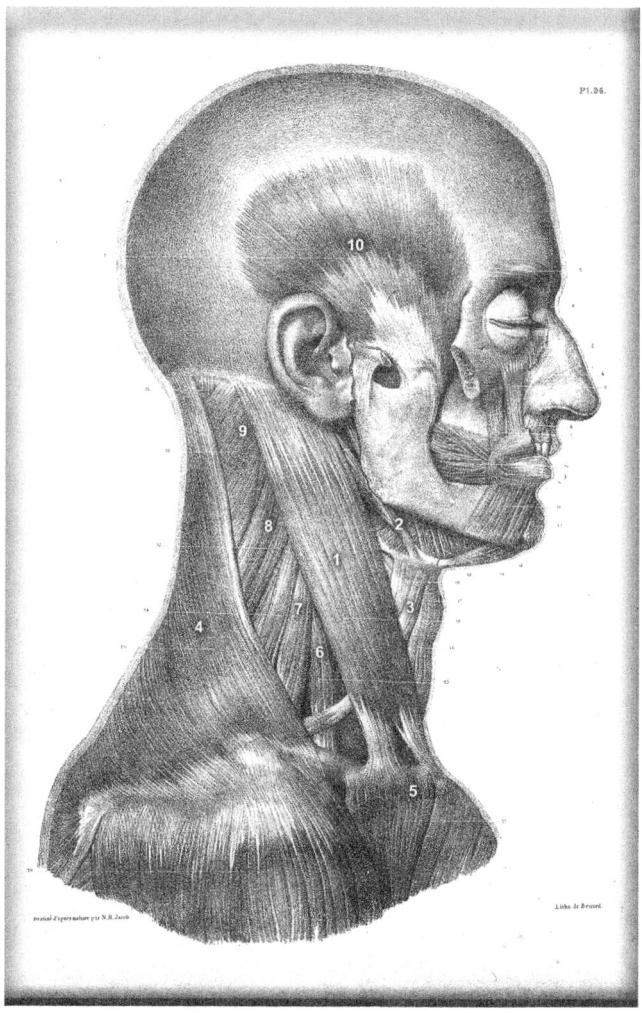

Credit
Muscles of the head and neck: an écorché seen in profile. Lithograph by N.H Jacob, 1831/1854..
Credit: Wellcome Collection. Attribution 4.0 International (CC BY 4.0). URL: https://wellcome-collection.org/works/a5t5ku22
License information
This work is used herein without restriction under copyright law.
Creative Commons Attribution (CC BY 4.0) terms and conditions https://creativecommons.org/licenses/by/4.0

Anatomy of the Upper Limb Veins

SUPERFICIAL VEINS AND MUSCLES

1. Cephalic vein
2. Basilic Vein
3. Suprascapular vein
4. External Jugular Vein
5. Anterior Jugular Vein
6. Dorsal Venous network of hand

Anatomy of the Upper Limb Veins

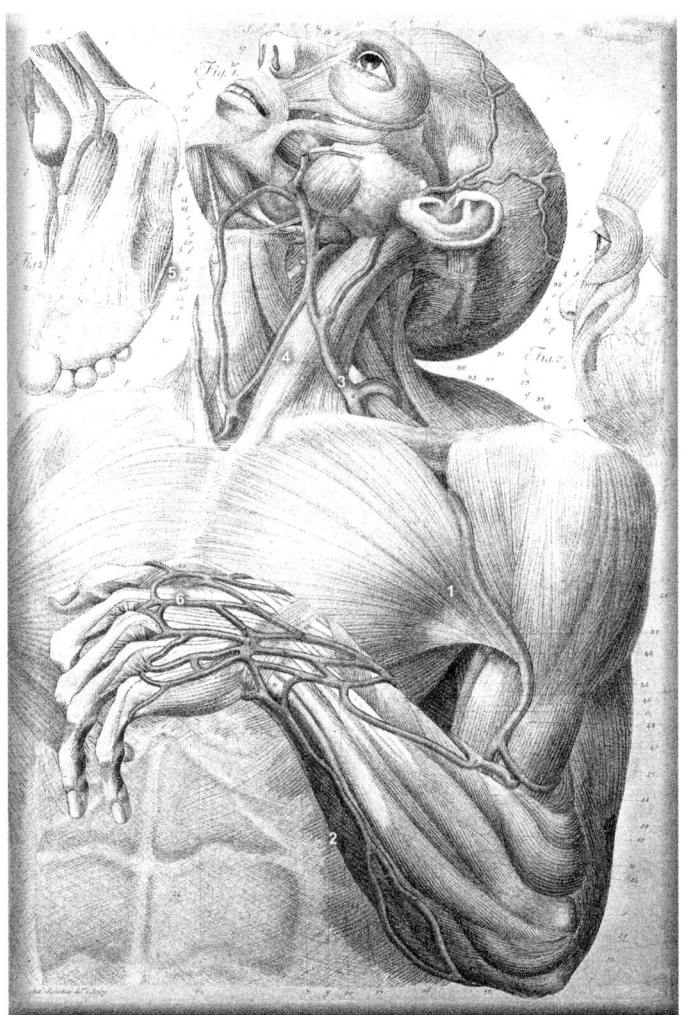

Credit
Muscles and blood-vessels of the head, neck, chest, arm and hand of an écorché, with two
details, showing the face and foot. Colour engraving by A. Serantoni, ca. 1816. Credit: Wellcome
Collection. Attribution 4.0 International (CC BY 4.0) URL: https://wellcomecollection.org/
works/ak5baehf
License information
This work is used herein without restriction under copyright law.
Creative Commons Attribution (CC BY 4.0) terms and conditions https://creativecommons.
org/licenses/by/4.0

Anatomy of the Root of Neck

FASCIA, NERVES, VEINS AND ARTERIES

1. Supraclavicular nerves
2. External Jugular Vein
3. Subclavian artery
4. Inferior belly of omohyoid m.
5. Suprascapular vein

Anatomy of the Root of Neck

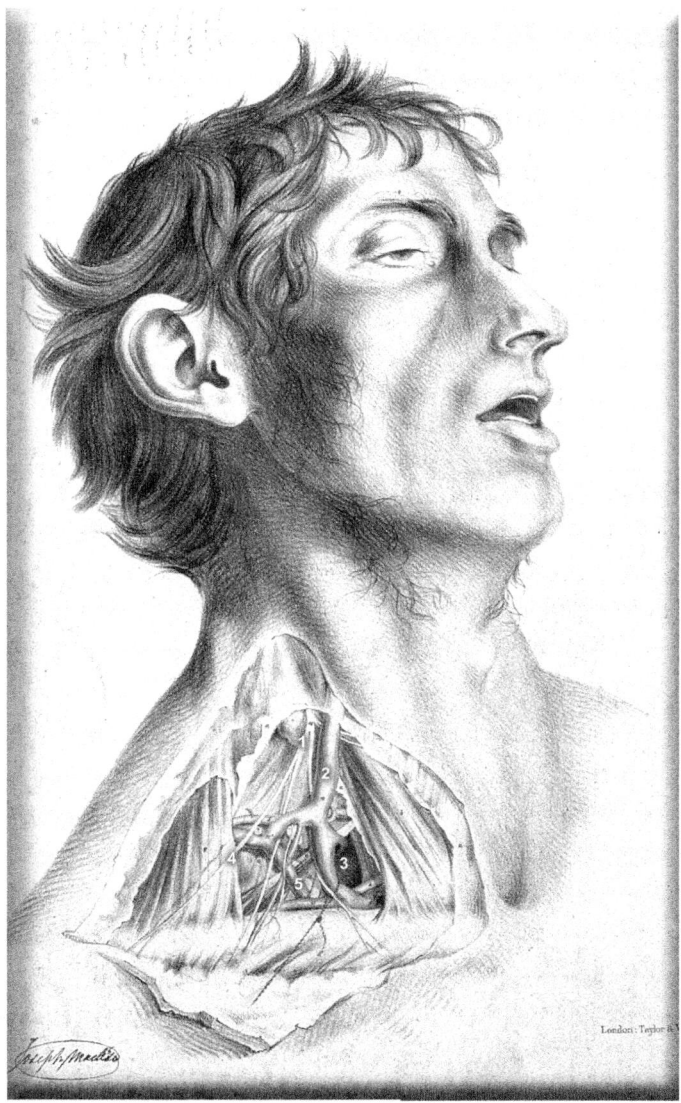

Credit
The circulatory system: two dissections of the neck of a man, with arteries, blood vessels and veins. Coloured lithograph by J. Maclise, 1841/1844. Credit: Wellcome Collection. Attribution 4.0 International (CC BY 4.0) URL: https://wellcomecollection.org/works/augte7tr
License information
This work is used herein without restriction under copyright law.
Creative Commons Attribution (CC BY 4.0) terms and conditions https://creativecommons.org/licenses/by/4.0

Anatomy of the Neck
MAIN ARTERIES & VEINS, WITH MUSCLES & FASCIA

1. Omohyoid m.
2. Subclavian artery
3. Common carotid artery
4. Thyrocervical trunk

Anatomy of the Neck

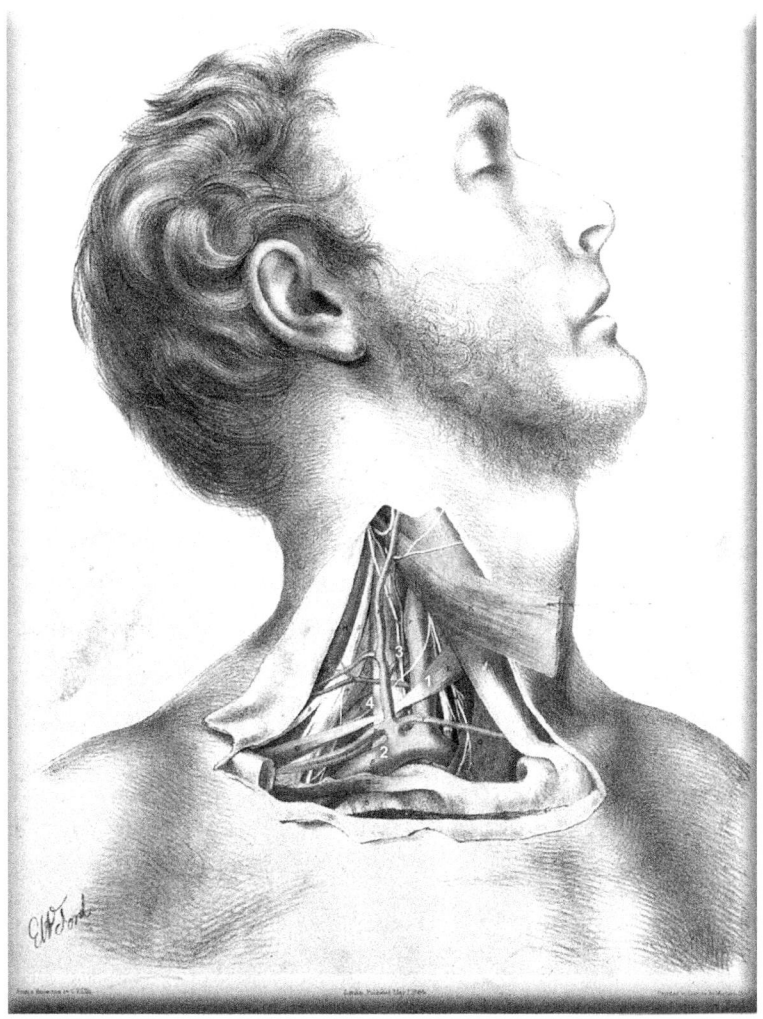

Credit
Dissection of the neck of a man, with the muscles and blood vessels indicated. Lithograph by
G.H. Ford, 1864. Credit: Wellcome Collection. Attribution 4.0 International (CC BY 4.0) URL:
https://wellcomecollection.org/works/m2zabqja

Anatomy of the Root of Neck

MAIN ARTERIES & VEINS, WITH MUSCLES & FASCIA

1. Common carotid aretry
2. Internal Jugular Vein
3. Vagus nerve

Anatomy of the Root of Neck

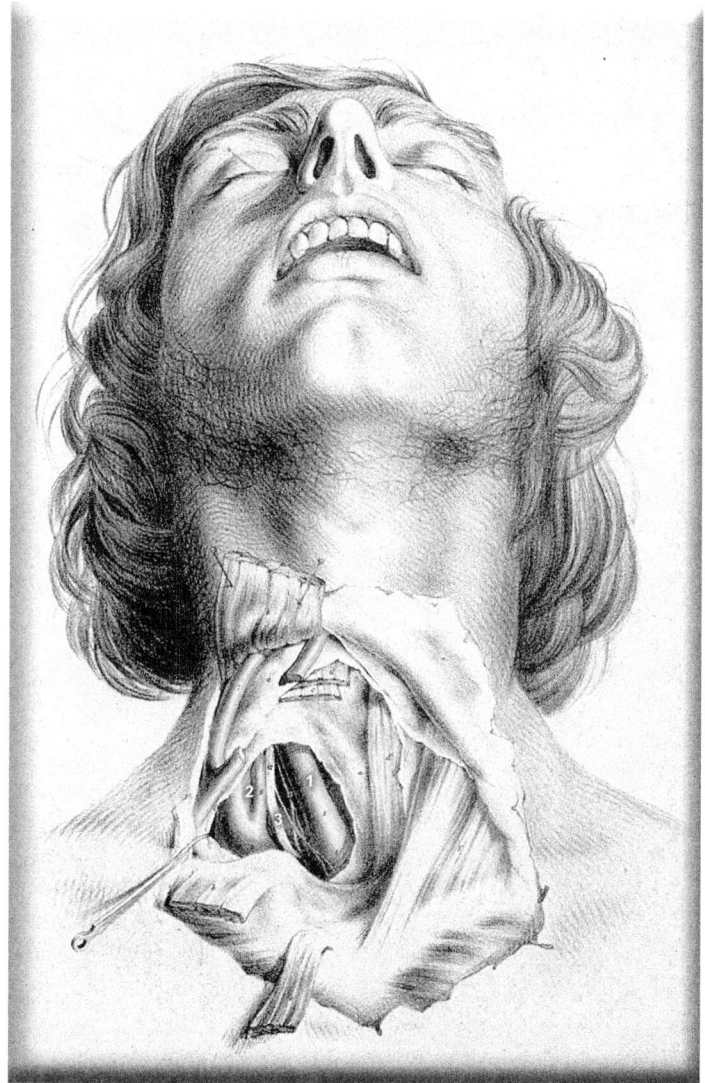

Credit
The circulatory system: two dissections of the neck of a man, with arteries, blood vessels and veins indicated in red and blue. Coloured lithograph by J. Maclise, 1841/1844. Credit: Wellcome Collection. Attribution 4.0 International (CC BY 4.0) URL: https://wellcomecollection.org/works/augte7tr
License information
This work is used herein without restriction under copyright law.
Creative Commons Attribution (CC BY 4.0) terms and conditions https://creativecommons.org/licenses/by/4.0

Anatomy of the Neck

CAROTID, JUGULAR, CERVICAL PLEXUS, NERVES

1. Common carotid artery
2. External carotid artery
3. Internal carotid artery
4. hypoglossal nerve
5. Ansa cervicalis
6. Internal jugular vein
7. cervical plexus
8. vagus nerve
9. subclavian artery

Anatomy of the Neck

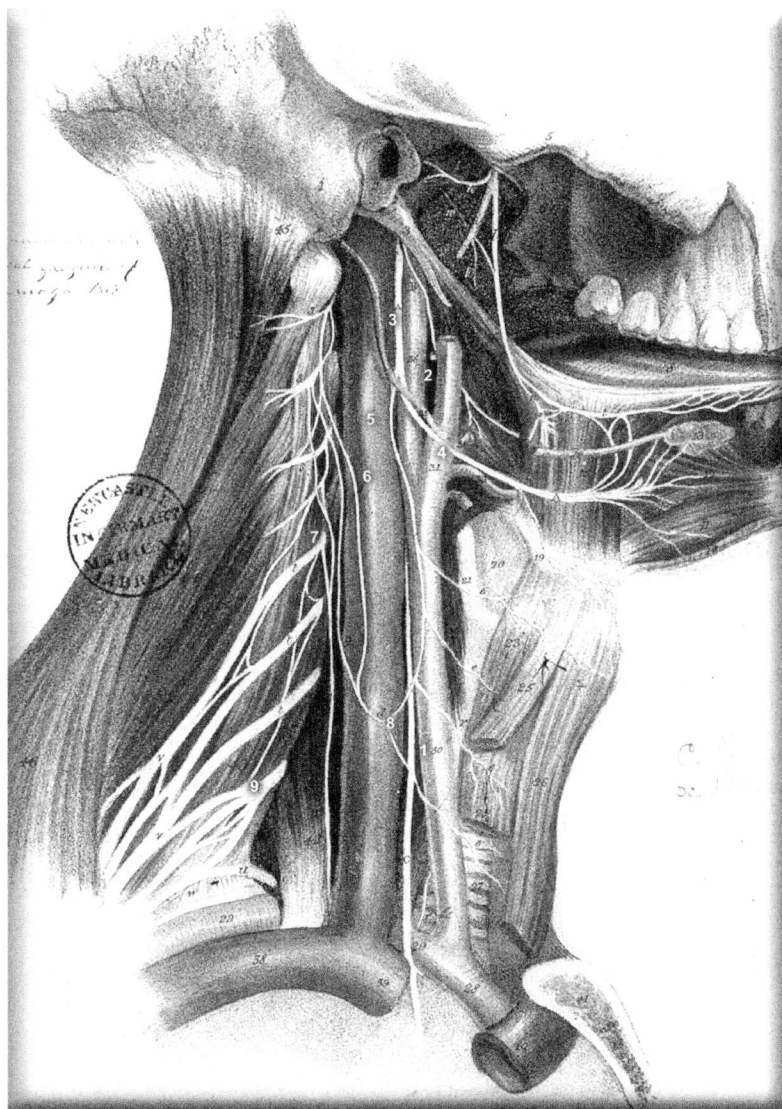

Credit
Nerves of the neck and mouth. Coloured lithograph by William Fairland, 1839, after W. Bagg after W.J.E. Wilson. Credit: Wellcome Collection. Attribution 4.0 International (CC BY 4.0)
URL: https://wellcomecollection.org/works/bemqyxm7
License information

Anatomy of the neck vessels

CAROTID, DEEP MUSCLES, NERVES

1. Common carotid artery
2. External carotid artery
3. Internal carotid artery
4. Superior thyroid artery
5. Hypoglossal nerve
6. Digastric m.
7. Omo-hyoid m.

Anatomy of the neck vessels

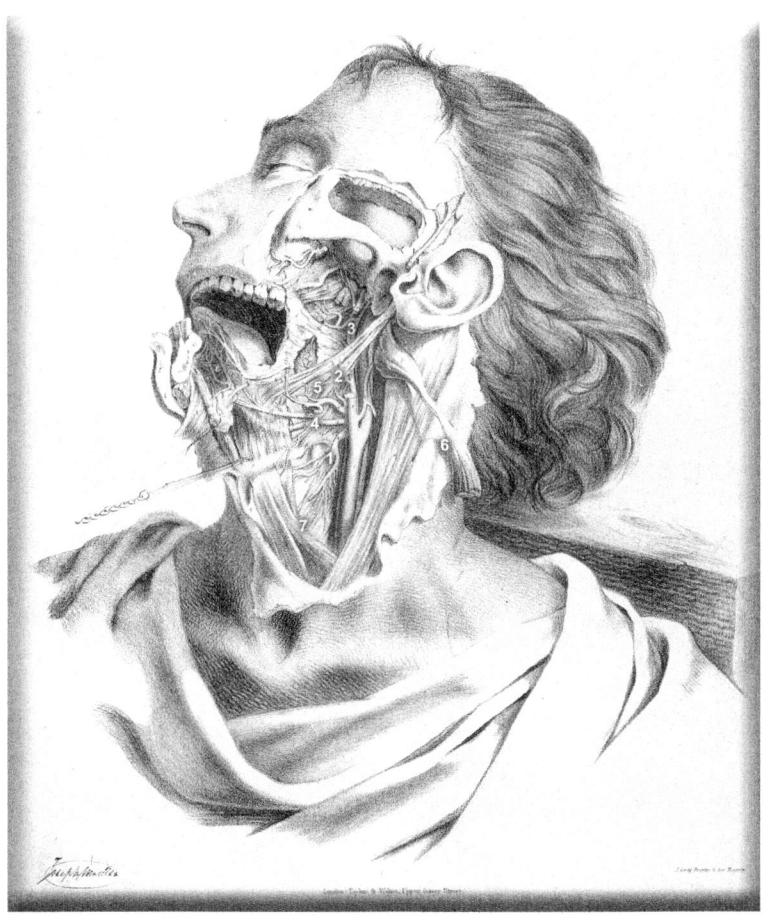

Credit
The circulatory system: partial dissection of the neck, jaw and face of a man, with arteries and blood vessels indicated in red. Coloured lithograph by J. Maclise, 1841/1844. Credit: Wellcome Collection. Attribution 4.0 International (CC BY 4.0) URL: https://wellcomecollection.org/works/h26qbysy

License information
This work is used herein without restriction under copyright law.
Creative Commons Attribution (CC BY 4.0) terms and conditions https://creativecommons.org/licenses/by/4.0

Anatomy of the Head and Neck

SUPERFICIAL AND DEEP VEINS

1. External Jugular Vein.
2. Transverse cervical nerves
3. Facial vein
4. Digastric muscle

Anatomy of the Head and Neck

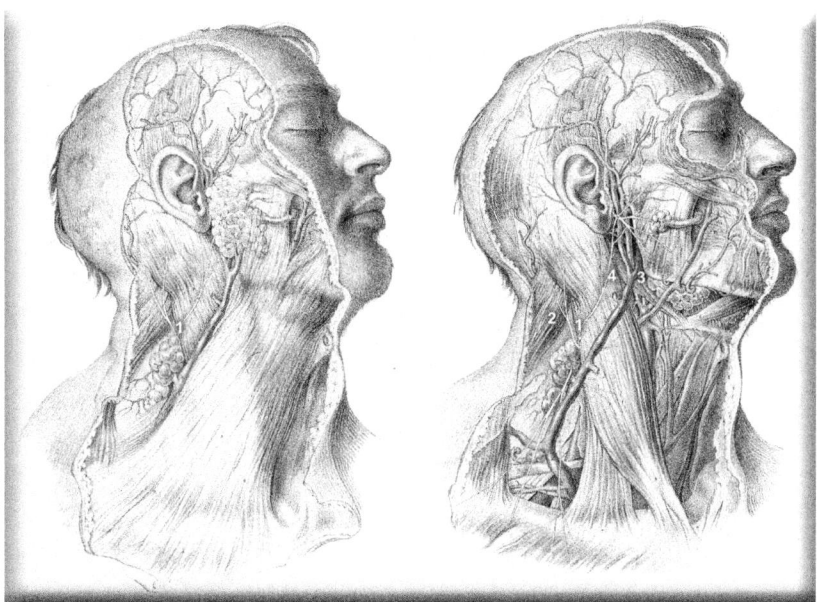

Credit
Blood-vessels of the head and neck. Coloured lithograph by J. Maclise, 1851. Credit: Wellcome Collection. Attribution 4.0 International (CC BY 4.0) URL: https://wellcomecollection.org/works/dgpzayxa

License information
This work is used herein without restriction under copyright law.
Creative Commons Attribution (CC BY 4.0) terms and conditions https://creativecommons.org/licenses/by/4.0

Anatomy of the Aortic Arch

AORTIC ARCH BRANCHES VARIATIONS

1. Left coronary artery.
2. Rigt coronary artery.
3. Variation 1: left CCA and Left Subclavian with one origin from aorta.
4. Variation 2: Left CCA originating from right brachicephalic trunk.
5. Variation 3: Right brachiochephalic originating distal to left subclavian.
6. Variation 4: Left CCH originating from right brachocephalic and left vertebral originating directly from aorta.
7. Variation 5: Left CCA originating from right brachiocephalic and right CCA originating directly from aorta
8. Variation 6.

Anatomy of the Aortic Arch

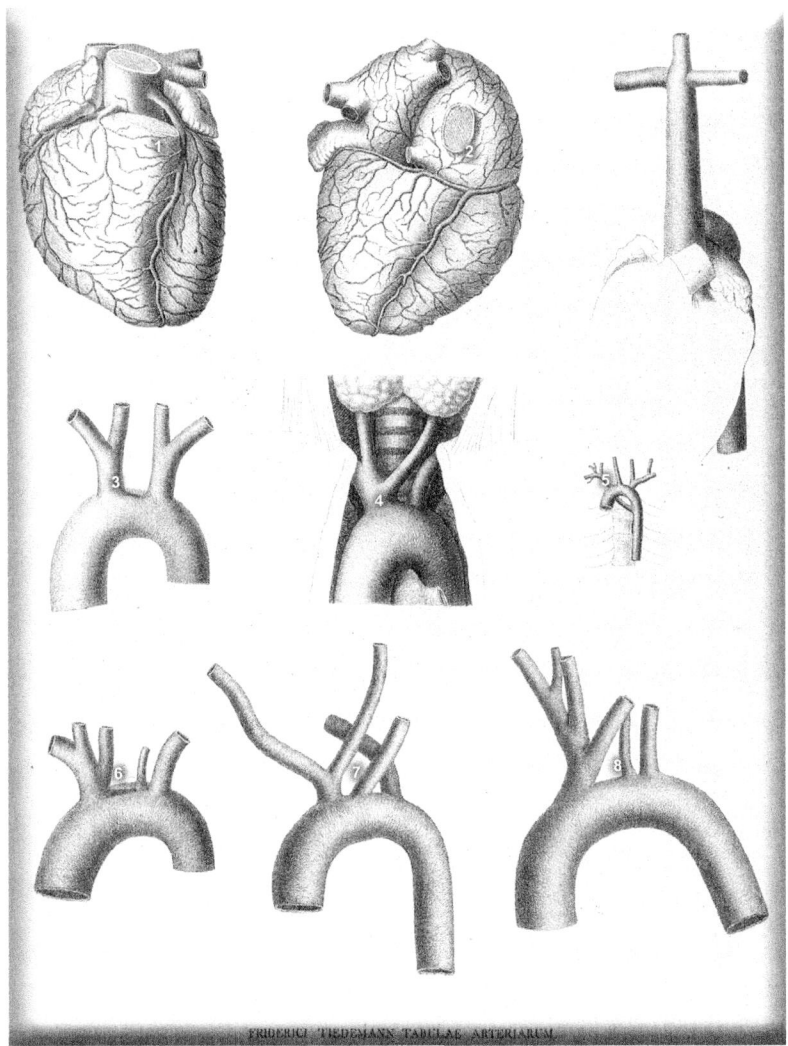

Credit
The heart, arteries of the neck and the aortic arch (?): nine figures, with arteries indicated in red.
Coloured lithograph by J. Roux, 1822.. Credit: Wellcome Collection. Attribution 4.0 International (CC BY 4.0) URL: https://wellcomecollection.org/works/abemhssg
License information
This work is used herein without restriction under copyright law.
Creative Commons Attribution (CC BY 4.0) terms and conditions https://creativecommons.org/licenses/by/4.0

Anatomy of the Circulatory System

CIRCULATORY SYSTEM HEAD TO TOES

1. Carotid arteries.
2. Aorta
3. Iliac Arteries.
4. Femoral arteries
5. Tibial arteries

Anatomy of the Circulatory System

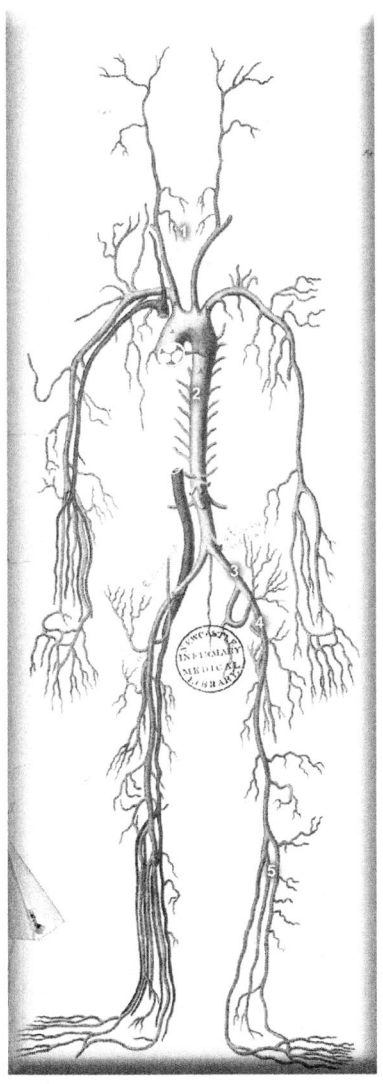

Credit
Blood-vessels and their role in circulation of blood. Coloured lithograph by William Fairland, 1837. Credit: Wellcome Collection. Attribution 4.0 International (CC BY 4.0) URL: https://well-comecollection.org/works/b9rrtk8e
License information
This work is used herein without restriction under copyright law.
Creative Commons Attribution (CC BY 4.0) terms and conditions https://creativecommons.org/licenses/by/4.0

Anatomy of the Chest and Abdomen

VESSELS IN CHEST AND ABDOMEN

1. Descending aorta.
2. Oesophagus
3. Celiac axis
4. Superior mesenteric artery

Anatomy of the Chest and Abdomen

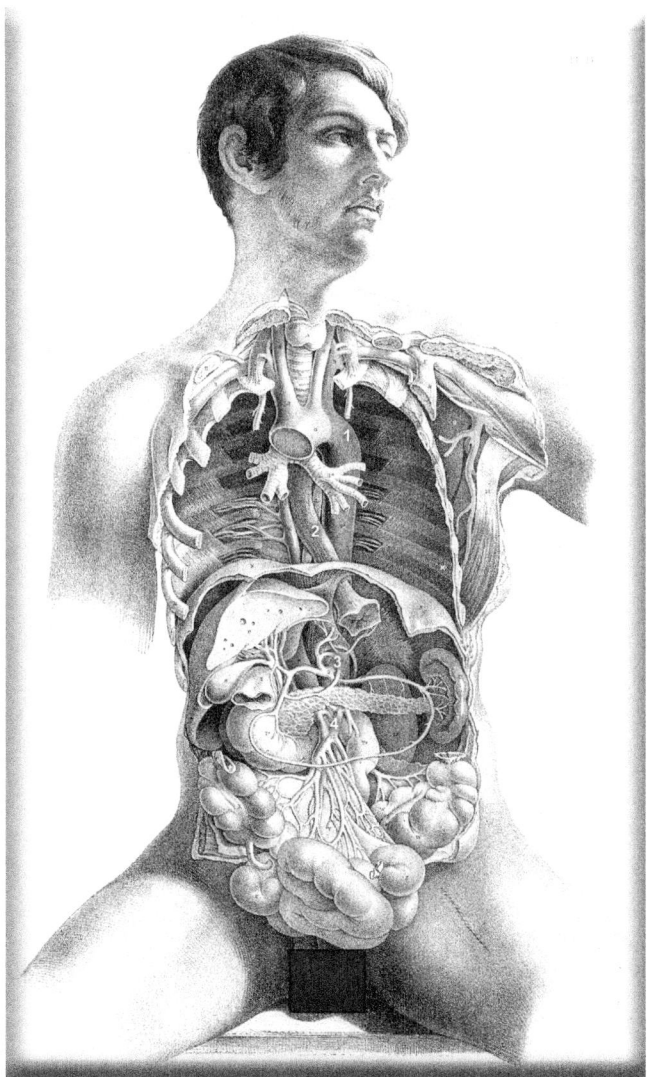

Credit
Dissection of the trunk of a seated white man showing the arteries and blood-vessels supplying the viscera of the thorax and abdomen. Coloured lithograph by L. M. (?) after J. Maclise, 1851. Credit: Wellcome Collection. Attribution 4.0 International (CC BY 4.0) URL: https://wellcome-collection.org/works/p9jwaxds

Anatomy of the Thoracic Aorta

THORACIC AORTA

1. Aortic valve.
2. Descending aorta
3. Oesophagus

Anatomy of the Thoracic Aorta

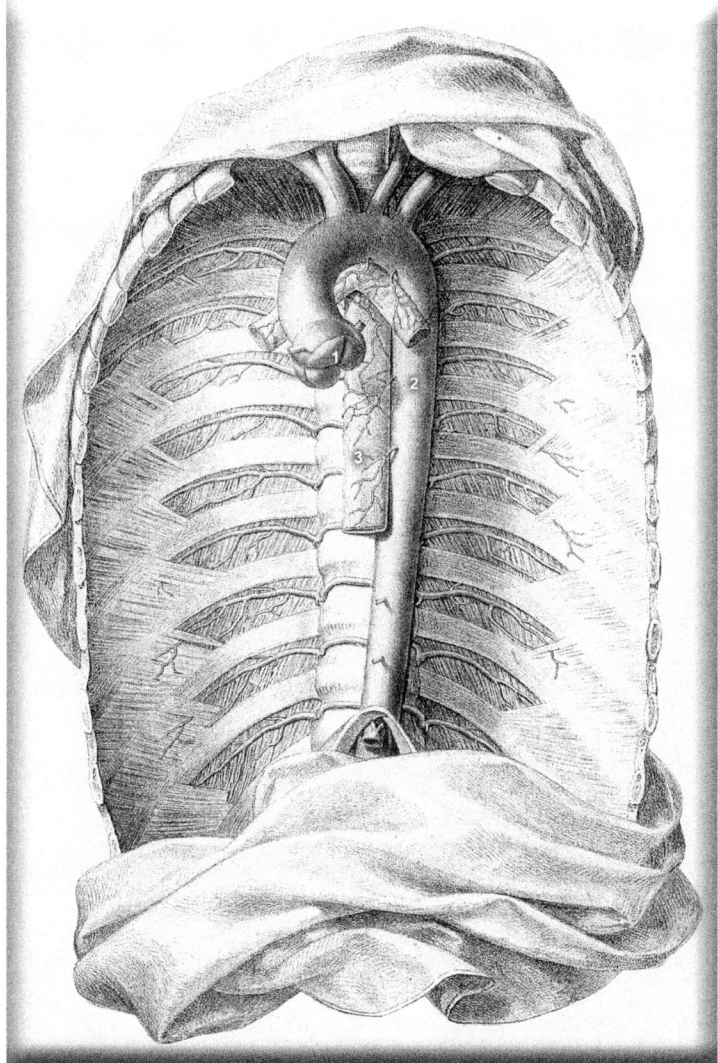

Credit
Dissection of the thorax, with the aortic arch, arteries and blood vessels indicated in red.
Coloured lithograph by J. Roux, 1822. Credit: Wellcome Collection. Attribution 4.0 International (CC BY 4.0) URL: https://wellcomecollection.org/works/gxqjz38k

Anatomy of the Abdominal Aorta

ABDOMINAL AORTA

1. Aortic valve.
2. Descending aorta
3. Oesophagus

Anatomy of the Abdominal Aorta

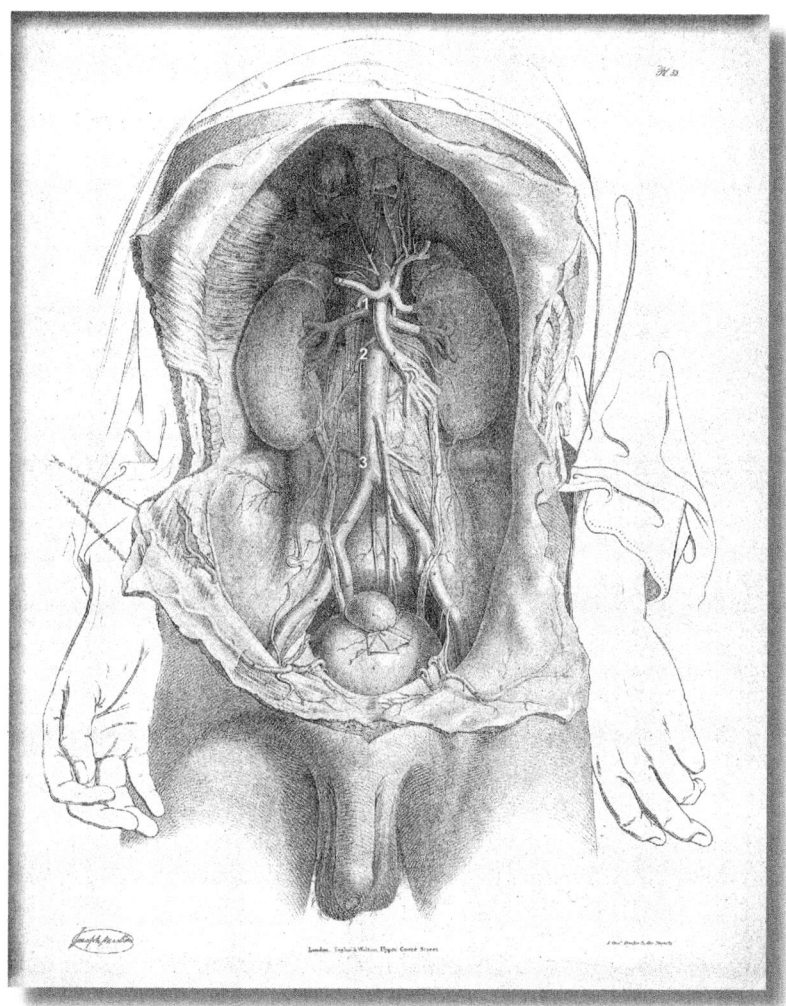

Credit
The circulatory system: dissection of the torso showing the kidneys and bladder, with the arteries and veins indicated in red and blue. Coloured lithograph by J. Maclise, 1841/1844. Credit: Wellcome Collection. Attribution 4.0 International (CC BY 4.0) URL: https://wellcomecollection.org/works/rqesdnyz
License information
This work is used herein without restriction under copyright law.
Creative Commons Attribution (CC BY 4.0) terms and conditions https://creativecommons.org/licenses/by/4.0

Anatomy of the Aorta

RETROPERITONEUM VESSELS & NERVES

1. Infrarenal aorta.
2. Inferior Vena Cava
3. Superior hypogastric plexus

Anatomy of the Aorta

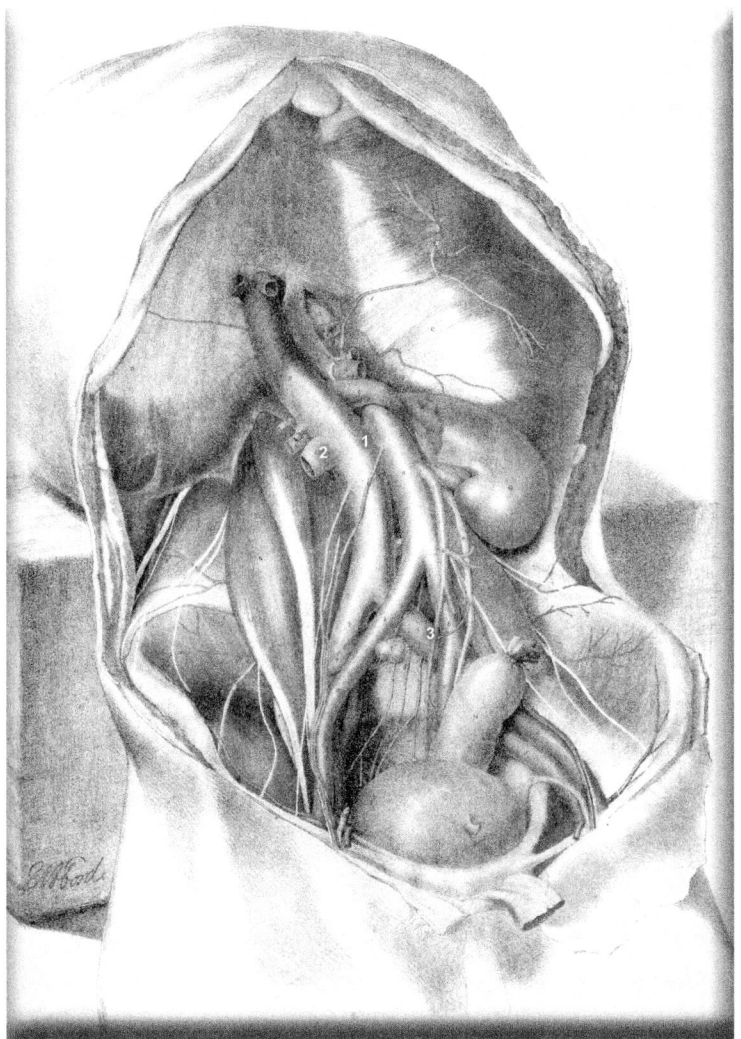

Credit
Deep Muscle of the Abdominal Parietes, and the Vessels of the Abdominal Cavity. Credit: Wellcome Collection. Attribution 4.0 International (CC BY 4.0) URL: https://wellcomecollection.org/works/k2gag2gh

Anatomy of the Pelvis

ILIAC ARTERIES AND NERVES

1. Aorta
2. Left external iliac artery
3. Left internal iliac artery
4. Splanchic plexus

Anatomy of the Pelvis

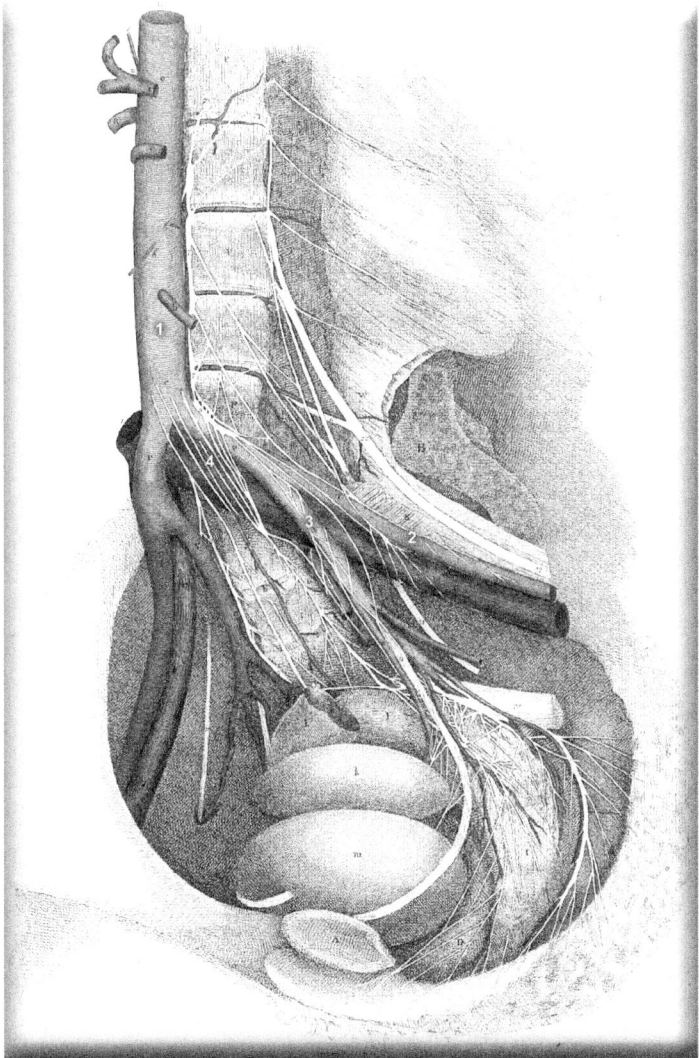

Credit
Abdominal cavity: dissection, with blood-vessels and nerves indicated in red and blue. Coloured line engraving by W.H. Lizars, 1822/1826. Credit: Wellcome Collection. Attribution 4.0 International (CC BY 4.0) URL: https://wellcomecollection.org/works/g4vrxnzg
License information
This work is used herein without restriction under copyright law.
Creative Commons Attribution (CC BY 4.0) terms and conditions https://creativecommons.org/licenses/by/4.0

Anatomy of the Axilla

VESSLES AND NERVES

1. External Jugular vein.
2. Subclavian artery.
3. Brachial plexus.
4. Brachial veins
5. Basilic vein

Anatomy of the Axilla

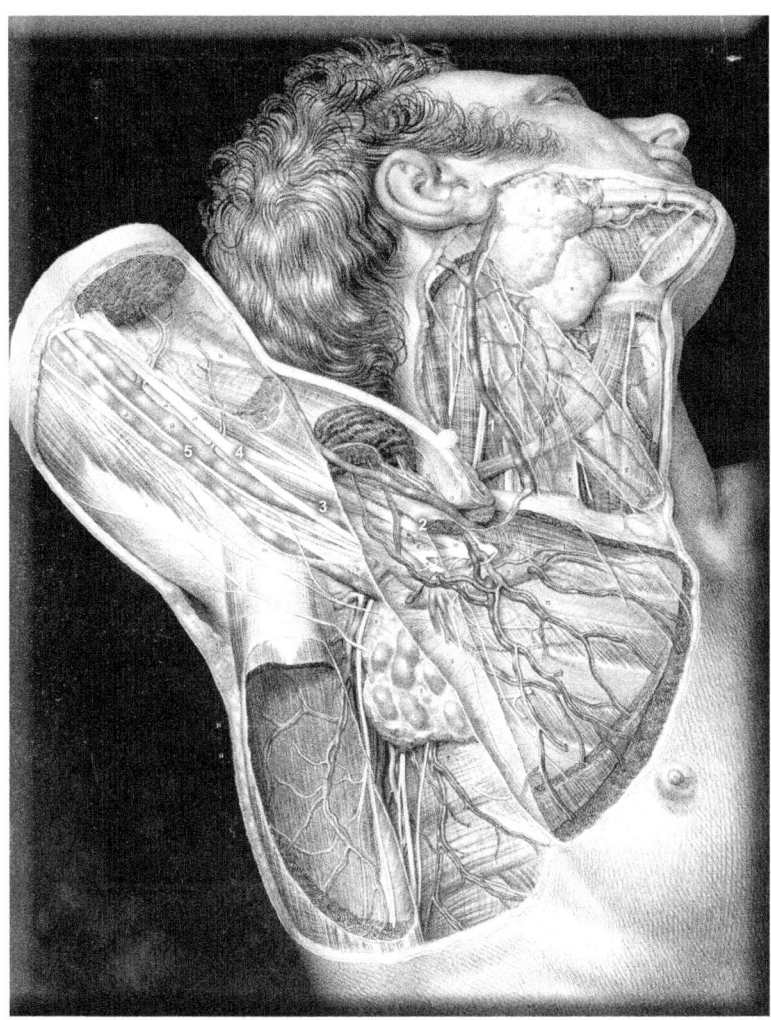

Credit
Plate 6, Surgical anatomy of the axilla. Credit: Wellcome Collection. Attribution 4.0 International (CC BY 4.0) URL: https://wellcomecollection.org/works/a72w8fzw
License information
This work is used herein without restriction under copyright law.
Creative Commons Attribution (CC BY 4.0) terms and conditions https://creativecommons.org/licenses/by/4.0

Anatomy of the Axillary Area

VEINS AND ARTERIES

1. Axillary vein.
2. Axillary artery.

Anatomy of the Axillary Area

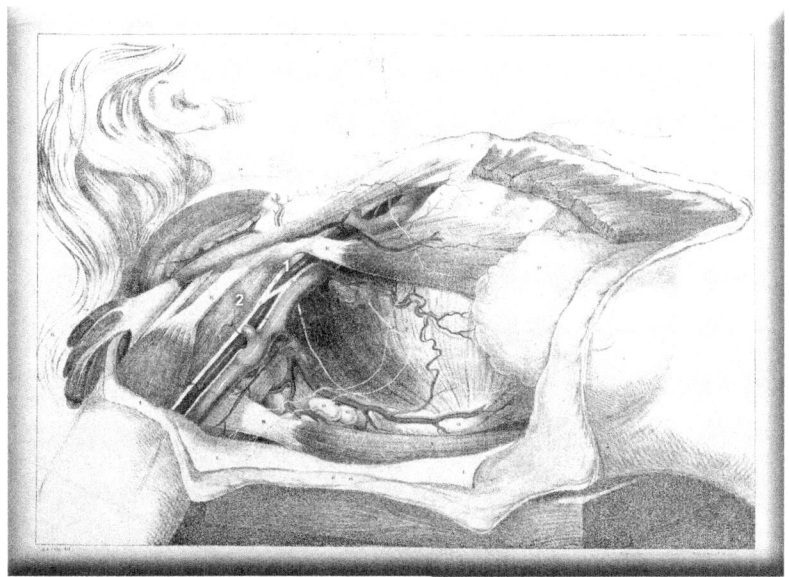

Anatomy of the Upper Arm

BRACHIAL VESSELS AND NERVES

1. Axillary artery.
2. Brachial Plexus.
3. Brachial artery.

Anatomy of the Upper Arm

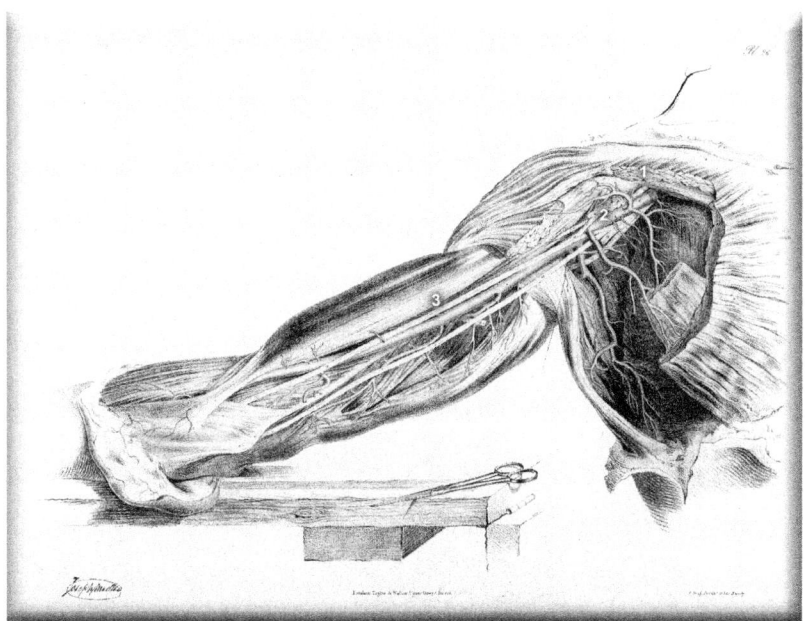

Credit
The circulatory system: dissection of the upper arm, shoulder and armpit, with arteries and blood vessels indicated in red. Coloured lithograph by J. Maclise, 1841/1844. Credit: Wellcome Collection. Attribution 4.0 International (CC BY 4.0) URL: https://wellcomecollection.org/works/bxg59wng
License information

Anatomy of the Arm

UPPER AND LOWER ARMS' ARTERIES AND NERVES

1. Brachial vein.
2. Brachial vein
3. Brachial aretry.
4. Median nerve.
5. Brachial artery.
6. Ulnar artery.
7. Radial artery.

Anatomy of the Arm

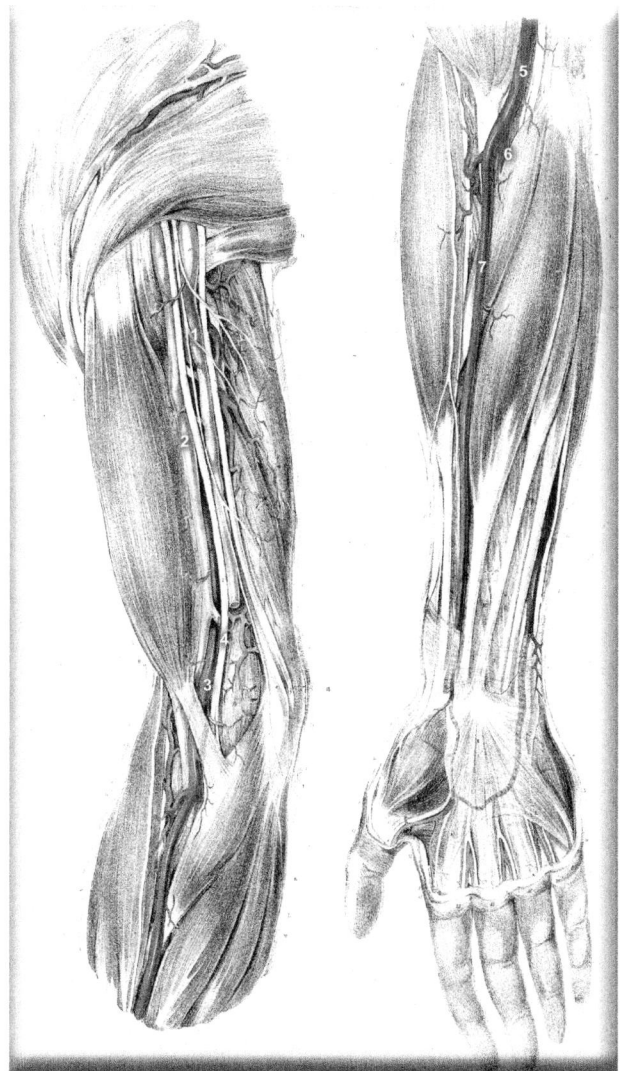

Credit
Vessels and muscles of the arm and hand: two figures showing dissections of a shoulder and upper arm, and a forearm and hand with palm facing upwards. Coloured lithograph by G.E. Madeley after A. A. Cane, 1834. Credit: Wellcome Collection. Attribution 4.0 International (CC BY 4.0) URL: https://wellcomecollection.org/works/cfcpxd3b
License information
This work is used herein without restriction under copyright law.
Creative Commons Attribution (CC BY 4.0) terms and conditions https://creativecommons.org/licenses/by/4.0

Anatomy of the Hand

TENDONS AND VESSELS

1. Radial artery.
2. Ulnar artery.
3. Radial artery.
4. Deep palmar arch.
5. Superfiical palmar arch.

Anatomy of the Hand

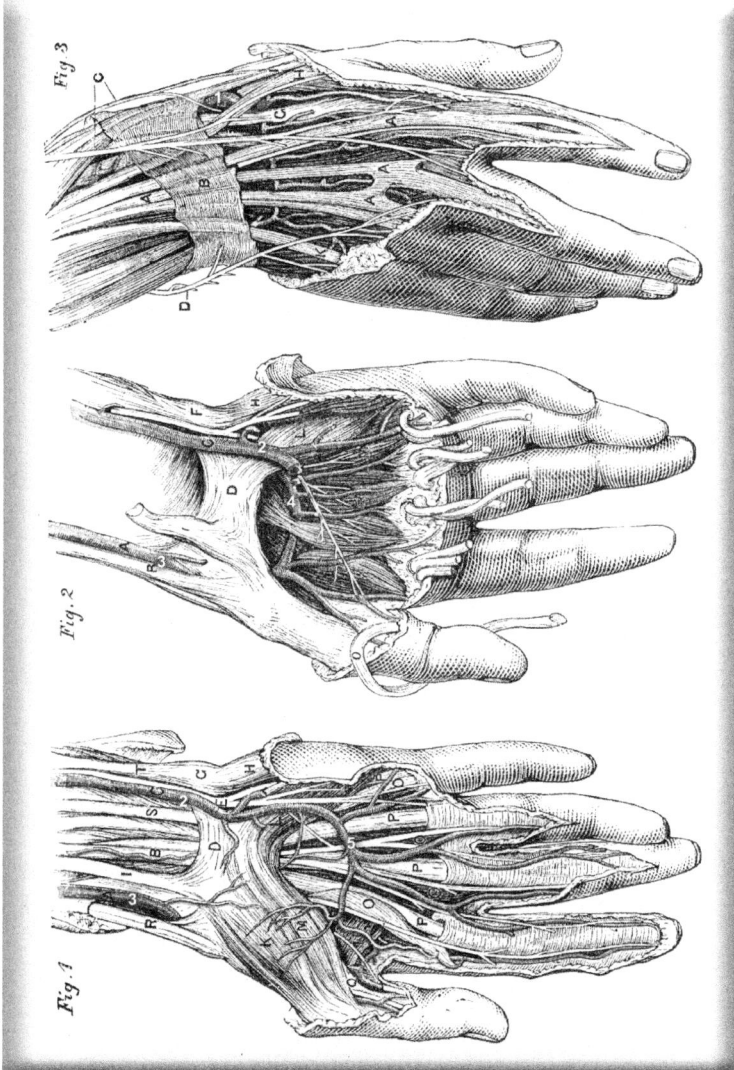

Credit
Dissection of the hand and fingers: three figures, showing the tendons and blood vessels. Colour wood engraving with letterpress, 1860/1900?. Credit: Wellcome Collection. Attribution 4.0 International (CC BY 4.0) URL https://wellcomecollection.org/works/bekzdah3
License information
This work is used herein without restriction under copyright law.
Creative Commons Attribution (CC BY 4.0) terms and conditions https://creativecommons.org/licenses/by/4.0

Anatomy of the Groin

EXTERNAL ILIACS AND EPIGASTRIC

1. External iliac artery.
2. External iliac vein.
3. Inferior epigastric a+v.
4. Obturator foramen.

Anatomy of the Groin

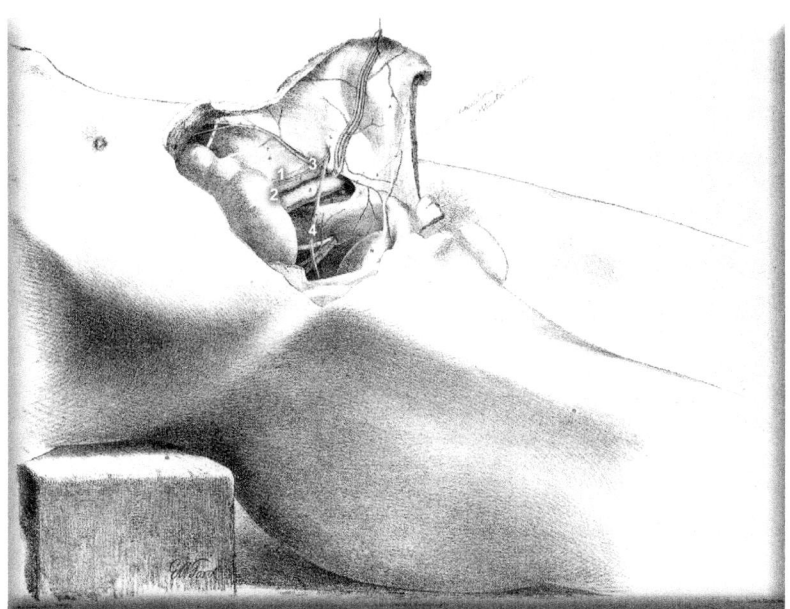

Anatomy of the Pelvis and Groin

VESSELS AND NERVES

1. Common iliac artery.
2. Common iliac vein.
3. Ureter.
4. Superficial femoral artery.
5. Femoral nerve.

Anatomy of the Pelvis and Groin

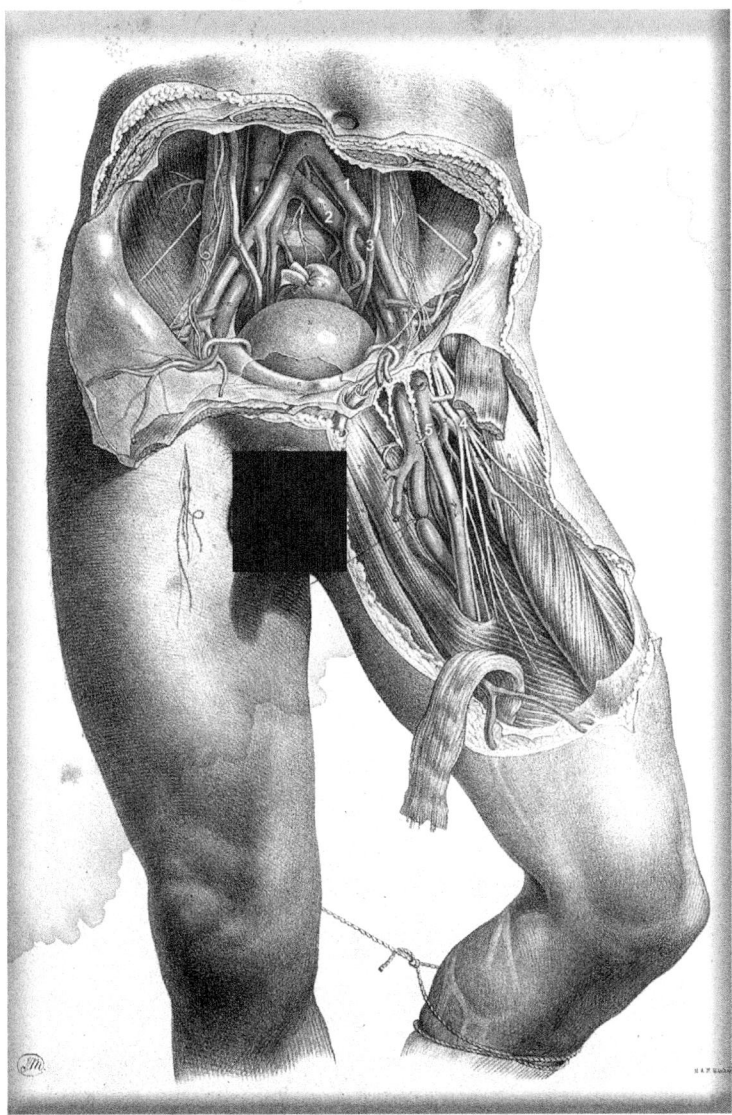

Credit
Dissection of the abdomen and thigh of a standing man, showing major blood-vessels. Coloured lithograph by J. Maclise, 1851. Credit: Wellcome Collection. Attribution 4.0 International (CC BY 4.0) URL: https://wellcomecollection.org/works/ac5x4m6m
License information
This work is used herein without restriction under copyright law.
Creative Commons Attribution (CC BY 4.0) terms and conditions https://creativecommons.org/licenses/by/4.0

Anatomy of the Thigh

FEMORAL ARTERIES

1. Common iliac artery.
2. Common femoral artery.
3. Profunda artery.
4. Superficial femoral artery.

Anatomy of the Thigh

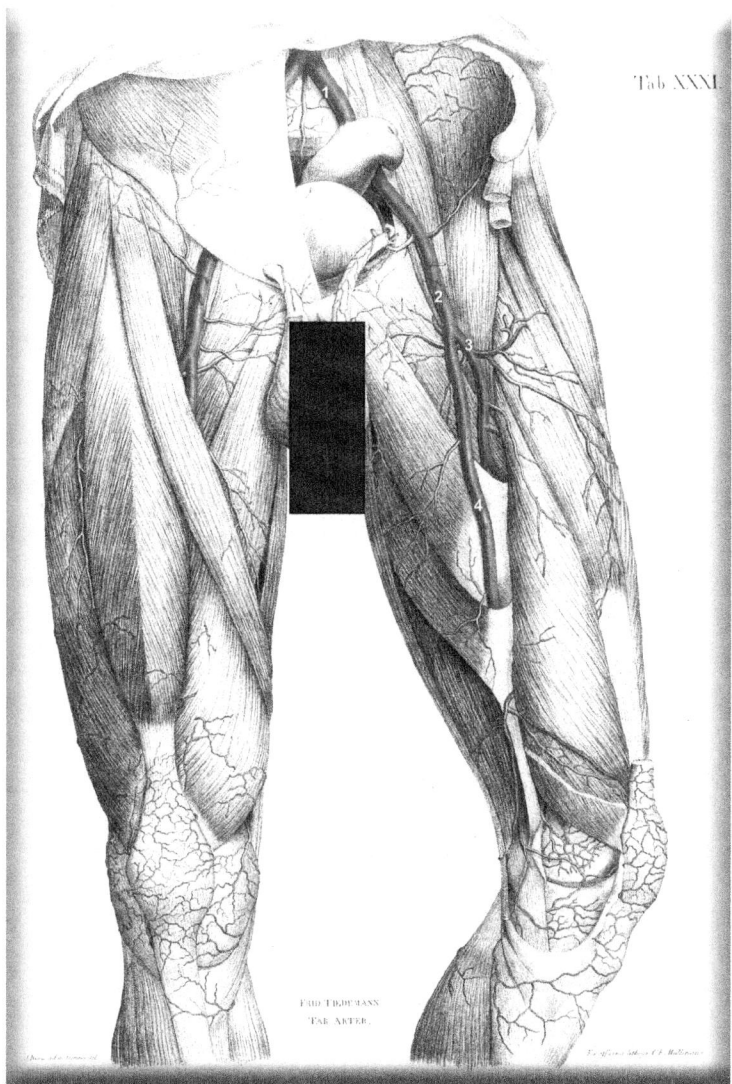

Credit
Dissection of the male genitalia, lower abdomen and thighs, with the arteries and blood vessels indicated in red. Coloured lithograph by J. Roux, 1822. Credit: Wellcome Collection. Attribution 4.0 International (CC BY 4.0) URL: https://wellcomecollection.org/works/by8excsr
License information
This work is used herein without restriction under copyright law.
Creative Commons Attribution (CC BY 4.0) terms and conditions https://creativecommons.org/licenses/by/4.0

Anatomy of the Popliteal Fossa, Leg and Foot

POPLITEAL VESSELS

1. Popliteal vein.
2. Sciatic nerve.
3. Common peroneal nerve.
4. Tibial nerve.
5. Popliteal vein.
6. Posterior tibial artery.
7. Deep plantar arch.

Anatomy of the Popliteal Fossa, Leg and Foot

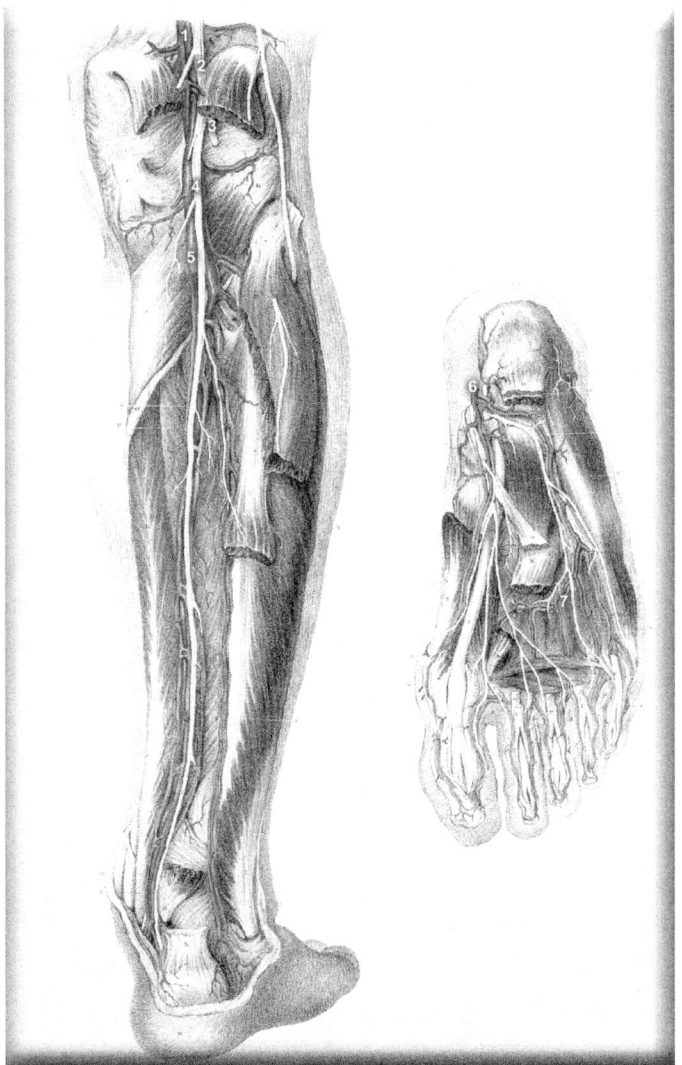

Credit
Blood vessels of the lower limb: two figures showing dissections of the leg and foot. Coloured
lithograph by G.E. Madeley after A. A. Cane, 1834. Credit: Wellcome Collection. Attribution 4.0
International (CC BY 4.0) URL: https://wellcomecollection.org/works/b6a3kt62
License information
This work is used herein without restriction under copyright law.
Creative Commons Attribution (CC BY 4.0) terms and conditions https://creativecommons.
org/licenses/by/4.0

Anatomy of the Posterior Leg

POPLITEAL AND TIBIAL ARTERIES

1. Popliteal artery.
2. Posterior tibial artery.
3. Peroneal artery.

Anatomy of the Leg

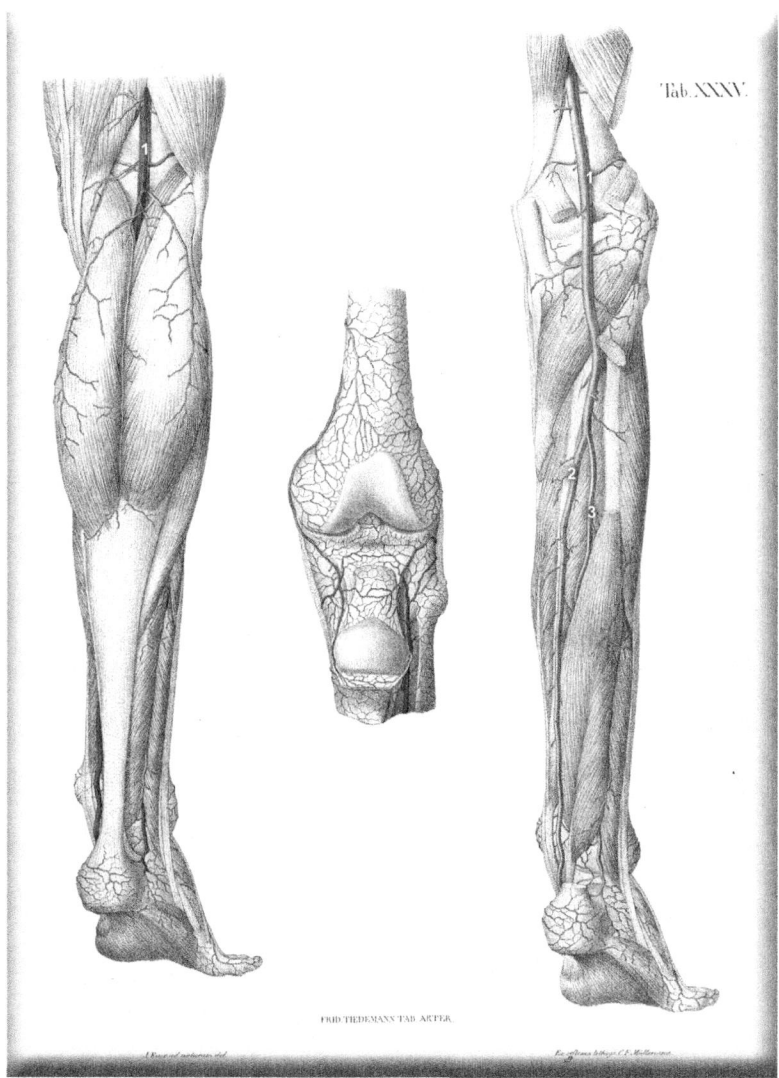

Credit
Dissections of the lower leg, knee joint and foot, back view: three figures, with the arteries and blood vessels indicated in red. Coloured lithograph by J. Roux, 1822. Credit: Wellcome Collection. Attribution 4.0 International (CC BY 4.0) URL: https://wellcomecollection.org/works/bbj2tc4a License information
This work is used herein without restriction under copyright law.
Creative Commons Attribution (CC BY 4.0) terms and conditions https://creativecommons.org/licenses/by/4.0

Anatomy of the Leg Veins

GREAT AND SHORT SAPHENOUS

1. Great saphenous vein.

Anatomy of the Leg Veins

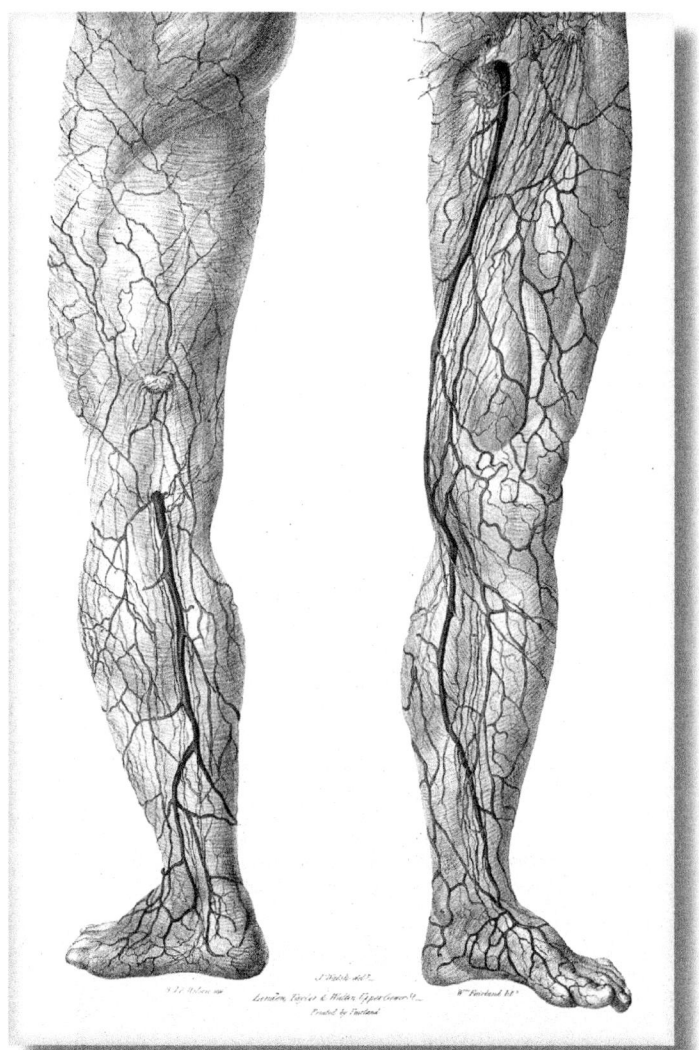

Credit
Veins and lymphatics of the leg: anterior and posterior views. Coloured lithograph by William Fairland, 1837, after J. Walsh after W.J.E. Wilson. Credit: Wellcome Collection. Attribution 4.0 International (CC BY 4.0) URL: https://wellcomecollection.org/works/xn5drus9

Anatomy of the Leg & Foot Veins

LOWER LEG & FOOT VEINS

1.   Great saphenous vein.

Anatomy of the Leg & Foot Veins

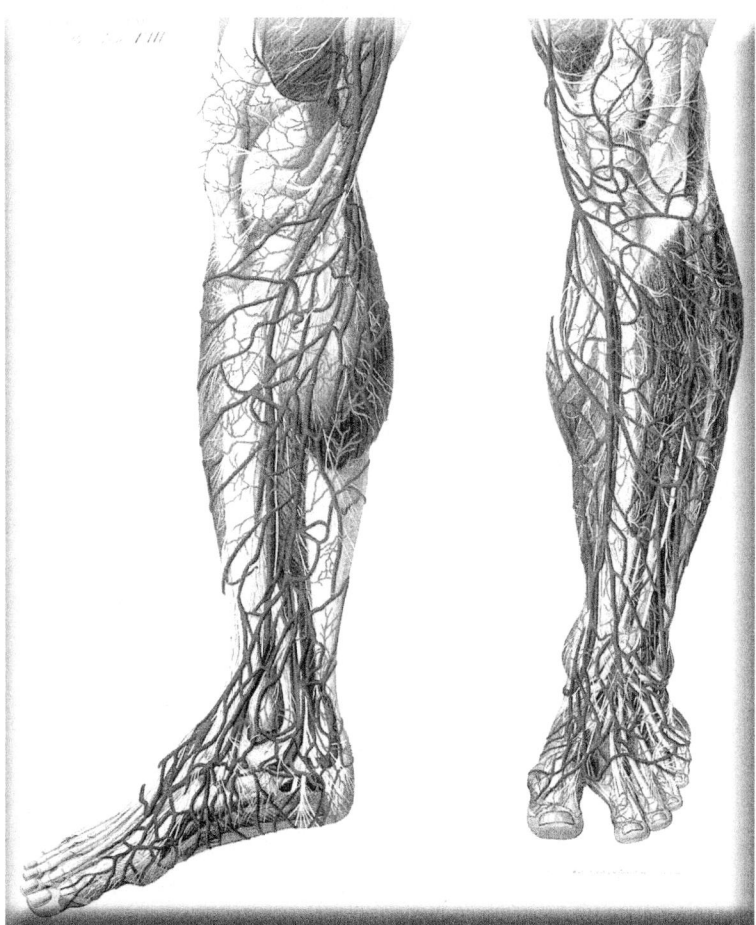

Credit
P. Mascagni, Anatomiae universae. 1823-32. Credit: Wellcome Collection. Attribution 4.0
International (CC BY 4.0) URL: https://wellcomecollection.org/works/jr7y4fhw

License information
This work is used herein without restriction under copyright law.
Creative Commons Attribution (CC BY 4.0) terms and conditions https://creativecommons.
org/licenses/by/4.0

Anatomy of the Foot

TENDONS AND ARTERIES

1. Anterior tibial artery.
2. Dorsalis pedis
3. Lateral plantar artery.
4. Deep plantar arch.
5. Plantar metatarsal artery.

Anatomy of the Foot

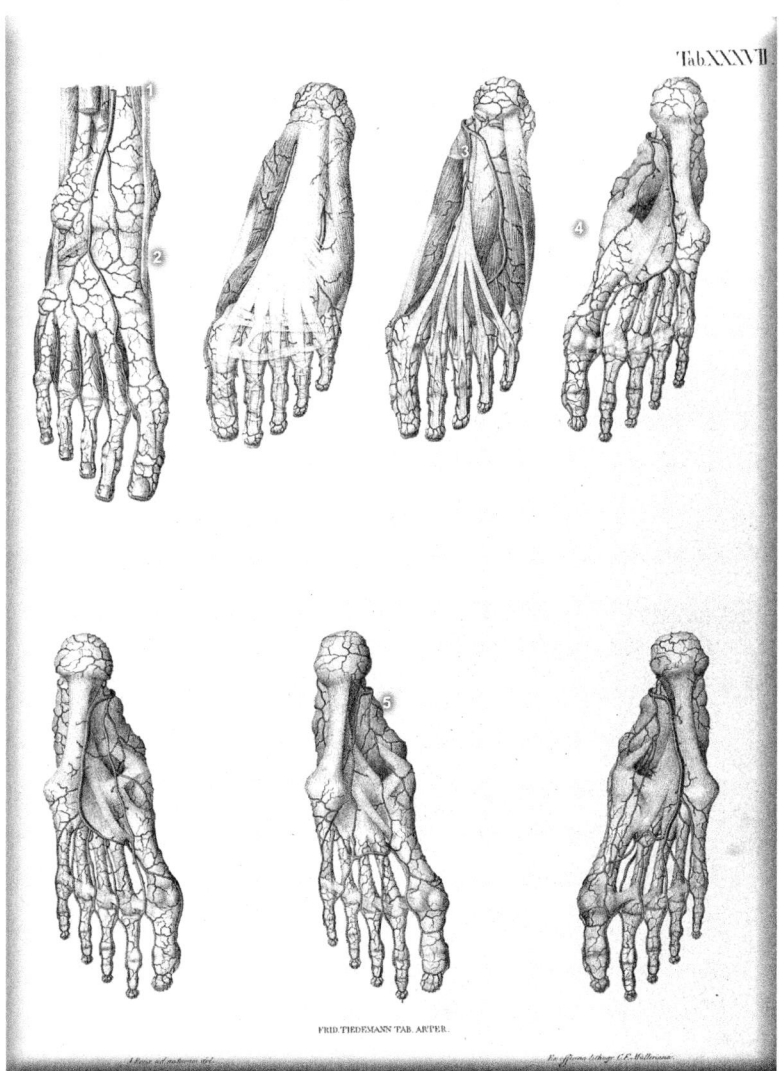

Tab.XXXVII.

FRID. THEDEMANN TAB. ARTER.

Credit
Dissections of the foot: seven figures, with the arteries and blood vessels indicated in red.
Coloured lithograph by J. Roux, 1822. Credit: Wellcome Collection. Attribution 4.0 International (CC BY 4.0) URL: https://wellcomecollection.org/works/bcpsnvyq
License information
This work is used herein without restriction under copyright law.
Creative Commons Attribution (CC BY 4.0) terms and conditions https://creativecommons.org/licenses/by/4.0

PART 2:
VASCULAR
OPERATIONS
PROFILE

OPERATION PROFILE:
CAROTID ENDARTERECTOMY

➤ ~70% Male
➤ ~75% Over 65 yrs
➤ ~25% diabetics
➤ ~30% with heart disease

➤ ~80% had mini stroke or stroke
➤ ~ 7% asymptomatic
➤ Average time from symptoms to procedure 10 days

➤ ~2% died and/or had a stroke within 30 days of the procedure
➤ ~5% readmission rate
➤ Average length of stay 2 days

REFERENCES:

• Vascular Services Quality Improvement Programme. 2019 Annual Report. URL: https://www.vsqip.org.uk/content/up-loads/2019/11/NVR-CEA-Infographic-2019.pdf. Accessed: June 2020

OPERATION PROFILE:
CAROTID ENDARTERECTOMY

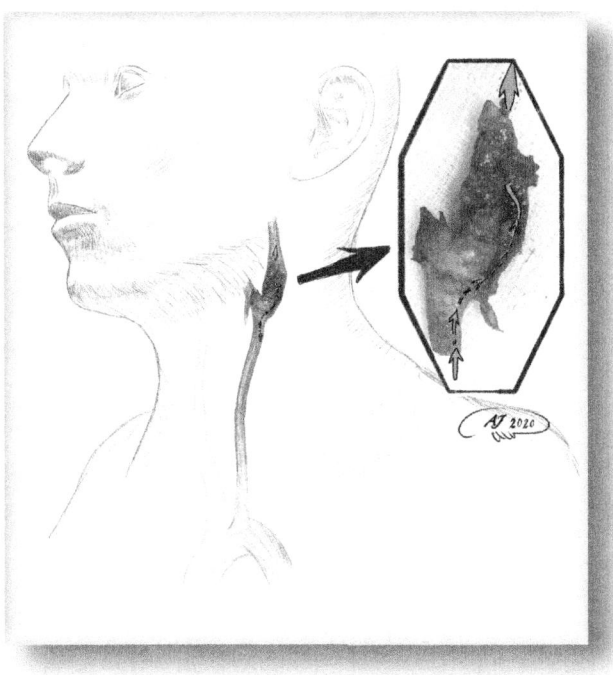

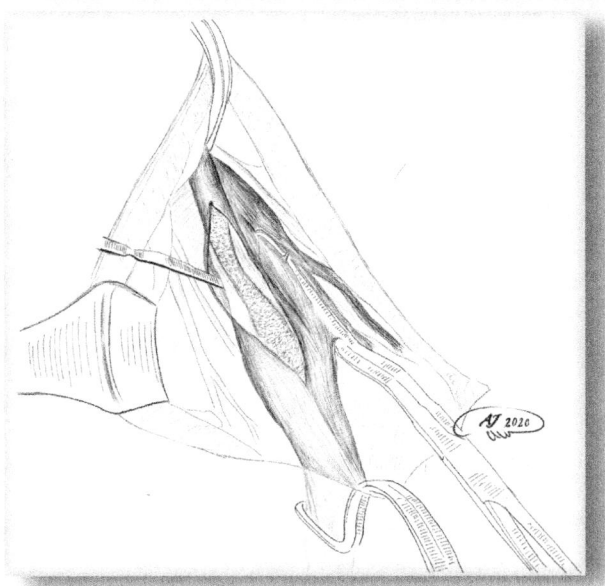

OPERATION PROFILE:
CAROTID ANEURYSM REPAIR

➤ Estimated incidence - 0.4% to 4.0% of all peripheral artery aneurysms.

➤ Untreated, stroke rate is nearly 50% and death rate ~ 70%.

➤ Majority are men

➤ Mean age of 50 to 60 years.

➤ Majority present with only a pulsatile neck mass just below the angle of the mandible without neurologic compromise.

➤ A small percentage suffer from TIA or stroke.

➤ All symptomatic patients should be considered for aneurysm repair.

➤ Asymptomatic aneurysms should be considered if the aneurysm is at least twice the size of the adjacent normal vessel or if there is a suspicion of an infected aneurysm.

➤ General operative approach is technically similar to that used for a standard carotid endarterectomy.

➤ Resection with primary end-to-end anastomosis (fig. 2a) or reversed greater saphenous vein interposition graft for a carotid aneurysm (fig. 2b) can be used.

➤ Endovascular treatment can also be considered where experience exists.

➤ Complications include death, stroke, TIA, myocardial events, cranial and peripheral nerve injury (greater auricular nerve} as well as postoperative neck hematomas.

REFERENCES:

• Fischer's Mastery of Surgery. 6th Edition. Lippincott Williams and Wilkins. 2012. ISBN 978-1-60831-740-0.

OPERATION PROFILE:
CAROTID ANEURYSM REPAIR

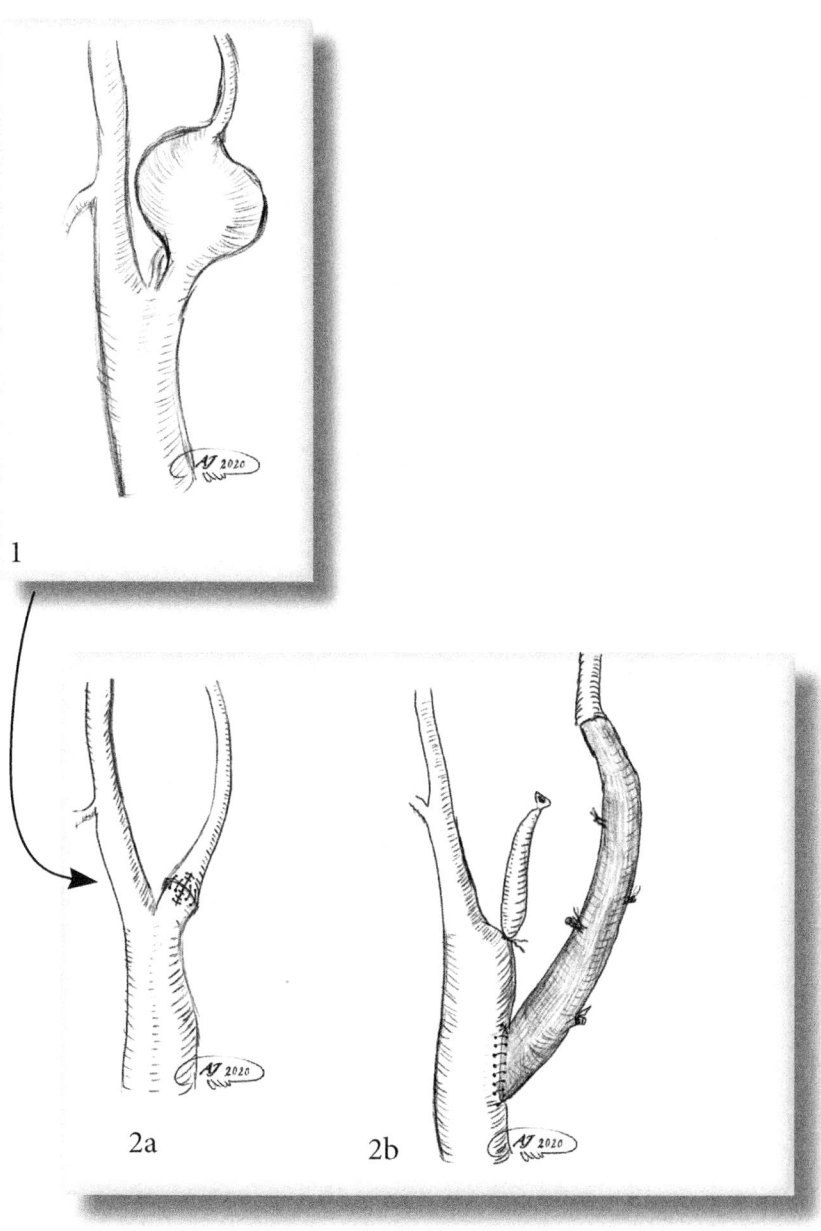

1

2a   2b

OPERATION PROFILE:
CAROTID BODY TUMOUR RESECTION

➤ Carotid body represents the largest mass of chemoreceptive tissue found anywhere in the body.
➤ Blood supply to the carotid body is usually derived from branches of ECA, and venous return occurs through tributaries of lingual and laryngopharyngeal veins.

➤ Affects mostly third or fourth decade of life
➤ No gender predominance
➤ When the tumor occurs in a familial pattern of inheritance, there is up to a 30% incidence of bilateral tumors, as opposed to 2-20% in nonfamilial cases.
➤ Tumours are highly vascular and often invade the adventitia of the adjacent carotid vessels .

➤ Most common presentation is incidentally noted asymptomatic neck mass.
➤ Almost 60% Presents with a painless neck mass, 10% with a painful mass, and a few with cranial nerve deficits.

➤ Once identified, all carotid body tumors should be removed, as most, if not all, will progress and become locally invasive.
➤
➤ An uncomplicated resection of a carotid body tumor is an extremely well-tolerated operation.
➤ Today, in experienced hands, a perioperative mortality of <0.5%, essentially no significant cerebrovascular sequelae, and a cranial nerve injury or other minor complication rate of no higher than 5% can be expected.

REFERENCES:
• Fischer's Mastery of Surgery. 6th Edition. Lippincott Williams and Wilkins. 2012. ISBN 978-1-60831-740-0.

OPERATION PROFILE:
Carotid Body Tumour Resection

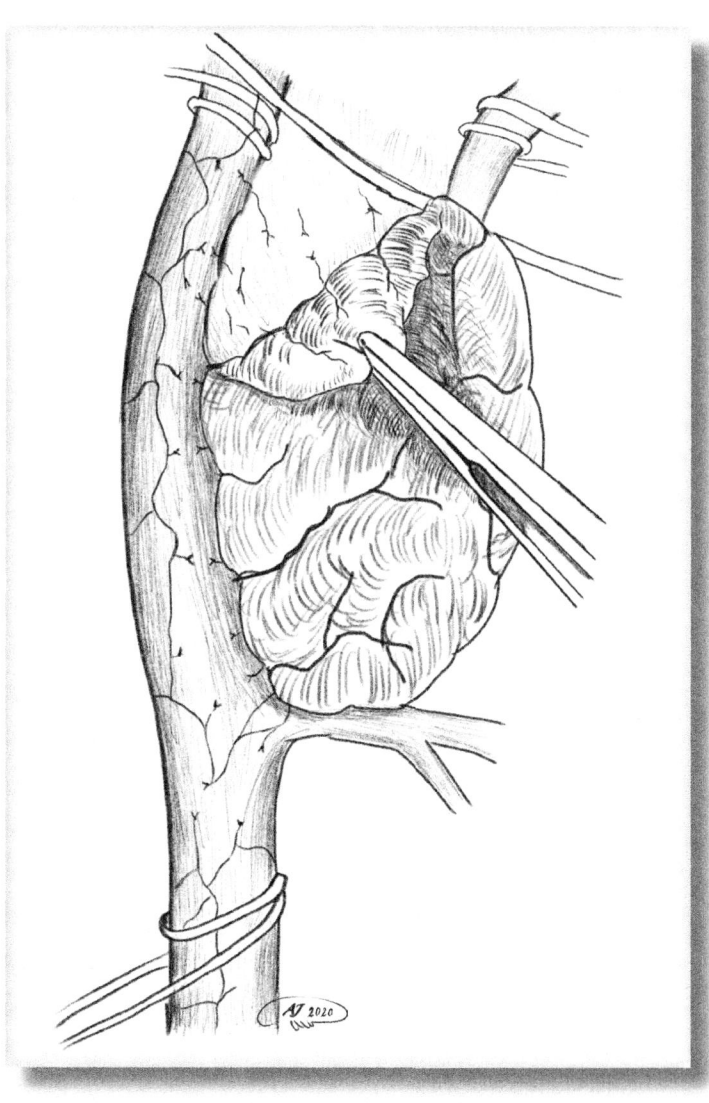

OPERATION PROFILE:
SUBCLAVIAN ARTERY ANGIOPLASTY AND STENTING

See page 403

OPERATION PROFILE:
SUBCLAVIAN ARTERY ANGIOPLASTY AND STENTING

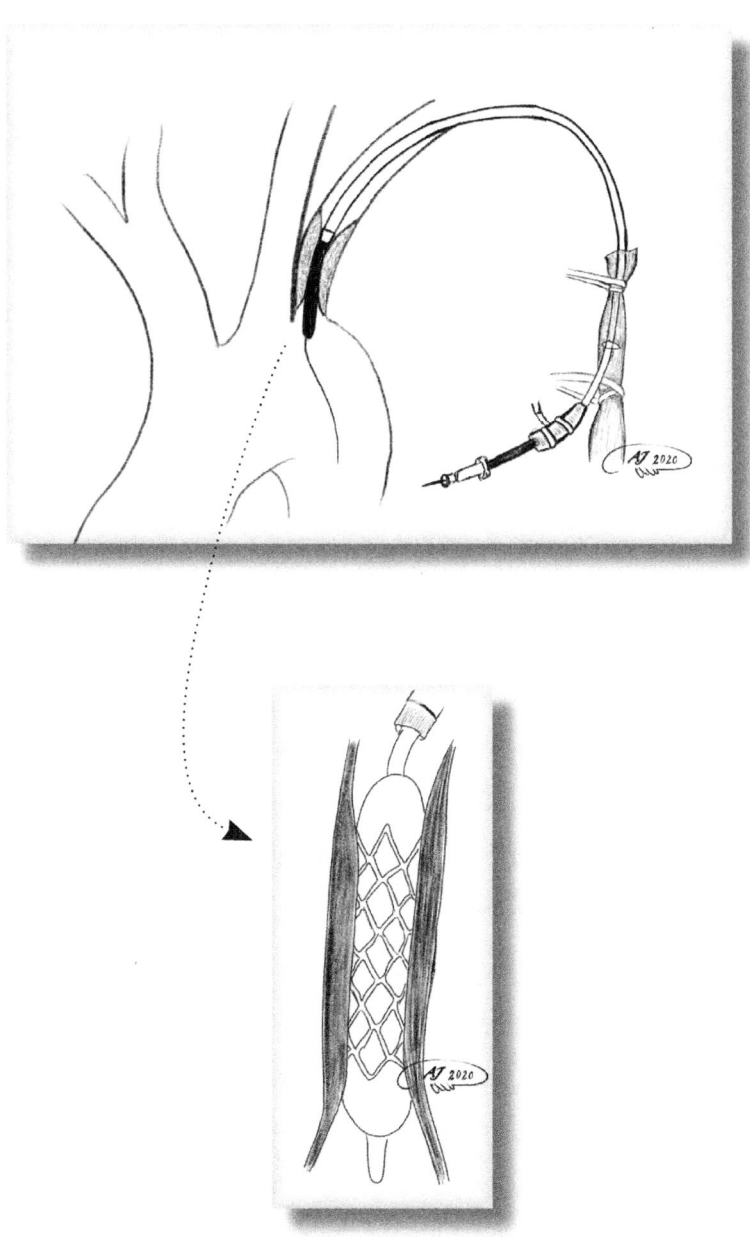

OPERATION PROFILE:
CAROTID SUBCLAVIAN BYPASS

➤ The results from direct reconstruction of the aortic arch branches are reasonably good.

➤ Primary graft patency of aortic arch branch reconstructions is 88% to 90% at 10 years.

➤ Direct arch reconstruction is effective at reducing the risk of ipsilateral neurologic events.

➤ The reported perioperative mortality ranges from 0% to 8% in surgical series published since 1990.

➤ See page 403

REFERENCES:

• Fischer's Mastery of Surgery. 6th Edition. Lippincott Williams and Wilkins. 2012. ISBN 978-1-60831-740-0.

OPERATION PROFILE:
CAROTID SUBCLAVIAN BYPASS

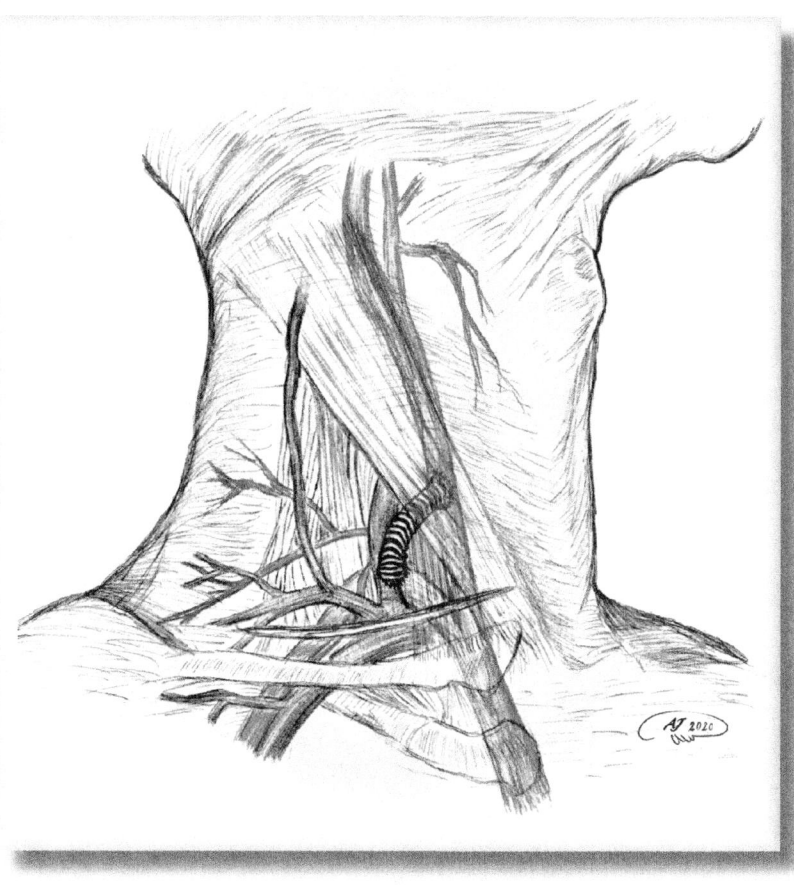

OPERATION PROFILE:
SUBCLAVIAN ANEURYSM REPAIR

➤ The results from direct reconstruction of the aortic arch branches are reasonably good.

➤ Primary graft patency of aortic arch branch reconstructions is 88% to 90% at 10 years.

➤ Direct arch reconstruction is effective at reducing the risk of ipsilateral neurologic events.

➤ The reported perioperative mortality ranges from 0% to 8% in surgical series published since 1990.

REFERENCES:

• Fischer's Mastery of Surgery. 6th Edition. Lippincott Williams and Wilkins. 2012. ISBN 978-1-60831-740-0.

OPERATION PROFILE:
SUBCLAVIAN ANEURYSM REPAIR

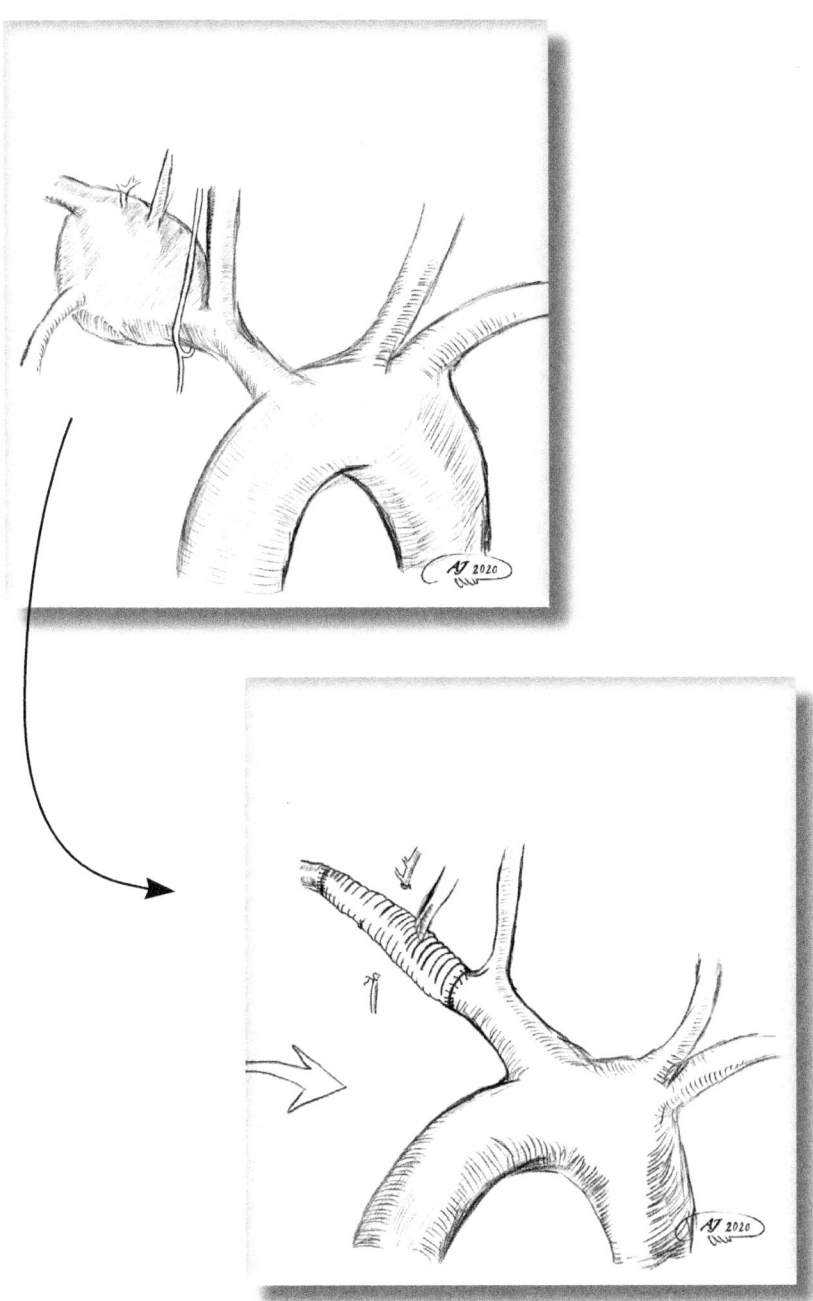

OPERATION PROFILE:
OPEN THORACIC ANEURYSM REPAIR

➤ See page 137

➤ Figure: Partial left heart bypass technique. Note the perfusion schemes to individual renal/visceral arteries while reconstructing the graft.

REFERENCES:

• Fischer's Mastery of Surgery. 6th Edition. Lippincott Williams and Wilkins. 2012. ISBN 978-1-60831-740-0.

OPERATION PROFILE:
OPEN THORACIC ANEURYSM REPAIR

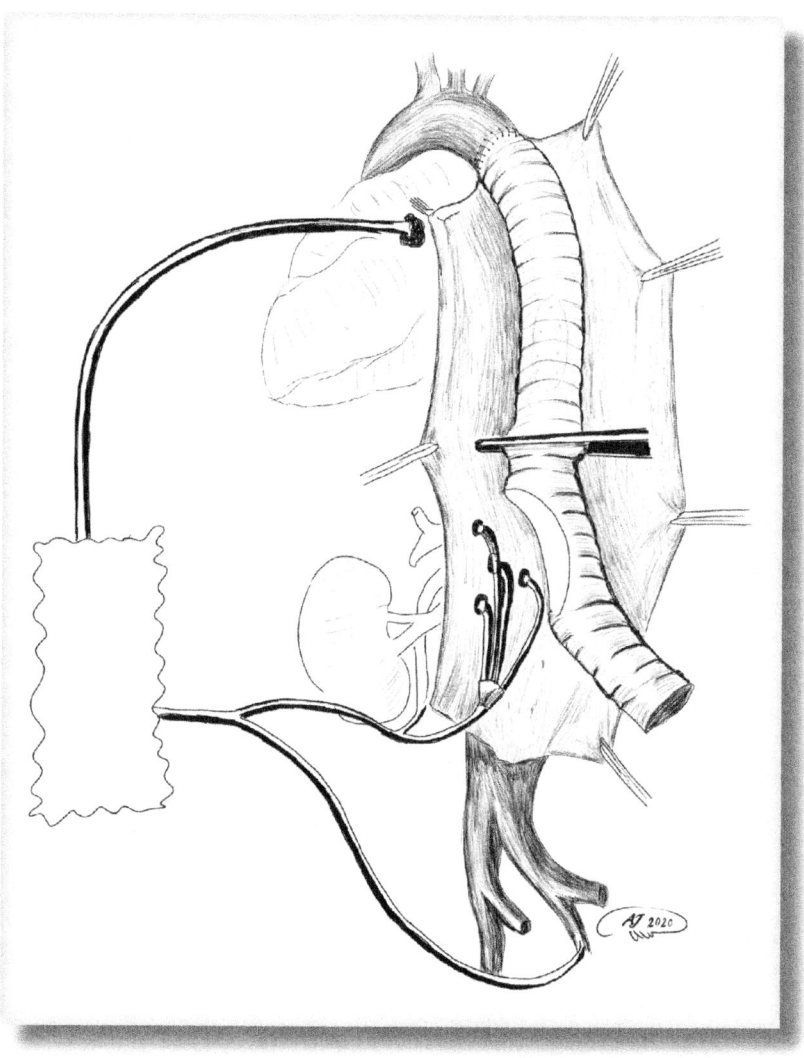

OPERATION PROFILE:
OPEN JUXTARENAL ANEURYSM REPAIR

➤ See page 116
➤ Figure: type IV thoracoabdorninal aneurysm repair. Note the beveled anastomosis and the reconstructed left renal artery bypass.

➤ ~90% Male
➤ ~80% Over 65 yrs
➤ ~80% hypertension
➤ ~80% are current or ex-smokers

OPEN REPAIR:
➤ ~14.7% died in hospital
➤ ~11% readmission rate
➤ Average length of stay 9 days

ENDOVASCULAR REPAIR:
➤ ~2.4% died in hospital
➤ ~9% readmission rate
➤ Average length of stay 4 days

REFERENCES:
• Fischer's Mastery of Surgery. 6th Edition. Lippincott Williams and Wilkins. 2012. ISBN 978-1-60831-740-0.
• Vascular Services Quality Improvement Programme. 2019 Annual Report. URL: https://www.vsqip.org.uk/content/up-loads/2019/11/NVR-CEA-Infographic-2019.pdf. Accessed: June 2020

OPERATION PROFILE:
OPEN JUXTARENAL ANEURYSM REPAIR

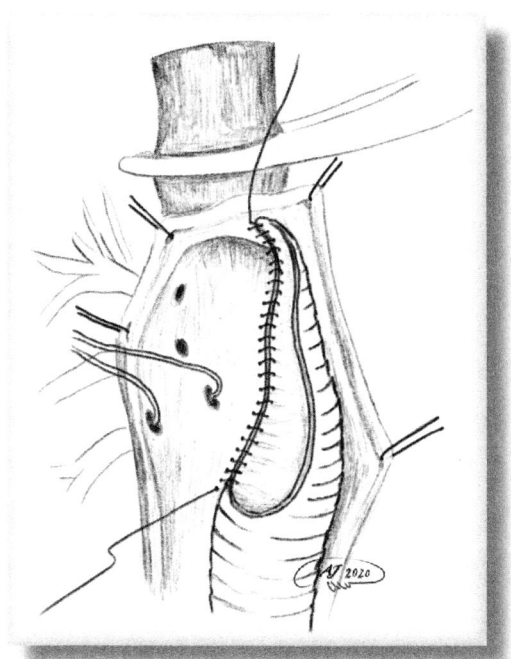

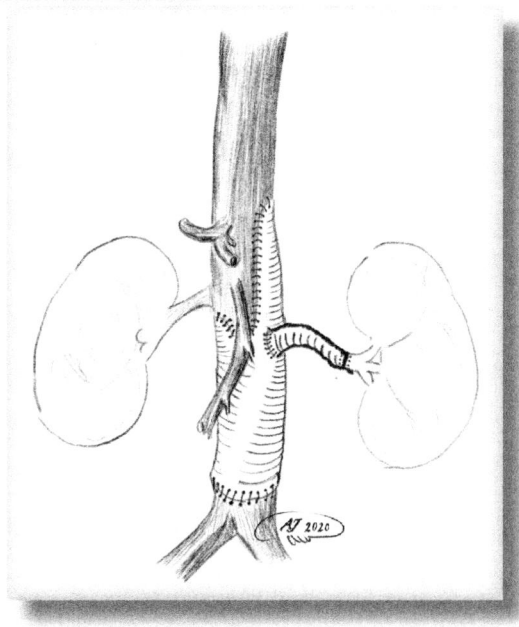

OPERATION PROFILE:
OPEN INFRARENAL ANEURYSM REPAIR

- ➤ ~90% Male
- ➤ ~75% Over 65 yrs
- ➤ ~70% hypertension
- ➤ ~85% are current or ex-smokers

- ➤ ~3.2% died in hospital
- ➤ ~6% readmission rate
- ➤ Average length of stay 7 days

REFERENCES:

• Vascular Services Quality Improvement Programme. 2019 Annual Report. URL: https://www.vsqip.org.uk/content/up-loads/2019/11/NVR-CEA-Infographic-2019.pdf. Accessed: June 2020

OPERATION PROFILE:
OPEN INFRARENAL ANEURYSM REPAIR

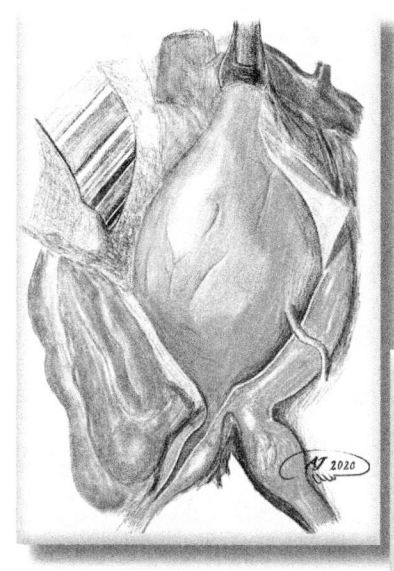

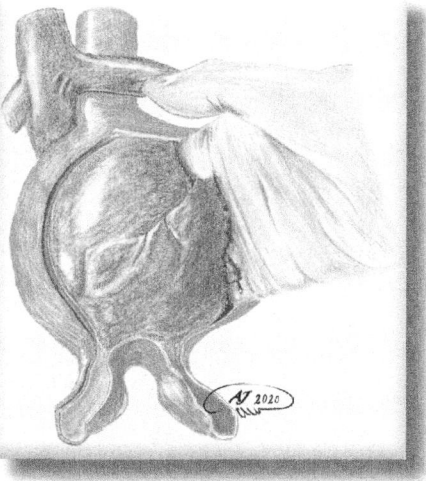

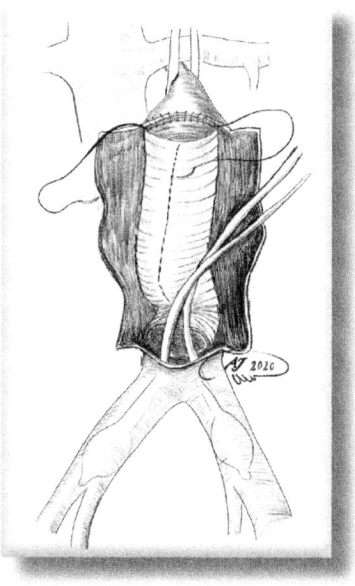

OPERATION PROFILE:
ENDOVASCULAR ANEURYSM REPAIR

- ➤ ~90% Male
- ➤ ~75% Over 65 yrs
- ➤ ~70% hypertension
- ➤ ~85% are current or ex-smokers

- ➤ ~0.4% died in hospital
- ➤ ~6% readmission rate
- ➤ Average length of stay 2 days

REFERENCES:

- Vascular Services Quality Improvement Programme. 2019 Annual Report. URL: https://www.vsqip.org.uk/content/up-loads/2019/11/NVR-CEA-Infographic-2019.pdf. Accessed: June 2020

OPERATION PROFILE:
ENDOVASCULAR ANEURYSM REPAIR

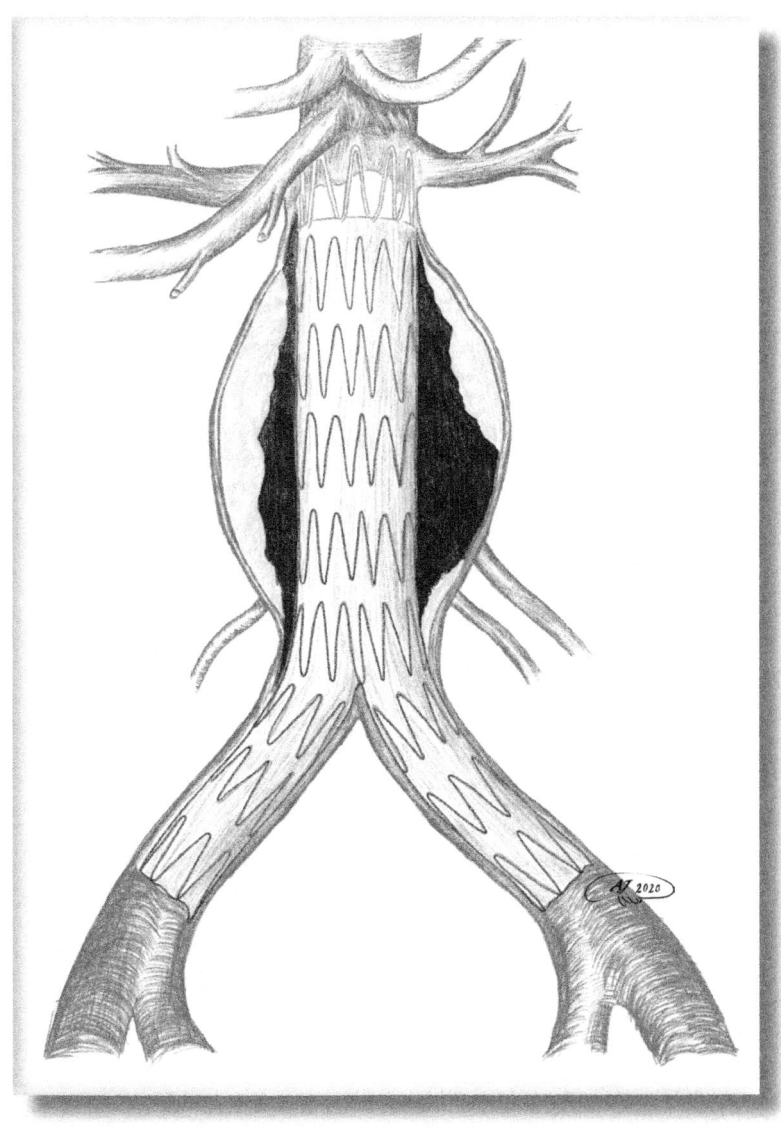

OPERATION PROFILE:
AORTO-BIFEMORAL BYPASS FOR BLOACKAGE

GENERAL PROFILE FOR LOWER LIMB BYPASSES
➤ ~75% Male
➤ ~65% Over 65 yrs
➤ ~35% diabetes
➤ ~90% are current or ex-smokers

AORT BIFEM/ILIAC BYPASS
➤ Percent of lower limb bypasses: elective 8%; emergecny 3.8%
➤ In hospital mortality: elective 2.7%; emergecny 10.3%

REFERENCES:

• Vascular Services Quality Improvement Programme. 2019 Annual Report. URL: https://www.vsqip.org.uk/content/up-loads/2019/11/NVR-CEA-Infographic-2019.pdf. Accessed: June 2020

OPERATION PROFILE:
AORTO-BIFEMORAL BYPASS FOR BLOACKAGE

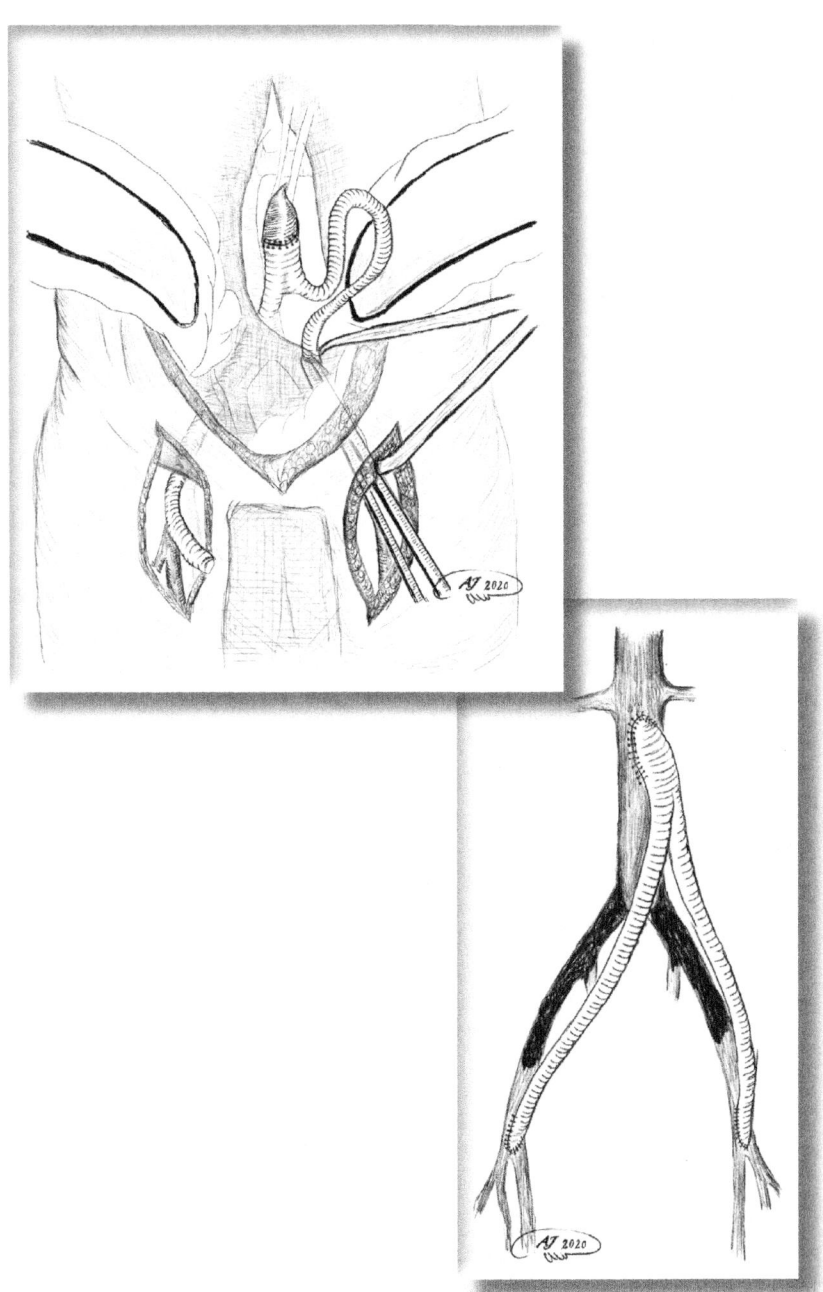

OPERATION PROFILE:
AORTIC ENDARTERECTOMY

GENERAL PROFILE FOR LOWER LIMB BYPASSES
➤ ~75% Male
➤ ~65% Over 65 yrs
➤ ~35% diabetes
➤ ~90% are current or ex-smokers

AORTIC ENDARTERECTOMY
➤ Figure: The plaque is mobilized and a secure end point distally in both iliac arteries is achieved.

REFERENCES:

• Vascular Services Quality Improvement Programme. 2019 Annual Report. URL: https://www.vsqip.org.uk/content/up-loads/2019/11/NVR-CEA-Infographic-2019.pdf. Accessed: June 2020

OPERATION PROFILE:
AORTIC ENDARTERECTOMY

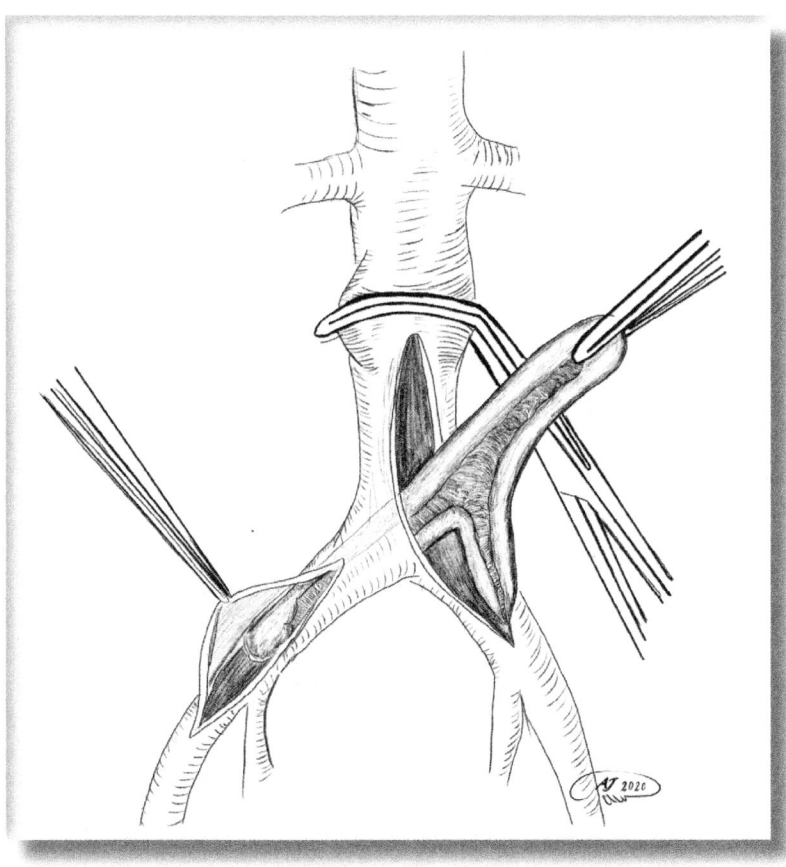

OPERATION PROFILE:
AXILLO-FEMORAL BYPASS

GENERAL PROFILE FOR LOWER LIMB BYPASSES
➤ ~75% Male
➤ ~65% Over 65 yrs
➤ ~35% diabetes
➤ ~90% are current or ex-smokers

AXILLARY FEMORAL BYPASS
➤ FOR MORE DETAILS, SEE PAGE 243

REFERENCES:

• Vascular Services Quality Improvement Programme. 2019 Annual Report. URL: https://www.vsqip.org.uk/content/uploads/2019/11/NVR-CEA-Infographic-2019.pdf. Accessed: June 2020

OPERATION PROFILE:
AXILLO-FEMORAL BYPASS

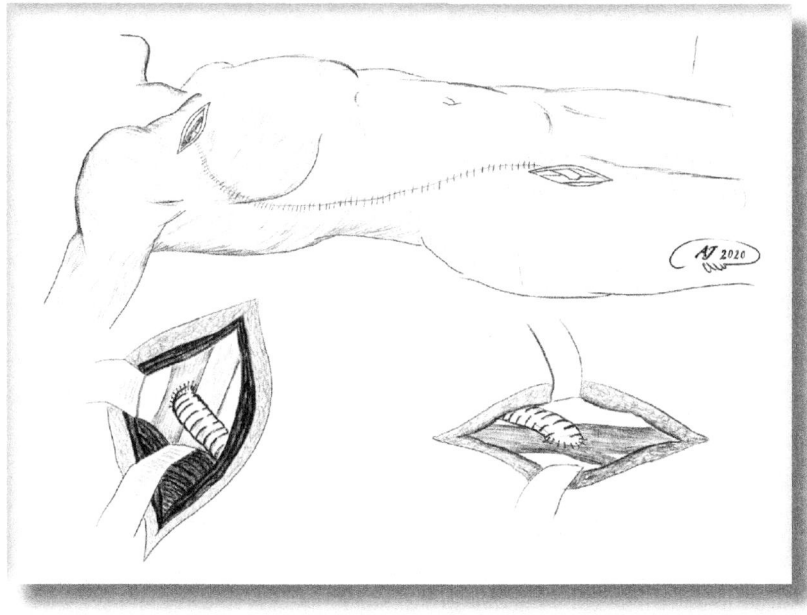

OPERATION PROFILE:
FEMO-POP BYPASS USING VEIN

GENERAL PROFILE FOR LOWER LIMB BYPASSES
➤ ~75% Male
➤ ~65% Over 65 yrs
➤ ~35% diabetes
➤ ~90% are current or ex-smokers

FEMORAL POPLITEAL/TIBIAL BYPASS
➤ Percent of lower limb bypasses: elective 53%; emergecny 9%
➤ In hospital mortality: elective 0.8%; emergecny 3.9%

REFERENCES:

• Vascular Services Quality Improvement Programme. 2019 Annual Report. URL: https://www.vsqip.org.uk/content/up-loads/2019/11/NVR-CEA-Infographic-2019.pdf.   Accessed: June 2020

OPERATION PROFILE:
FEMO-POP BYPASS USING VEIN

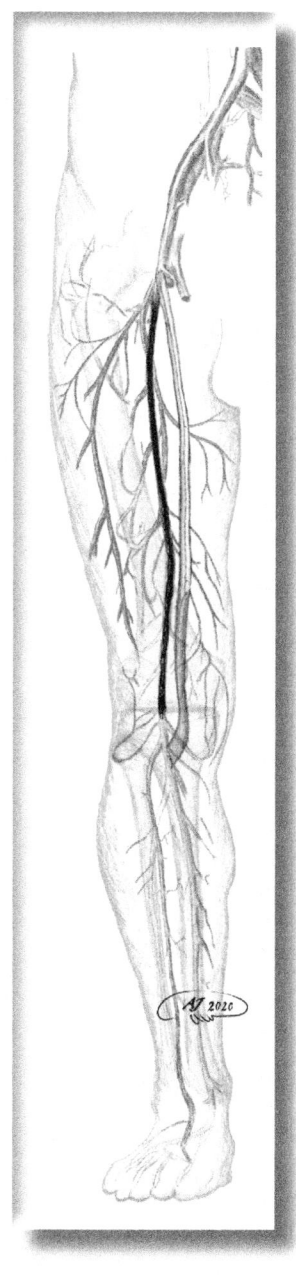

OPERATION PROFILE:
FEM-POP BYPASS USING A PROSTHESIS

GENERAL PROFILE FOR LOWER LIMB BYPASSES
➤ ~75% Male
➤ ~65% Over 65 yrs
➤ ~35% diabetes
➤ ~90% are current or ex-smokers

FEMORAL POPLITEAL/TIBIAL BYPASS
➤ Percent of lower limb bypasses: elective 53%; emergecny 9%
➤ In hospital mortality: elective 0.8%; emergecny 3.9%

REFERENCES:

• Vascular Services Quality Improvement Programme. 2019 Annual Report. URL: https://www.vsqip.org.uk/content/uploads/2019/11/NVR-CEA-Infographic-2019.pdf. Accessed: June 2020

OPERATION PROFILE:
FEM-POP BYPASS USING A PROSTHESIS

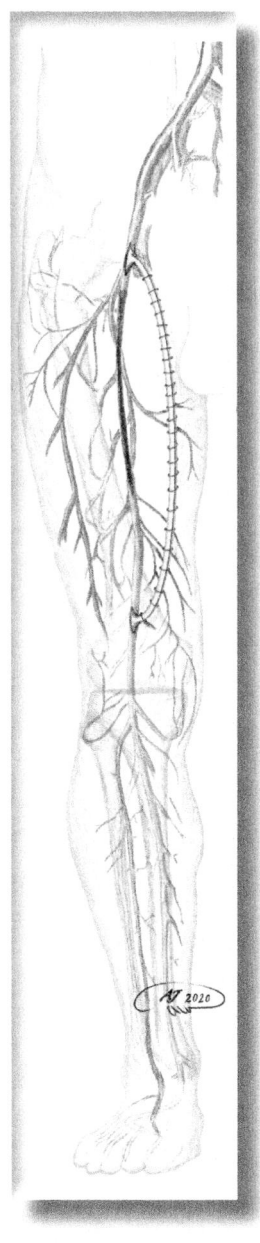

OPERATION PROFILE:
SARTURIOUS FLAP

➤ See page 137

➤ Figure: A sartorious flap is created and used to cover a repaired infected CFA.

REFERENCES:

• Fischer's Mastery of Surgery. 6th Edition. Lippincott Williams and Wilkins. 2012. ISBN 978-1-60831-740-0.

OPERATION PROFILE:
SARTURIOUS FLAP

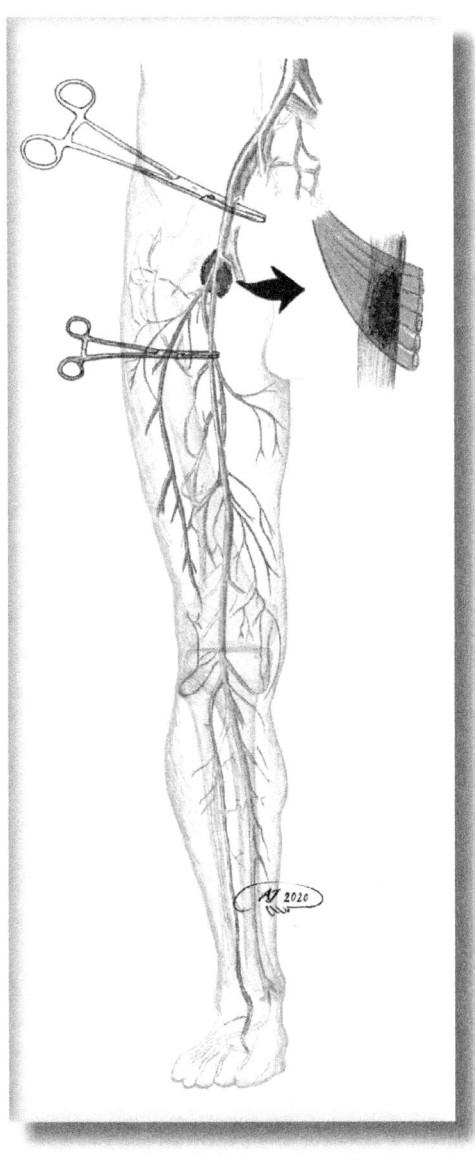

OPERATION PROFILE:
DISTAL (DP) BYPASS

In situ vein graft is used and tunneled at a gentle angle to avoid the resulting skin bridge from the two incisions (the DP exposure incision and the GSV harvesting incision).

See page 24.

OPERATION PROFILE:
DISTAL (DP) BYPASS

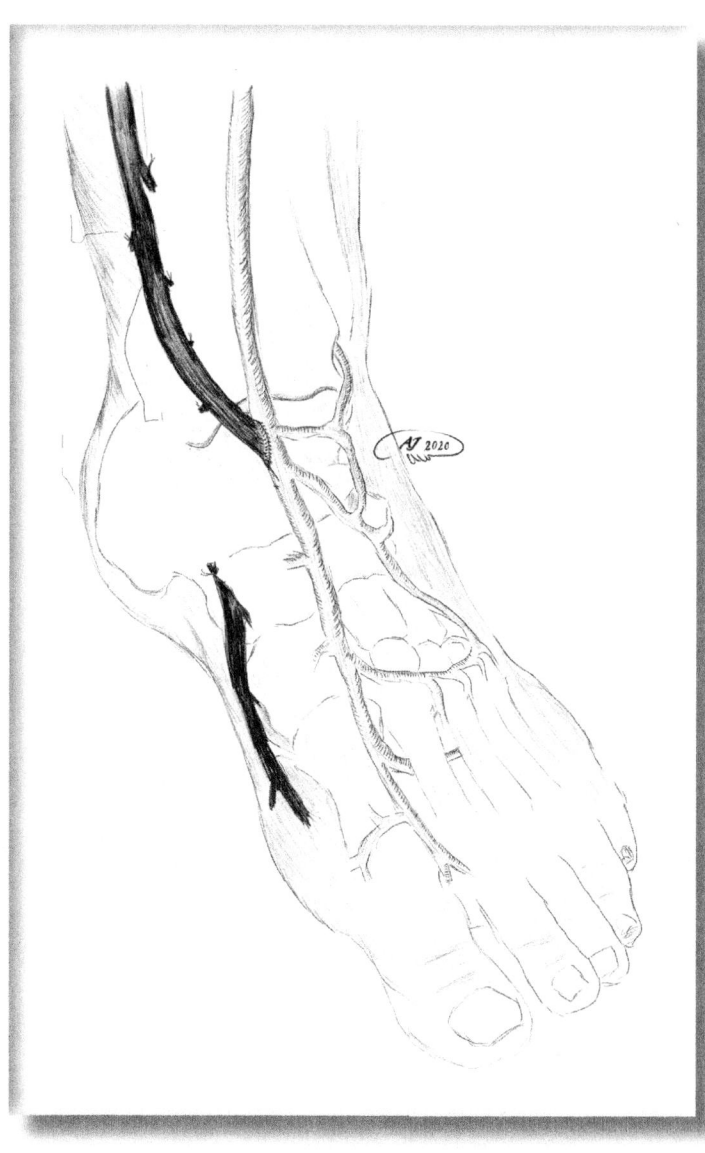

OPERATION PROFILE:
ABOVE KNEE AMPUTATION

- ➤ ~70% Male
- ➤ ~70% Over 65 yrs
- ➤ ~45% diabetics
- ➤ ~85% are current or ex-smokers

- ➤ ~11% died in hospital
- ➤ ~9% readmission rate
- ➤ Average length of stay 22 days

REFERENCES:

- Vascular Services Quality Improvement Programme. 2019 Annual Report. URL: https://www.vsqip.org.uk/content/up-loads/2019/11/NVR-CEA-Infographic-2019.pdf. Accessed: June 2020

OPERATION PROFILE:
ABOVE KNEE AMPUTATION

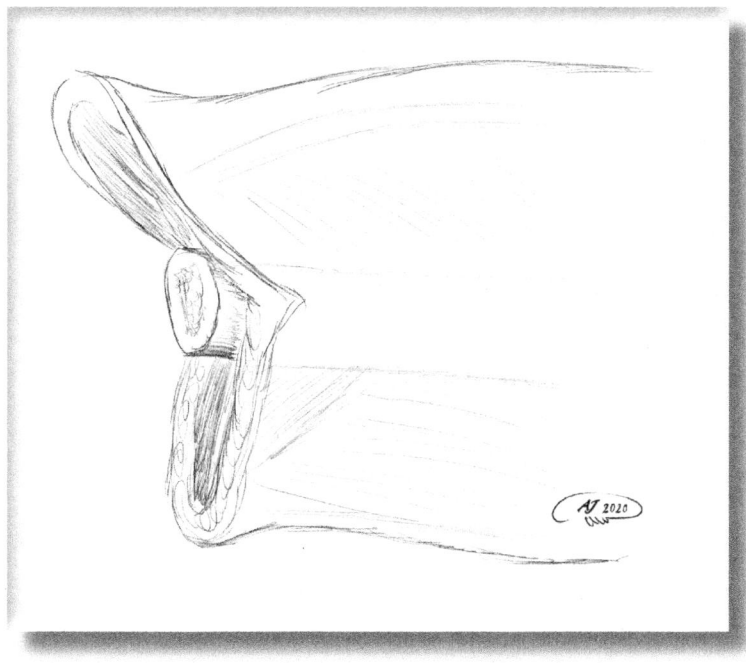

OPERATION PROFILE:
BELOW KNEE AMPUTATION

- ➤ ~70% Male
- ➤ ~70% Over 65 yrs
- ➤ ~45% diabetics
- ➤ ~85% are current or ex-smokers

- ➤ ~4.7% died in hospital
- ➤ ~11% readmission rate
- ➤ Average length of stay 24 days

REFERENCES:

- Vascular Services Quality Improvement Programme. 2019 Annual Report. URL: https://www.vsqip.org.uk/content/up-loads/2019/11/NVR-CEA-Infographic-2019.pdf. Accessed: June 2020

OPERATION PROFILE:
BELOW KNEE AMPUTATION

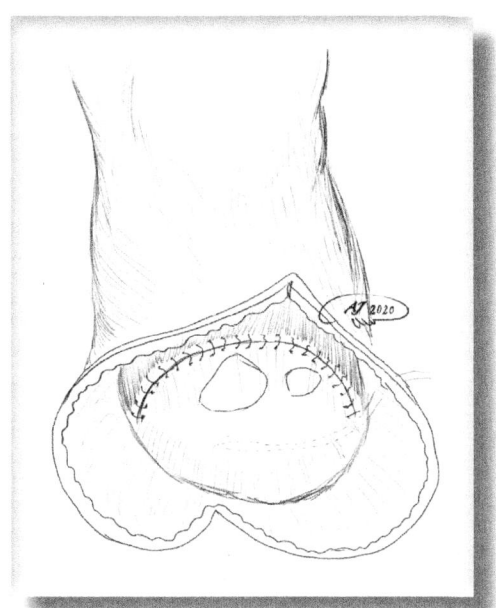

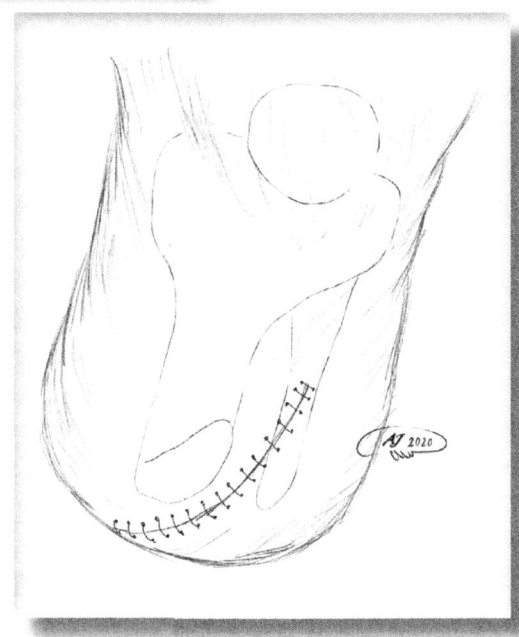

OPERATION PROFILE:
TOE AMPUTATION

Digital amputation of the first toe with a plantar flap.

Ray amputation of the third toe with a "racquet" incision.

REFERENCES:
- Fischer's Mastery of Surgery. 6th Edition. Lippincott Williams and Wilkins. 2012. ISBN 978-1-60831-740-0.

OPERATION PROFILE:
TOE AMPUTATION

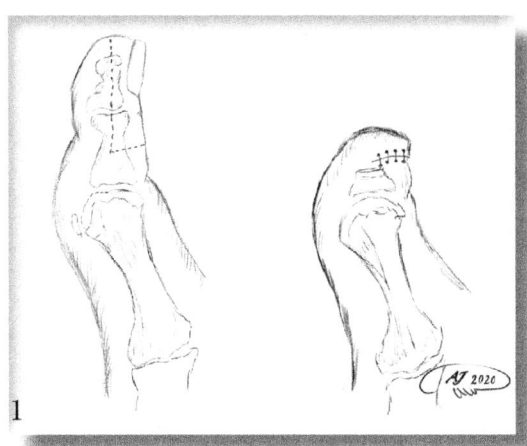

1

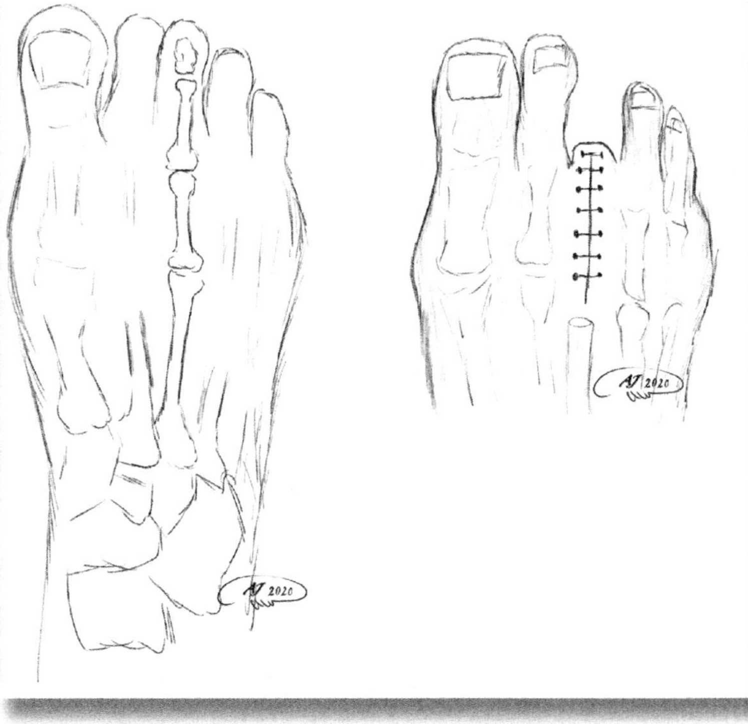

2

APPENDICES

APPENDIX 1:
FACTS AND FIGURES IN
HAEMODYNAMICS AND
ULTRASONOGRAPHY

Peripheral Circulation Pressure Profiles

1- PRESSURE GRADIENTS - WRIST TO FINGER

Age	Mean	SD	Cuff size	No.
23-54	9.5 mmHg	6.8	3.8 cm	14

2- PRESSURE GRADIENTS - FINGURE TO ARM

Age	Mean	SD	Cuff size	No.
<50	8.9 mmHg	11.0	2.4 cm	40
>50	5.2 mmHg	11.9	2.4 cm	40
17-31	9.3 mmHg	6.8	2.4 cm	10
43-57	-0.5 mmHg	6.6	2.4 cm	14

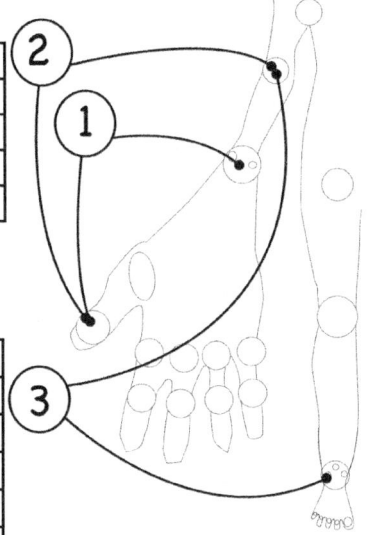

3- PRESSURE RATIO - LOWER LIMB TO ARM

(ADULTS)

Level	Ratio	Cuff size
Upper thigh	> 0.8	15.5 cm
	> 0.9	12 cm
Above knee	> 0.8	15.5 cm
	> 0.9	12 cm
Below Knee	> 0.8	15.5 cm
	> 0.9	12 cm
Above Ankle	> 0.8	13 cm
	> 0.97	12.5 cm
	> 1.0	12 cm
Toe	> 0.7	2 cm

REFERENCES:
- Angiology . 1978 Aug;29(8):601-6. PMID: 686496
- J Vasc Surg . 1996 Aug;24(2):258-65. PMID: 8752037
- Circulation. 1978 Nov;58(5):902-8. PMID: 699258
- Scand J Clin Lab Invest. 1976 Nov;36(7):627-32. PMID: 1019573
- Med Biol Eng Comput. 1997 Jul;35(4):425-7. PMID: 9327624
- Int Arch Occup Environ Health. 2008 Apr;81(5):625-32. PMID: 17901974

Peripheral Circulation Pressure Profiles

PWV	6.8-8.3

PWV	5.20

PWV	4.00

PWV	5.00
PWV25	6.40
PWV65	8.60
PWV40U	7.41
PWV40T	6.71

PWV	4.90
INF(- fore-arm)	3.1 (SD 0.7)

INF (hand)	9.3 (SD 2.1)

INF (digits)	15 - 40

PWV	8.80

INF (Calf)	3.6 (SD 1.3)
ReactInf	28.9 (SD 5.4)

INF (Foot)	1.2 (SD 0.8)
ReactInf	12.2 (SD 4.0)

- PWV: Pressure Wave Velocity (m/s)
- PWV25: Pressure Wave Velocity - age 25 (m/s)
- PWV65: Pressure Wave Velocity - age 65 (m/s)
- PWV20U: Pressure Wave Velocity - age 20 Untrained (m/s)
- PWV20T: Pressure Wave Velocity - age 20 Trained (m/s)
- PWV40U: Pressure Wave Velocity - age 40 Untrained (m/s)
- PWV40T: Pressure Wave Velocity - age 40 Trained (m/s)
- INF: Mean Arterial Inflow to 100mg of tissue (mL/min)
- ReactInf: Reactive Hyperaemia - Maximal inflow to 100mg of tissue (mL/min)

Peripheral Circulation Duplex Profiles

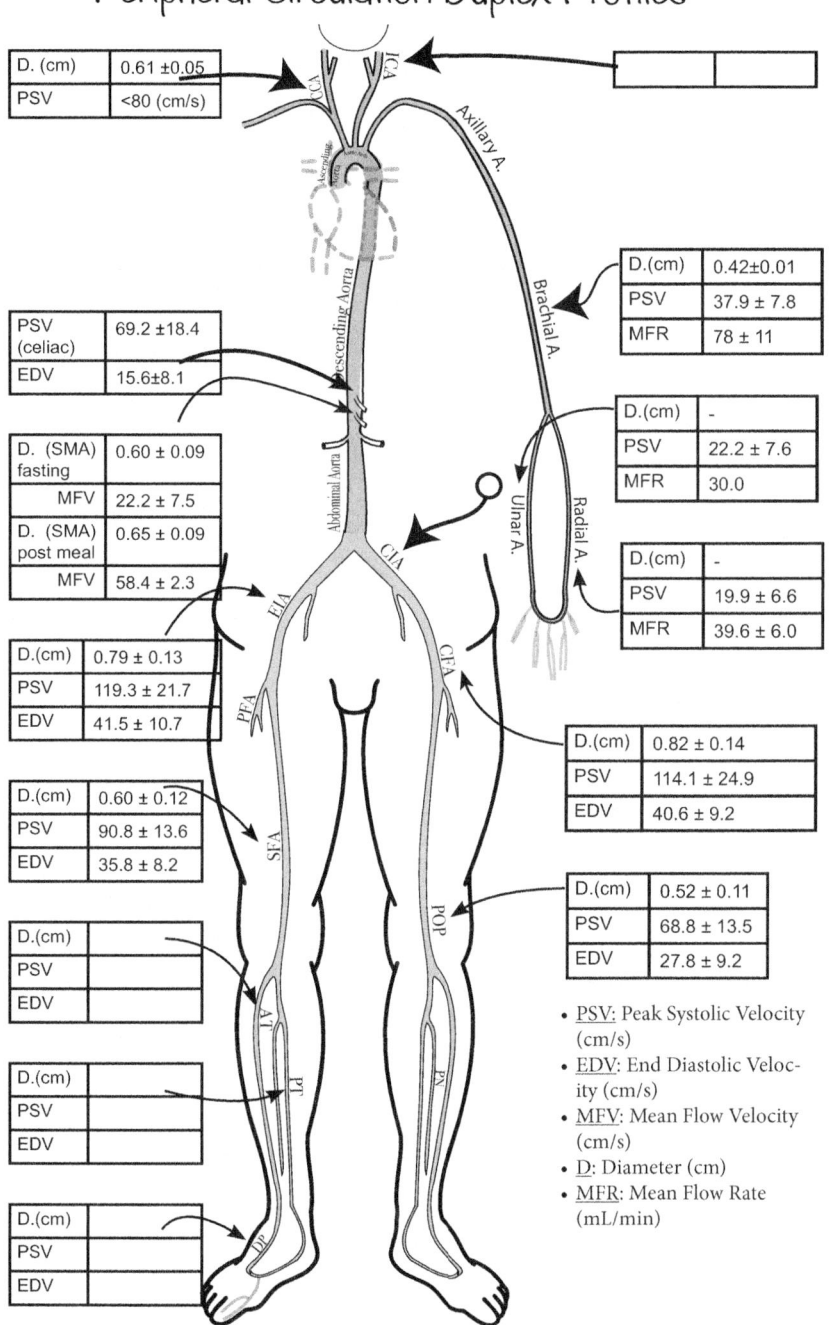

D. (cm)	0.61 ±0.05
PSV	<80 (cm/s)

PSV (celiac)	69.2 ±18.4
EDV	15.6±8.1

D. (SMA) fasting	0.60 ± 0.09
MFV	22.2 ± 7.5
D. (SMA) post meal	0.65 ± 0.09
MFV	58.4 ± 2.3

D.(cm)	0.79 ± 0.13
PSV	119.3 ± 21.7
EDV	41.5 ± 10.7

D.(cm)	0.60 ± 0.12
PSV	90.8 ± 13.6
EDV	35.8 ± 8.2

D.(cm)	
PSV	
EDV	

D.(cm)	
PSV	
EDV	

D.(cm)	
PSV	
EDV	

D.(cm)	0.42±0.01
PSV	37.9 ± 7.8
MFR	78 ± 11

D.(cm)	-
PSV	22.2 ± 7.6
MFR	30.0

D.(cm)	-
PSV	19.9 ± 6.6
MFR	39.6 ± 6.0

D.(cm)	0.82 ± 0.14
PSV	114.1 ± 24.9
EDV	40.6 ± 9.2

D.(cm)	0.52 ± 0.11
PSV	68.8 ± 13.5
EDV	27.8 ± 9.2

- PSV: Peak Systolic Velocity (cm/s)
- EDV: End Diastolic Velocity (cm/s)
- MFV: Mean Flow Velocity (cm/s)
- D: Diameter (cm)
- MFR: Mean Flow Rate (mL/min)

Peripheral Circulation Oxygen Saturation Profile

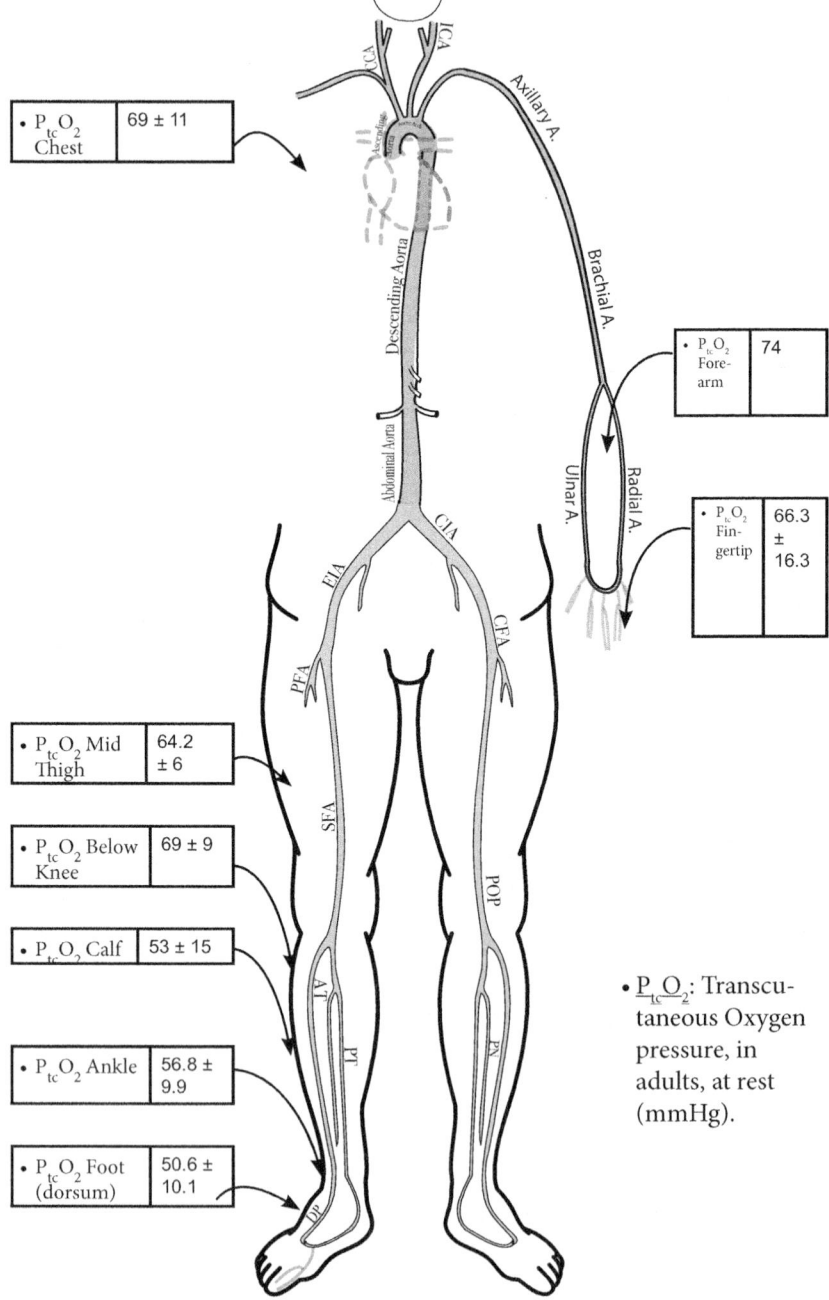

$P_{tc}O_2$ Chest	69 ± 11

$P_{tc}O_2$ Fore-arm	74

$P_{tc}O_2$ Fin-gertip	66.3 ± 16.3

$P_{tc}O_2$ Mid Thigh	64.2 ± 6

$P_{tc}O_2$ Below Knee	69 ± 9

$P_{tc}O_2$ Calf	53 ± 15

$P_{tc}O_2$ Ankle	56.8 ± 9.9

$P_{tc}O_2$ Foot (dorsum)	50.6 ± 10.1

• $\underline{P_{tc}O_2}$: Transcutaneous Oxygen pressure, in adults, at rest (mmHg).

Facts and Figures in Ultrasound Sonography

Sound Levels:

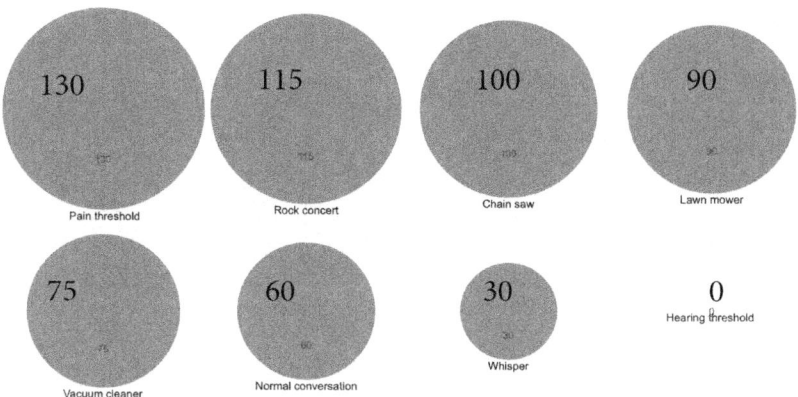

Attenuation Levels:

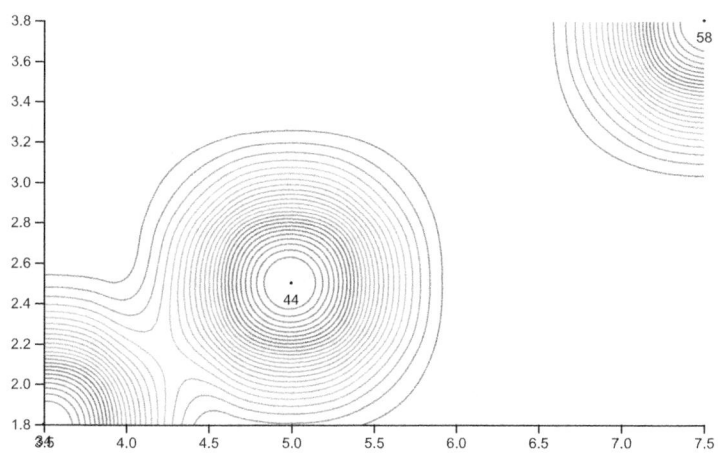

With Sound Frequency (MHz - x axis) being 3.5, 5, and 7.5, the average attenuation Coefficient for soft tissue (dB/cm - y axis) is 1.8, 2.5, and 3.8; and the intensity reduction in 1cm path (% - values of bubbles) is 34, 44, and 58.

Facts and Figures in Ultrasound Sonography

Pulse Round-Trip Travel Time for Various Reflector Depths

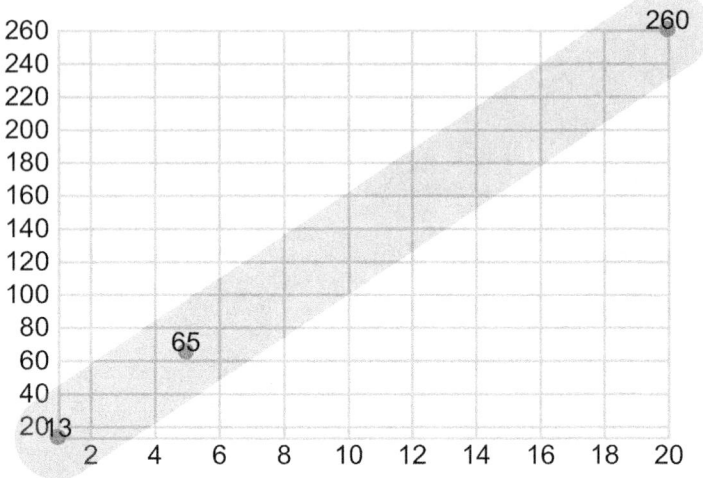

With depth (cm - x axis) being 1, 5, and 20, the pulse round travel time (μs - y axis) is 13, 65, and 260.

Sound parameters in tissues

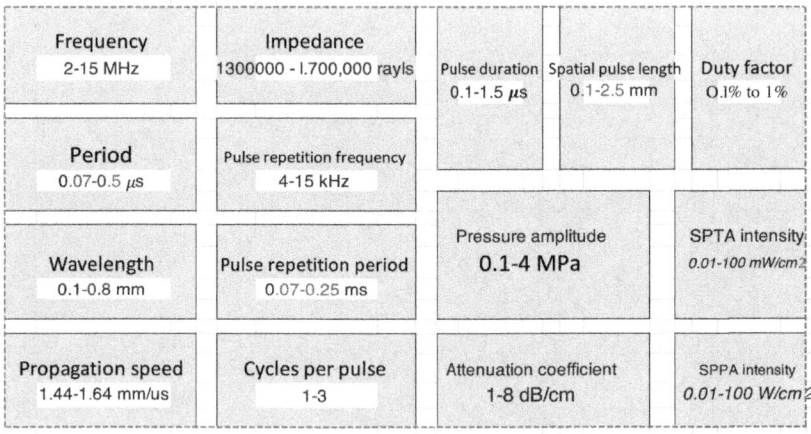

Frequency	Impedance	Pulse duration	Spatial pulse length	Duty factor
2-15 MHz	1300000 - 1.700,000 rayls	0.1-1.5 μs	0.1-2.5 mm	0.1% to 1%

Period	Pulse repetition frequency			
0.07-0.5 μs	4-15 kHz			

Wavelength	Pulse repetition period	Pressure amplitude		SPTA intensity
0.1-0.8 mm	0.07-0.25 ms	0.1-4 MPa		0.01-100 mW/cm2

Propagation speed	Cycles per pulse	Attenuation coefficient	SPPA intensity
1.44-1.64 mm/us	1-3	1-8 dB/cm	0.01-100 W/cm2

Transducer Element Thickness for Various Operating Frequencies

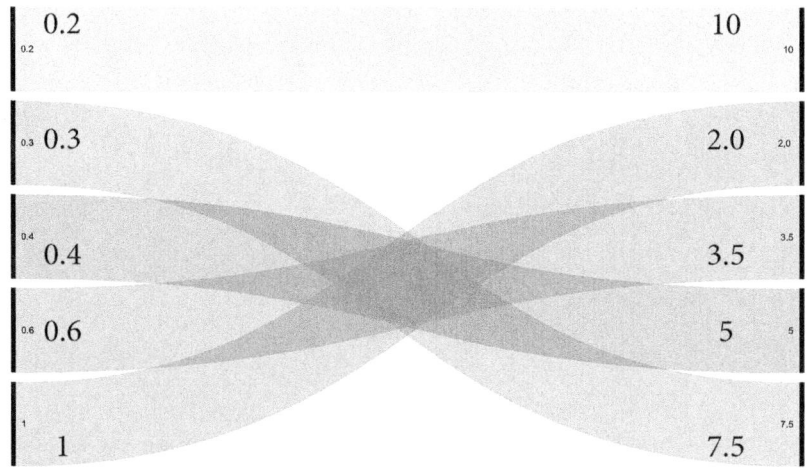

* Each element thickness (mm - left axis) produces specific frequency (MHz - right axis).

Near-Zone length (NZL) for Unfocused Elements

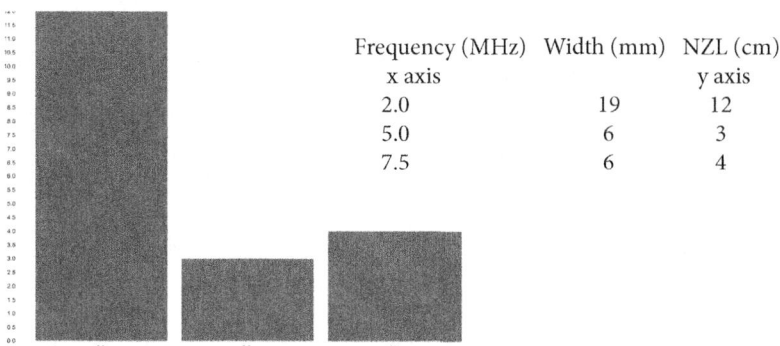

Frequency (MHz) x axis	Width (mm)	NZL (cm) y axis
2.0	19	12
5.0	6	3
7.5	6	4

Imaging Depth and Axial Resolution in Tissue

Frequency (MHz) (x axis)	Imaging Depth (em) (y axis)	Axial Resolullon (mm) (value)
3.5	17	0.44
5	12	0.31
7.5	8	0.2
10	6	0.15

Gain (Decibels) and Corresponding Power and Amplitude Ratios (the output power divided by input power)

Gain (dB) Ratio	Power Ralio	Amplitude
1	1.3	1.1
5	3.2	1.8
10	10	3.2
20	100	10
40	10000	100

Doppler Frequency Shifts for Various Scatter Speeds towards the Sound Source at a Zero Doppler Angle

Incldenl Frequency (MHz)	Scatter Speed (cm/s)	Reflecled Frequency (MHz)	Doppler Shiff (kHz)
5	50	5.0032	3.2
10	50	10.0065	6.5

Doppler Frequency Shifts for Various Angles and Scatter Speeds toward the Sound Source of Frequency 5 MHz

Scatter Speed (cm/s)	Angle (degrees)	Doppler Shiff (kHz)
100	0	6.5
100	30	5.6
100	60	3.2
300	30	17
300	30	9.7

Doppler Signal in carotid stenosis

Stenosis degree (NASECT. %)	PSA (ICA) (cm/s)	PSV(ICA)/EDV(CCA) (ratio)	PSV(ICA)/PSV(CCA) (ratio)
<50	<125	<8	<2
50-69%	>125	8-10	2-4
70-79%	>230	14-21	>4
>90%	>400	>30	>5

Duplex System Parameters

- **MODES**:
  - » B Mode: Echo amplitude is presented as brightness on a two dimensional cross-sectional display.
  - » CF Mode: Color Doppler Blood Flow
  - » PW Mode: Pulse Doppler mode. Pulsed wave has a sample volume located at a depth down the beam determined by the time that the gate opens.
  - » M Mode: A B mode presentation of changing reflector position (motion) vs. time (used in echocardiography).
  - » CW Mode: Continuous Wave Doppler mode. Continuous wave is not pulsed, has no range resolution, and detects flow anywhere in the beam.
  - » Advanced Modes:
    - ▷ 3D mode.
    - ▷ 4D mode.
    - ▷ PDI mode: Energy Doppler mode. Under this mode, a sampling area key is used to select the position of energy sampling box; the size of energy sampling box is regulated usually using a trackball. A column on the screen show the energy level.
    - ▷ B/B mode.
    - ▷ 4B mode.

- **B MODE PARAMETERS**:
  - » Gain:
    - ▷ Gain controls make total gain of two-dimensional gray image increase or decrease, thus obtaining brighter or darker image.
    - ▷ Amplification (overall gain) is the process by which small voltages are enhanced to larger ones.
    - ▷ Compensation (swept gain) is the equalisation of received echo amplitude differences caused by different attenuations for different reflector depths. This is known as swept gain , depth gain compensation (DGC), or time gain compensation (TGC).
  - » Depth:
    - ▷ Depth controls increase depth to display structures with deeper distances.
    - ▷ Depth is related to the probe in use and is usually dis-

played in D (cm) on screen.
  ▷ Generally speaking, the larger the depth range is, the lower the frame frequency is.
» <u>Frequency:</u>
  ▷ Frequency is related to the probe in use and is usually displayed in Freq (MHz) on screen.
  ▷ Generally speaking, the higher the frequency is, the poorer the penetrability is and the higher the resolution is.
» <u>View area:</u>
  ▷ Generally speaking, the higher the view area is, the poorer the penetrability is and the lower the frame frequency is.
» <u>Dynamic range:</u>
  ▷ Dynamic range is the ratio (in decibels) of largest to smallest power that a system can handle; ratio of the largest to smallest intensity of echoes encountered.
  ▷ Dynamic range controls how does echo intensity change to grey gradient, and therefore can optimise the tissue texture of different anatomical structures.
  ▷ Selecting different dynamic range values will change the display effect of image grey scale; the dynamic range is displayed in DR (dB) on screen.
» <u>Edge (image) enhancement:</u>
  ▷ A signal image processing function that improves the display of tissue boundaries.
  ▷ This is part of processing and postprocessing functions which include persistence (averaging sequential frames together), frame averaging, smoothing, and fill-in interp - lation (filling in missing pixel information).
» <u>Rejection:</u>
  ▷ The elimination of small-amplitude voltages.
  ▷ Rejection function eliminates low-level echo caused by noise by rejecting the echo signal with low amplitude so as to reduce the influence of noise on ultrasonic image
  ▷ Different rejection values to change the display effect of low-level echo of image on screen.
» <u>Image inversion:</u>
  ▷ Black/white inversion switches from white echo on black background to black echo on white background format.
  ▷ Up/Down inversion obtains the ultrasonic image in line with actual anatomical position through vertically inverting the image.
» <u>Focus:</u>

▷ The near field (Fresnel zone) is the region of the beam from the transducer surface to the focus. The far field (Fraunhofer zone) is the region beyond the focus.

▷ Focusing is the process of using lenses and electronic phasing of the driving voltages to change the beam focus area.

▷ Focusing enhance the resolution of assigned area and obtain distinct image of the area you're interested in.

▷ The focus position is usually marked with a symbol on the screen scale (such as a triangle); the focus number is usually marked with the number of triangular symbol at screen scale with maximum number being defined (for example 4); when the number of triangular marker is 0, the focus is usually set as automatic dynamic focusing.

» Frame average:

▷ This is a postprocessing function that implements filtering treatment to multi-frame image in time area and reduces the speckle noise so as to obtain more smooth and mild image.

▷ Generally, the stronger the frame average treatment is, the poorer the instantaneity is (instantaneity is the quality of being instant or immediate).

» Acoustic Output:

▷ This is measured using pressure (compression, rarefaction - mmHg or MPa), power (mW), and intensity (mW/cm^2).

▷ Regulation of acoustic power should comply with ALARA (As Low As Reasonably Achievable) principle. The acoustic power is usually displayed in percentage in sub-menu on screen.

▷ Intensity is not uniform across a beam but usually is highest at the centre and decreasing away from the centre.

» Line density:

▷ Line density of two-dimensional image of B Mode balances the transverse spatial resolution and frame frequency to obtain proper optimal image.

▷ Increases the number of scan lines per frame decreases the frame rate.

▷ The line density value is usually displayed in sub-menu on screen in two grades, standard (Std) and high density (High).

- COLOR BLOOD FLOW (CF) AND PULSE WAVE (PW) MODE PARAM-
  ETERS:
  - » Sampling box:
    - ▷ This determines the position and size of color Doppler image displayed under CF/PDI mode on B image.
    - ▷ The fundamental variables for sampling are:
      - ➤ Packet size is number of pulses used to generate one color Doppler image scan line.
      - ➤ Line density is the number of scan lines per color frame.
      - ➤ Maximum depth
      - ➤ Frame rate. Increasing any of the above (a, b, c) decreases frame rate.
      - ➤ Echo vs. color threshold. The echo strength level at which the instrument chooses to play a gray-scale or color coded, Doppler-shifted echo at each pixel location.
  - » Gain:
    - ▷ In CF mode, this magnifies or decreases the overall i - tensity of echo treated in color blood flow window so as to obtain ideal color image.
    - ▷ The gain is displayed in Gn (dB) on screen. The gain value will increase or decrease with 1dB.
  - » Frequency:
    - ▷ In CF mode, this allows for adaptation to the demands of the tissue with different movement speeds.
    - ▷ Generally, the frequency of CF/PDI mode increased when observing a low-speed blood flo .
    - ▷
  - » Frame average:
    - ▷ In CF mode, this implement filtering treatment to mu - ti-frame color image and reduces the speckle noise so as to obtain more smooth and mild image.
    - ▷ The higher frame average value makes the display time of color image longer, which strengthens the visibility of fluid.
  - » Colour map:
    - ▷ The direction of color blood flow map is defined as re toward the probe and blue away from the probe.
    - ▷ Colour maps represents the hue (change of colour based on frequency of light received), saturation (the amount of hue present in a mix with white), and luminance (brightness of a presented hue and saturation.

» Angle steer:
  ▷ This enables the operator to meet the angle requirement needed by ultrasonic Doppler effect, without moving the probe, through steering the color sampling box.
  ▷ The angel steer function can usually steer leftward (15°), middle (0 °) or rightward (15°).
  ▷ With proper angle incorporation, the Doppler equation is solved to present flow velocity in meters per second or centimetres per second on the vertical axis of the spectral display.
  ▷ Maximum Doppler shift occurs with zero Doppler angle. Maximum echo strength occurs with a 90-degree angle of incidence.
» Angle correct:
  ▷ In PW mode, angle correct estimates the speed of blood flow at the direction that forms certain angle. The angel value increases or decreases with 1°.
» Threshold:
  ▷ The threshold distributes the grade of grey scale range so as to select more color images or more grey images of B mode.
  ▷ The threshold restricts the low-level echo in inner wall of vessel covered by color blood flo , which is helpful to reduce the color overflow of vessel wall.
» Packet size:
  ▷ This is the number of pulses used to generate one color Doppler image scan line.
  ▷ Changing packet size enhances or reduces the color sensitivity and color average.
  ▷ Generally, the magnification of the size of sampling packet will enhance the quality of color image, but reduce frame frequency.
» Pulse repetition frequency (PRF):
  ▷ Pulse repetition frequency is the number of pulses per second; sometimes called pulse repetition rate.
  ▷ In general, the PRF has to be increased when observing a high-speed blood flo .
» Wall filte :
  ▷ This filter removes useless movement through filtering th low-speed color signal and eliminates the color artefact caused by breathing or other activities of the patient.
  ▷ Overly high wall-filter settings can artificially remove legi -

mate lower-frequency Doppler shifts.
» <u>Acoustic Output:</u>
  ▷ See above.
» <u>Line density:</u>
  ▷ See above.
» <u>Colour transparency:</u>
  ▷ Changing the transparency of color image allows the color image to observe the tissue structure behind color.
  ▷ The value of color transparency is usually displayed in on screen in ten grades.
» <u>Spatial filter</u>
  ▷ This filter reduces image pixel and makes the color image more smooth.
  ▷ The value of color transparency is usually displayed in on screen in five grades.
» <u>Baseline:</u>
  ▷ Baseline shift can be used to eliminate aliasing. Increased pulse repetition frequency and baseline shift may be necessary in extreme cases.
  ▷ The default base line is midpoint.
» <u>Sweep speed:</u>
  ▷ In PW mode, the sweep speed controls the update speed of frequency spectrogram to observe more or fewer frequency spectrum cycles on screen.

APPENDIX 2: ENDOVASCULAR TOOLS, CHARTS, TIPS AND TRICKS

Guidewires

COILED STAINLESS STEEL GUIDEWIRES

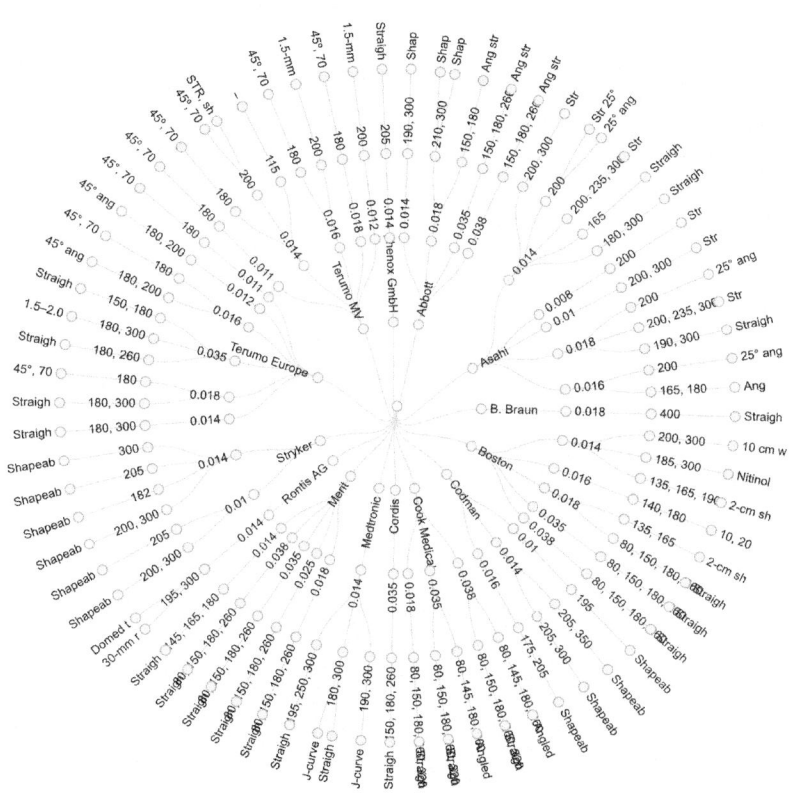

*Company, wire size (F), length (cm) and tip shape

REFERENCES:

- Endovascular Tody. Device Guide. June 2020. URL: https://evto-day.com/device-guide/european

Guidewires

HYDROPHILIC GUIDEWIRES

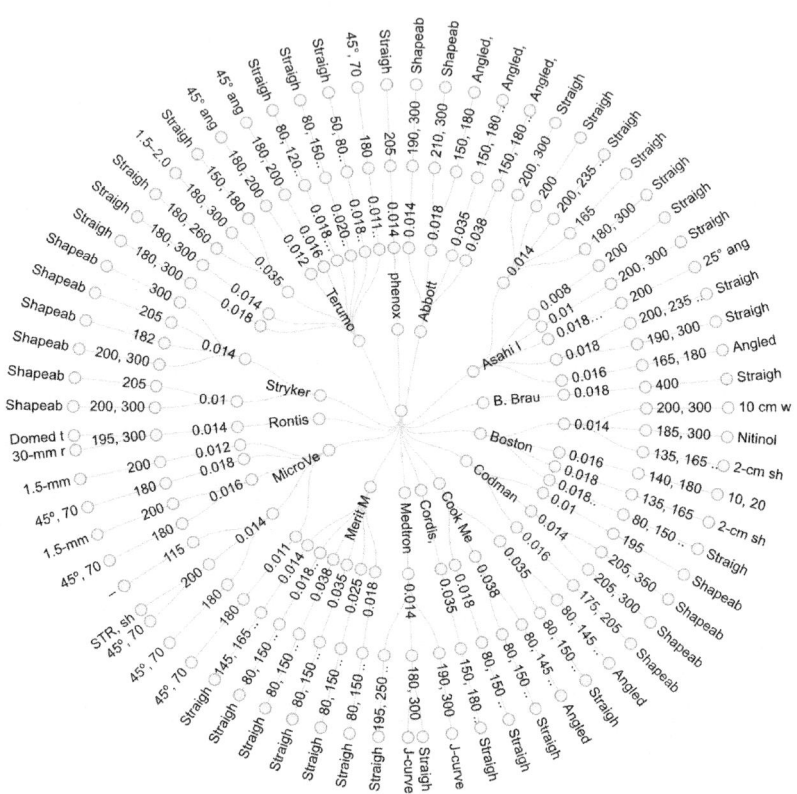

*Company, wire size (F), length (cm) and tip shape

REFERENCES:

- Endovascular Tody. Device Guide. June 2020. URL: https://evto-day.com/device-guide/european

Guidewires

MANDRIL/SPECIALTY GUIDEWIRES

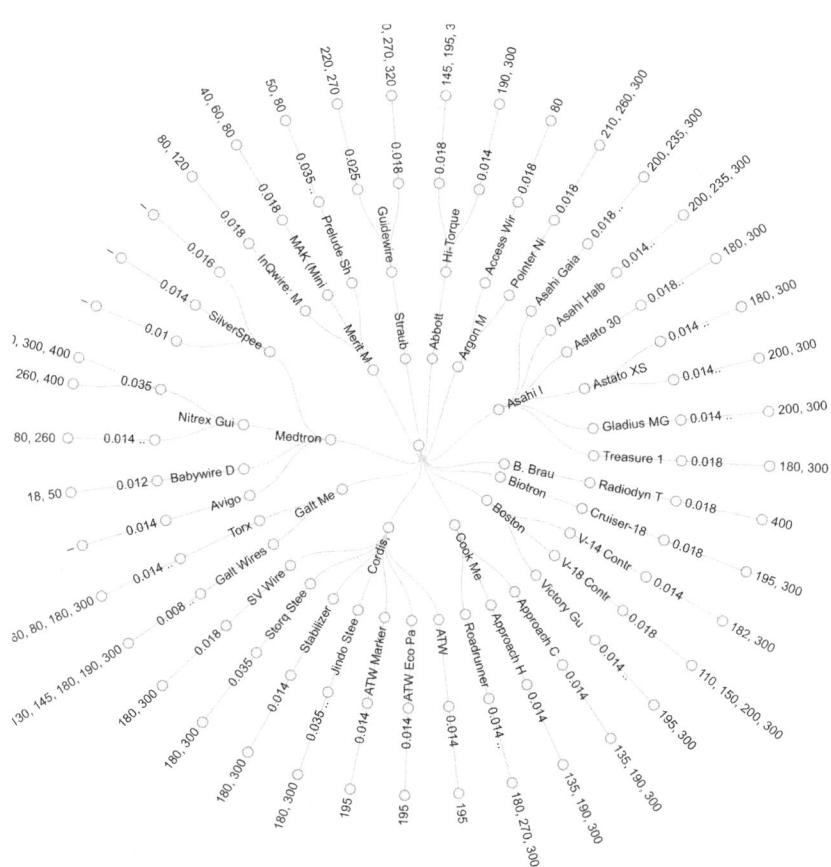

*Company, product name, wire size (F) and length (cm)

REFERENCES:

- Endovascular Tody. Device Guide. June 2020. URL: https://evto-day.com/device-guide/european

Catheters

ANGIOGRAPHIC CATHETERS: FLUSH

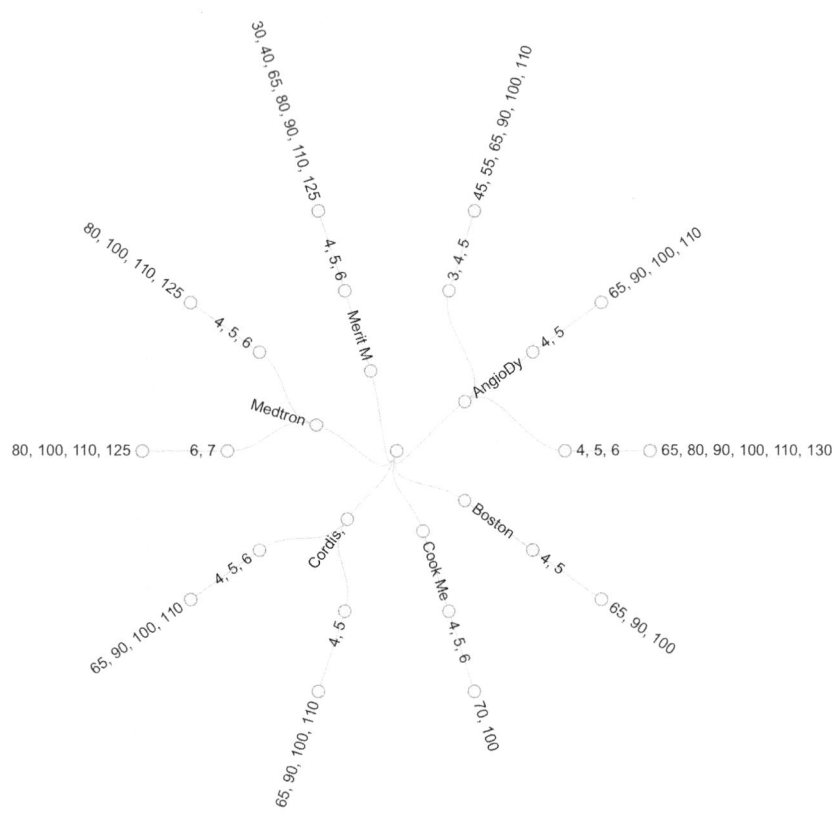

*Company, size (F) and length (cm)

REFERENCES:

- Endovascular Tody. Device Guide. June 2020. URL: https://evto-day.com/device-guide/european

Catheters

ANGIOGRAPHIC CATHETERS: FLUSH, RADIOPAQUE BANDS

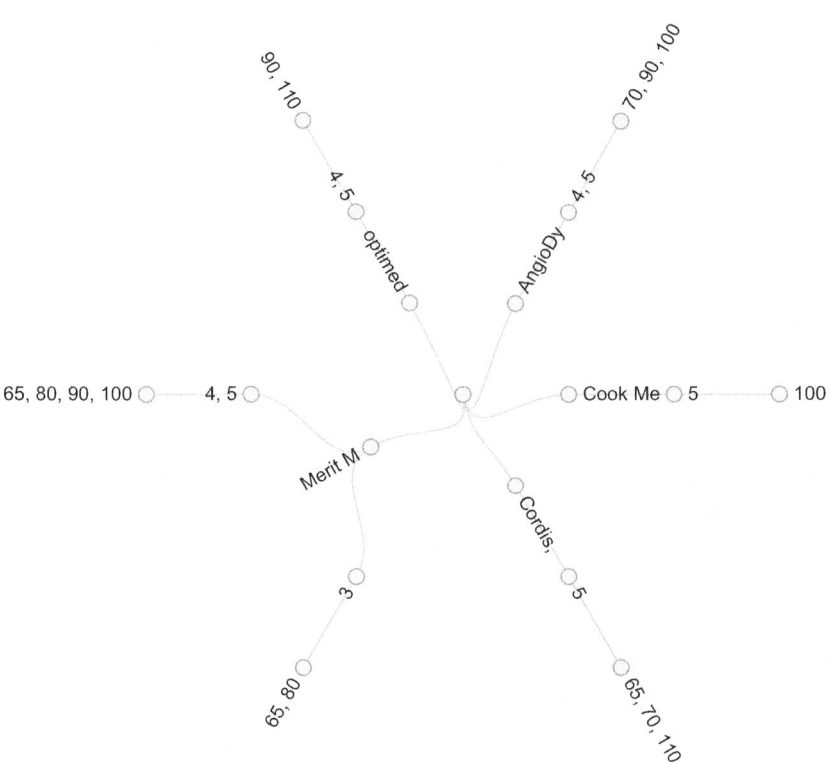

*Company, size (F) and length (cm)

REFERENCES:

- Endovascular Tody. Device Guide. June 2020. URL: https://evto-day.com/device-guide/european

Catheters

ANGIOGRAPHIC CATHETERS: SELECTIVE, HYDROPHILIC COATED

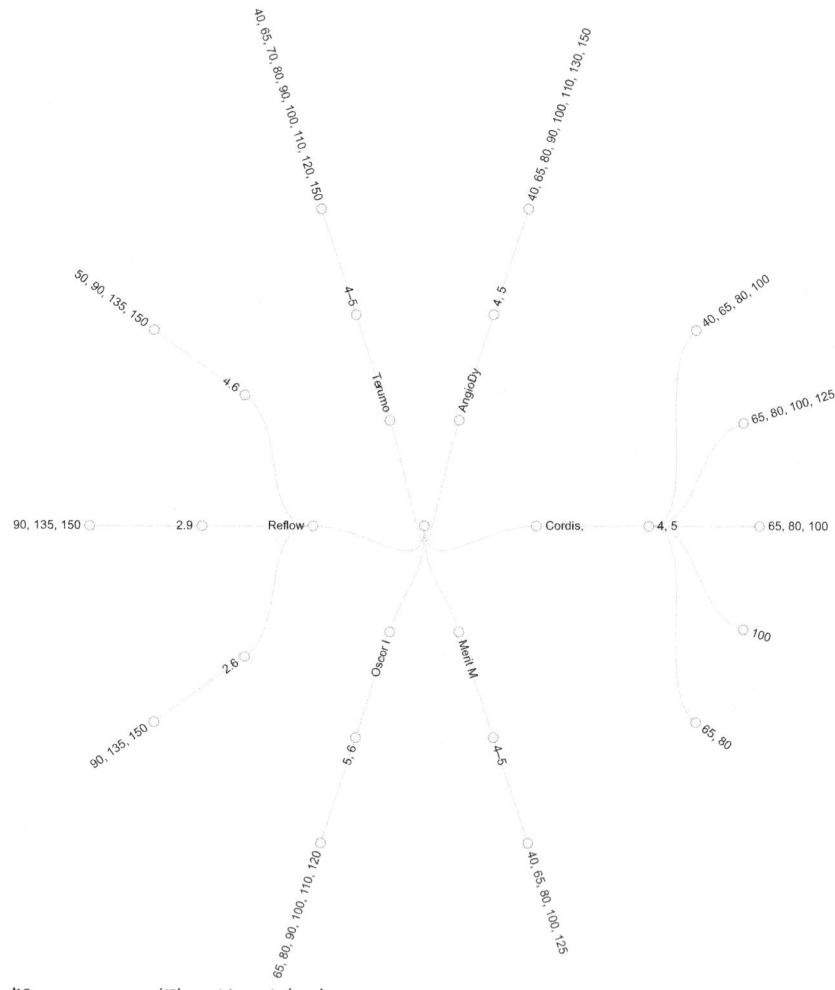

*Company, size (F) and length (cm)

REFERENCES:

- Endovascular Tody. Device Guide. June 2020. URL: https://evto-day.com/device-guide/european

Catheters

ANGIOGRAPHIC CATHETERS: SELECTIVE, NONHYDROPHILIC COATED

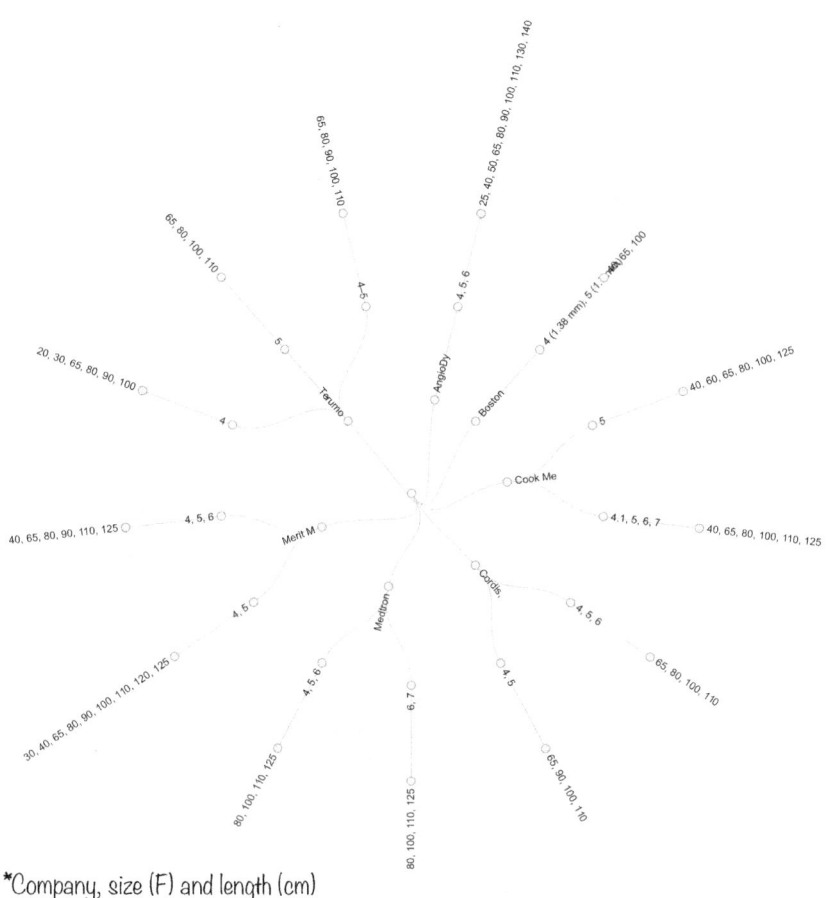

*Company, size (F) and length (cm)

REFERENCES:

- Endovascular Tody. Device Guide. June 2020. URL: https://evto-day.com/device-guide/european

Catheters

SPECIALTY CATHETERS

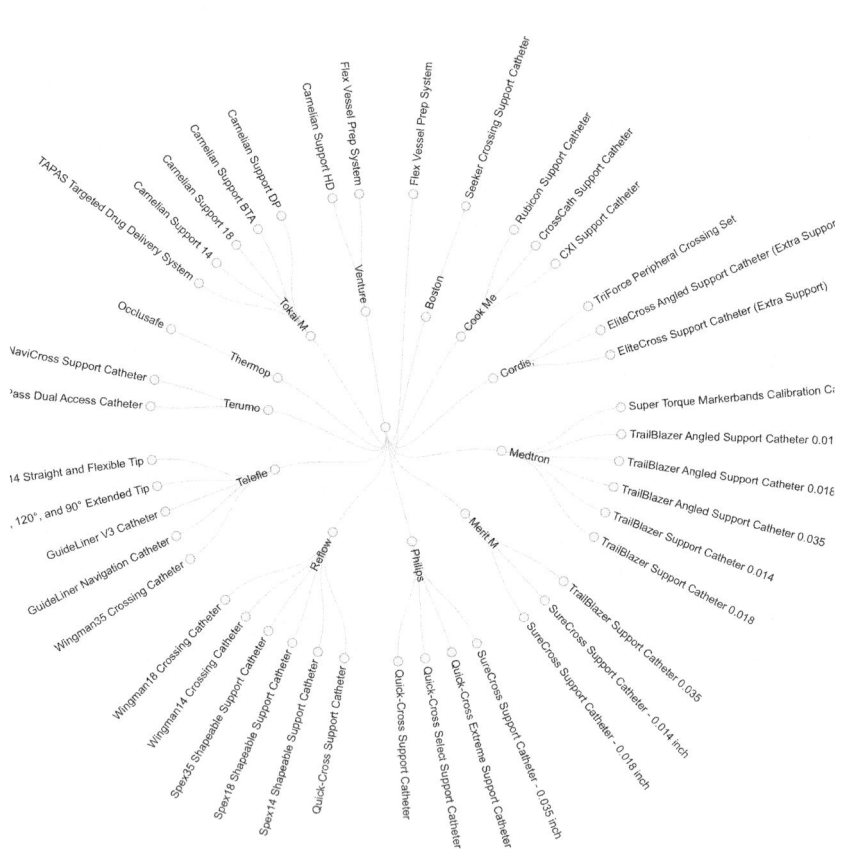

*Company and product name

REFERENCES:

- Endovascular Tody. Device Guide. June 2020. URL: https://evto-day.com/device-guide/european

Sheaths

STANDARD SHEATHS

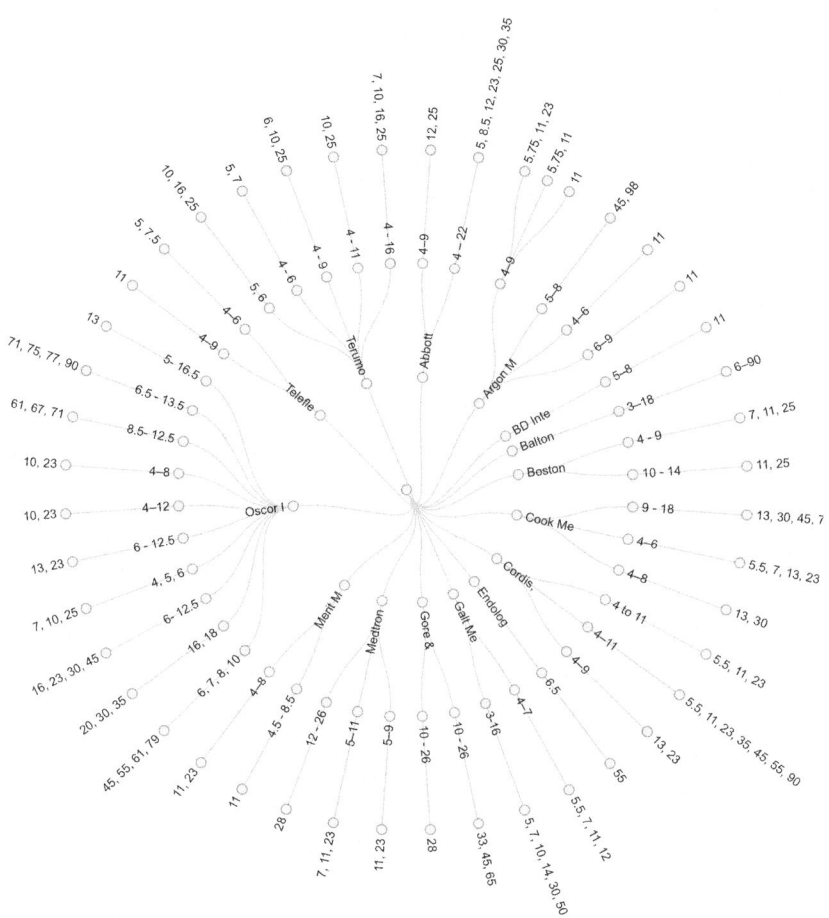

*Company, size (F) and length (cm)

REFERENCES:

- Endovascular Tody. Device Guide. June 2020. URL: https://evto-day.com/device-guide/european

Balloons

PTA Balloons

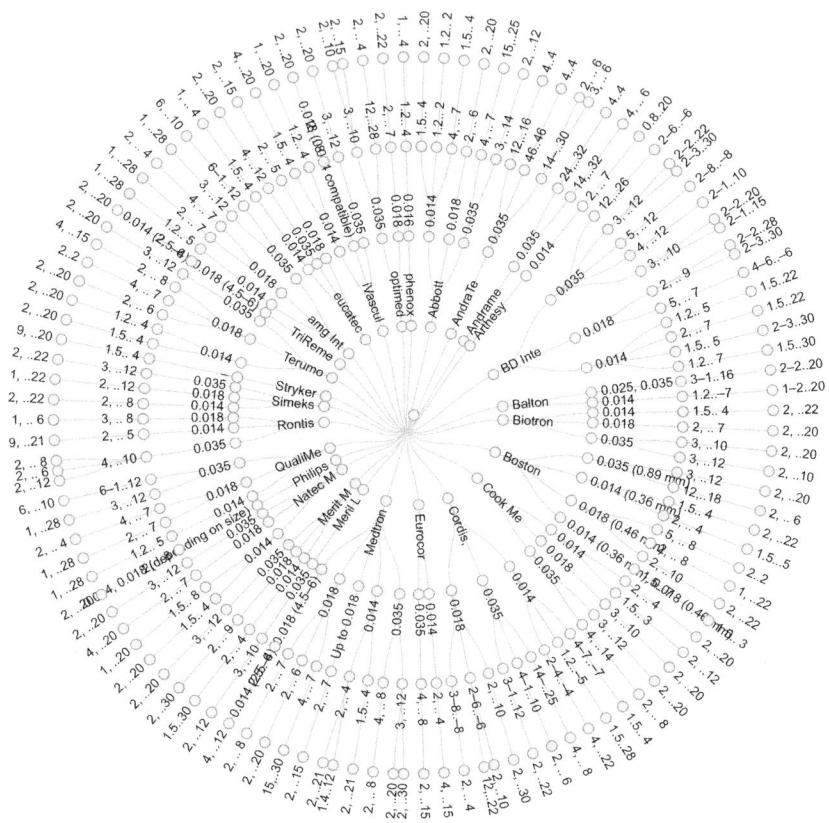

*Company, wire size (F), diameter range (F) and length range (cm)

References:

- Endovascular Tody. Device Guide. June 2020. URL: https://evto-day.com/device-guide/european

Balloons

DRUG COATED BALLOONS

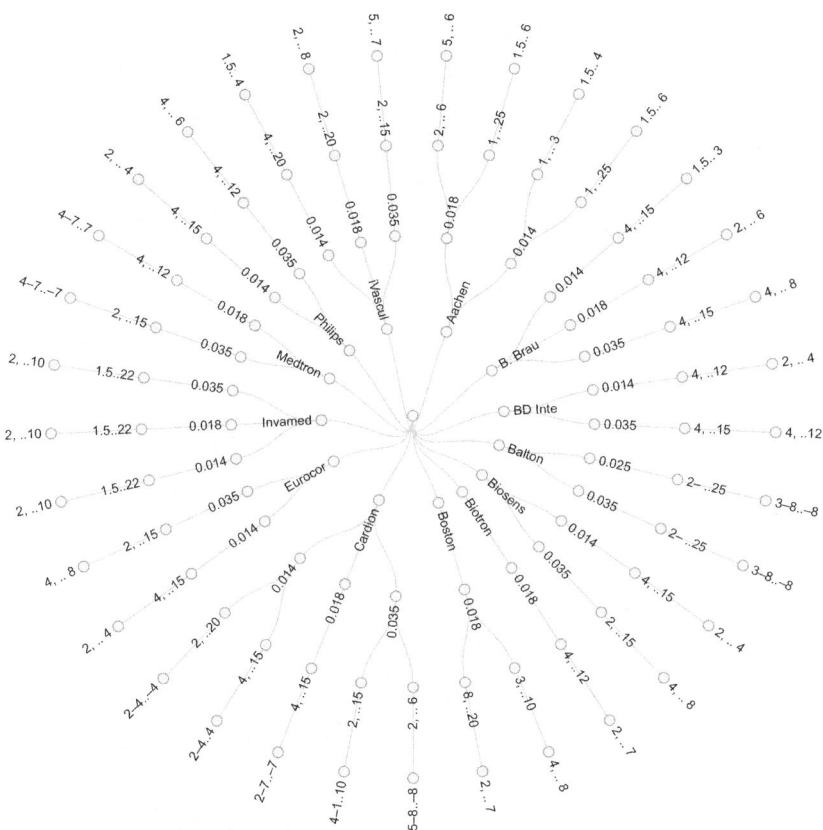

*Company, wire size (F), diameter range (F) and length range (cm)

REFERENCES:

- Endovascular Tody. Device Guide. June 2020. URL: https://evto-day.com/device-guide/european

Balloons

SPECIALTY BALLOONS

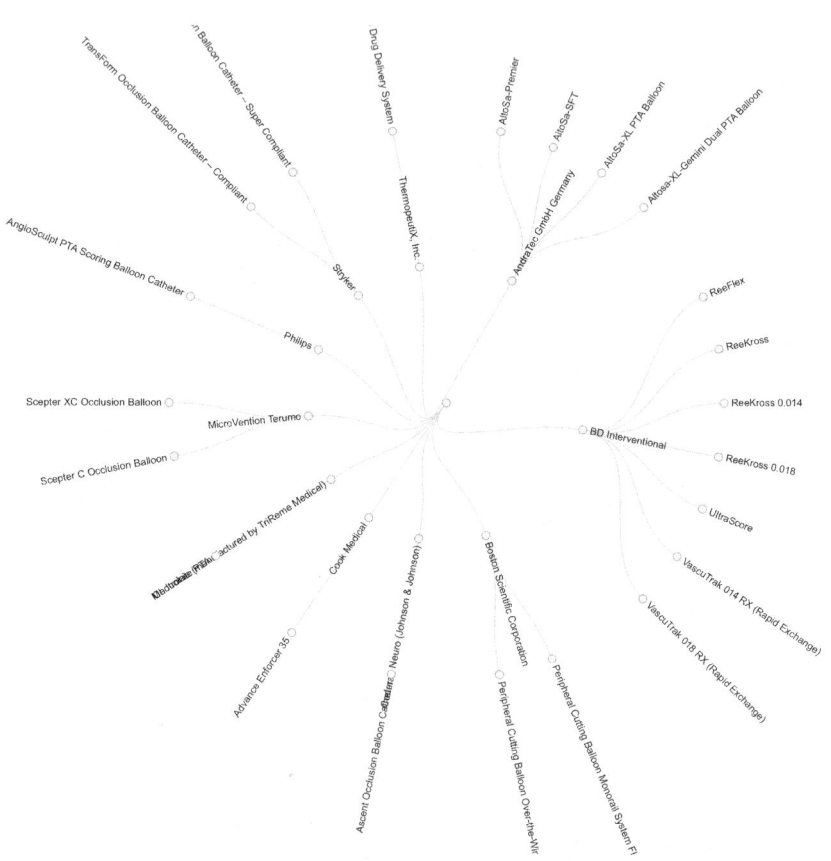

- TransForm Occlusion Balloon Catheter – Compliant
- ...n Balloon Catheter – Super Compliant
- Drug Delivery System
- AltoSa-Premier
- AltoSa-SFT
- AltoSa-XL FTA Balloon
- AltoSa-XL-Gemini Dual PTA Balloon
- AngioSculpt PTA Scoring Balloon Catheter
- Stryker
- ThermopeutiX, Inc.
- Andrax GmbH Germany
- ReeFlex
- Philips
- ReeKross
- Scepter XC Occlusion Balloon
- MicroVention Terumo
- ReeKross 0.014
- BD Interventional
- Scepter C Occlusion Balloon
- ReeKross 0.018
- UltraScore
- Electrosal... (PBM...actured by TriReme Medical)
- Cook Medical
- VascuTrak 014 RX (Rapid Exchange)
- VascuTrak 018 RX (Rapid Exchange)
- Advance Enforcer 35
- Ascent Occlusion Balloon Catheter
- ...Neuro (Johnson & Johnson)
- Boston Scientific Corporation
- Peripheral Cutting Balloon Over-the-Wir...
- Peripheral Cutting Balloon Monorail System FI...

*Company and product name

REFERENCES:

- Endovascular Tody. Device Guide. June 2020. URL: https://evto-day.com/device-guide/european

Stents

BALLOON-EXPANDABLE COVERED STENTS

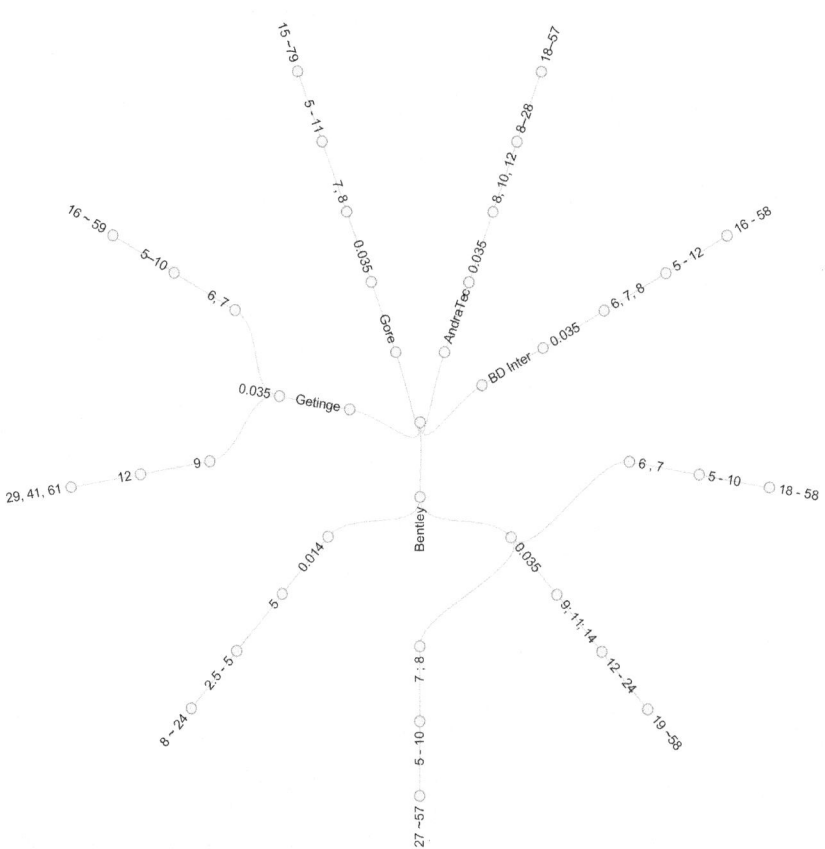

*Company, wire size (F) , introducer size (F), stent diameter (F) and stent length range (cm)

REFERENCES:

- Endovascular Tody. Device Guide. June 2020. URL: https://evto-day.com/device-guide/european

Stents

BALLOON-EXPANDABLE STENTS

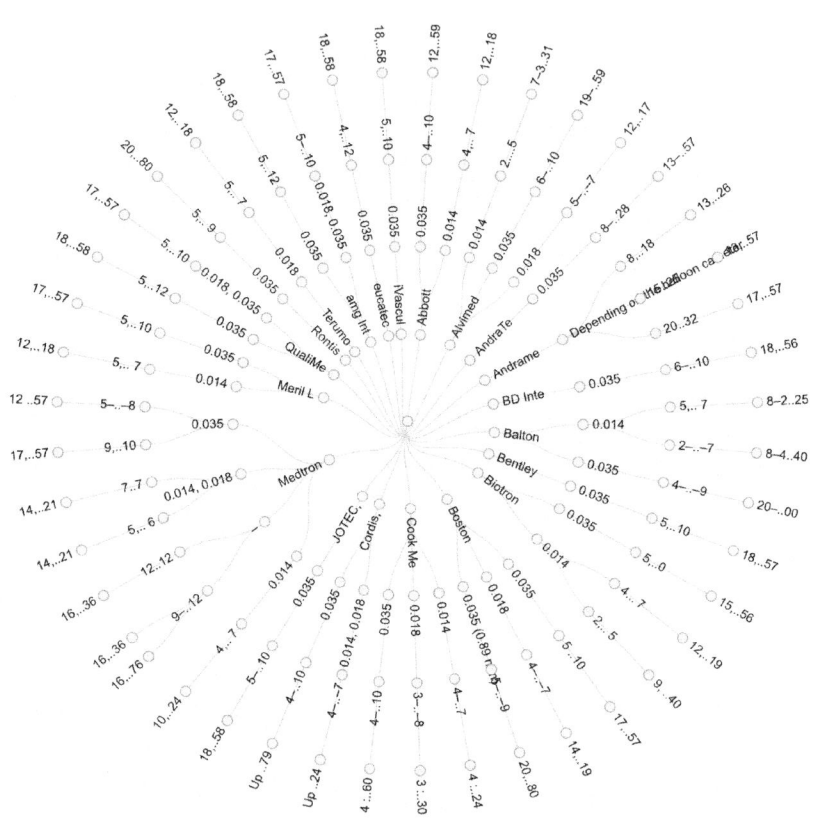

*Company, wire size (F), introducer size (F), stent diameter range (F) and stent length range (cm)

REFERENCES:

- Endovascular Tody. Device Guide. June 2020. URL: https://evto-day.com/device-guide/european

Stents

DRUG-ELUTING STENTS

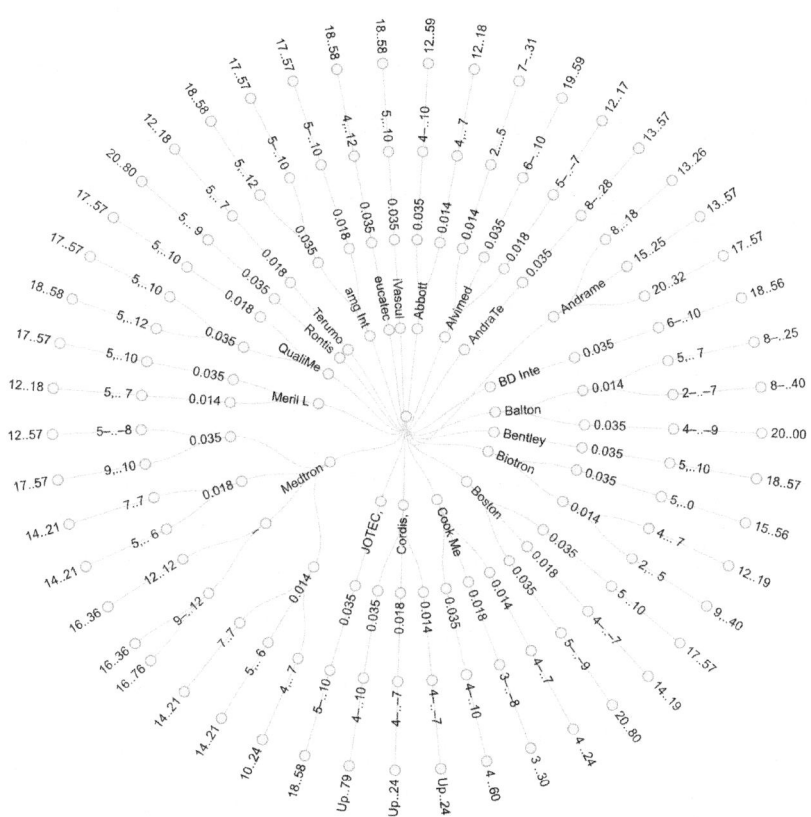

*Company, wire size (F), introducer size (F), stent diameter range (F) and stent length range (cm)

REFERENCES:

- Endovascular Tody. Device Guide. June 2020. URL: https://evto-day.com/device-guide/european

Stents

SELF-EXPANDING STENT GRAFTS

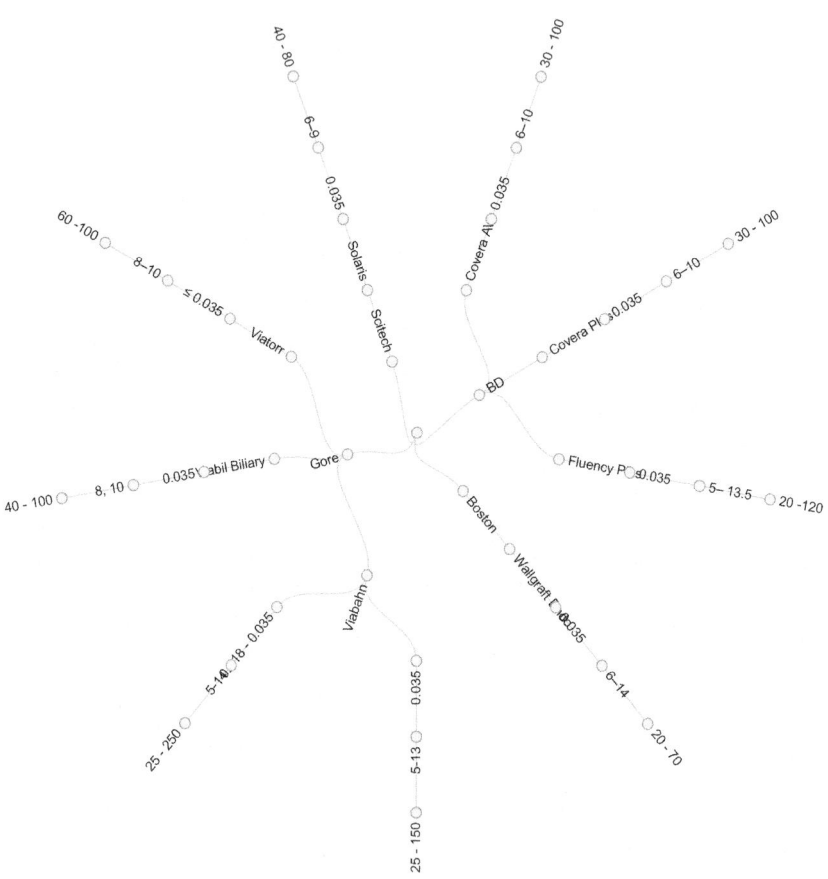

*Company, device name, wire size (F) , stent diameter range (F) and stent length range (cm)

REFERENCES:
- Endovascular Tody. Device Guide. June 2020. URL: https://evto-day.com/device-guide/european

Stents

SELF-EXPANDING STENT

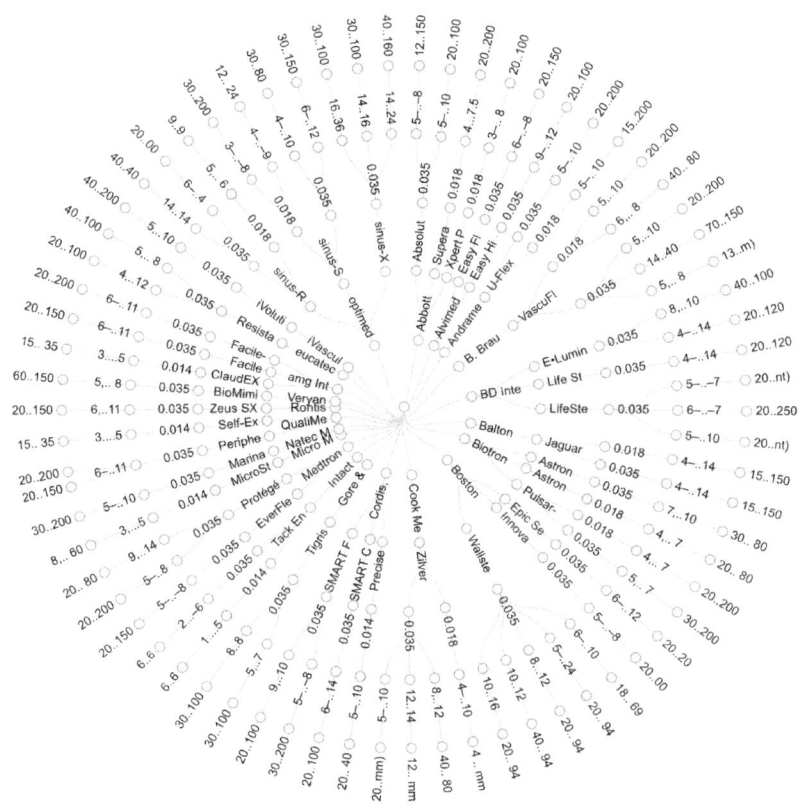

*Company, device name, wire size (F), stent diameter range (F) and stent length range (cm)

REFERENCES:

- Endovascular Tody. Device Guide. June 2020. URL: https://evto-day.com/device-guide/european

Stents

VENOUS STENTS

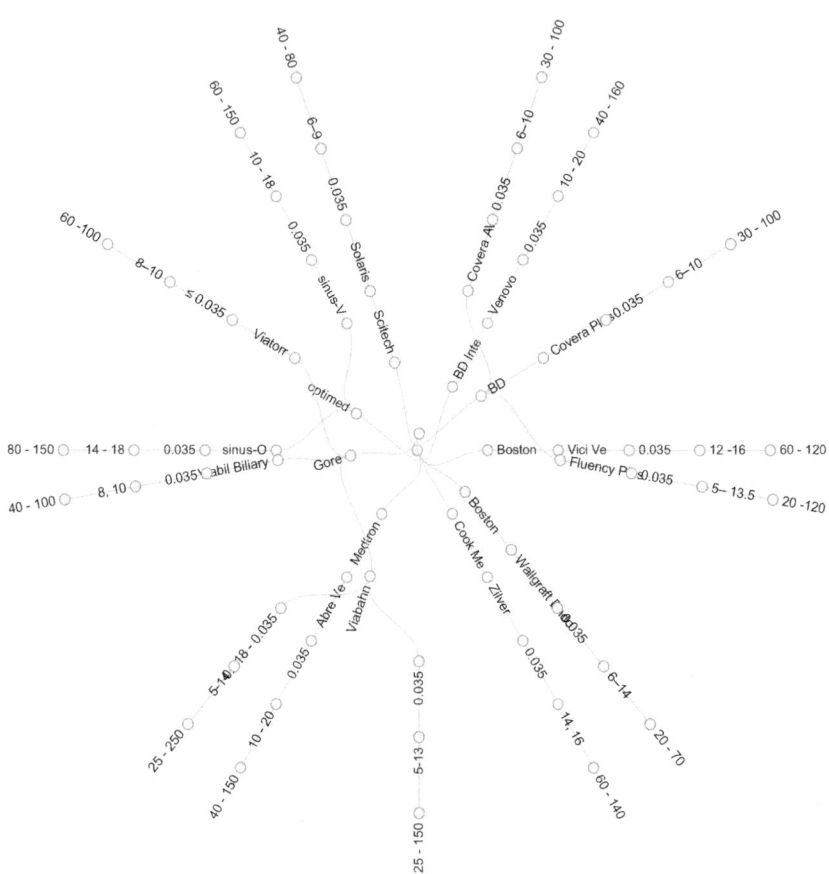

*Company, device name, wire size (F), stent diameter range (F) and stent length range (cm)

REFERENCES:

- Endovascular Tody. Device Guide. June 2020. URL: https://evto-day.com/device-guide/european

AAA Stent Grafts

MAIN PRODUCTS

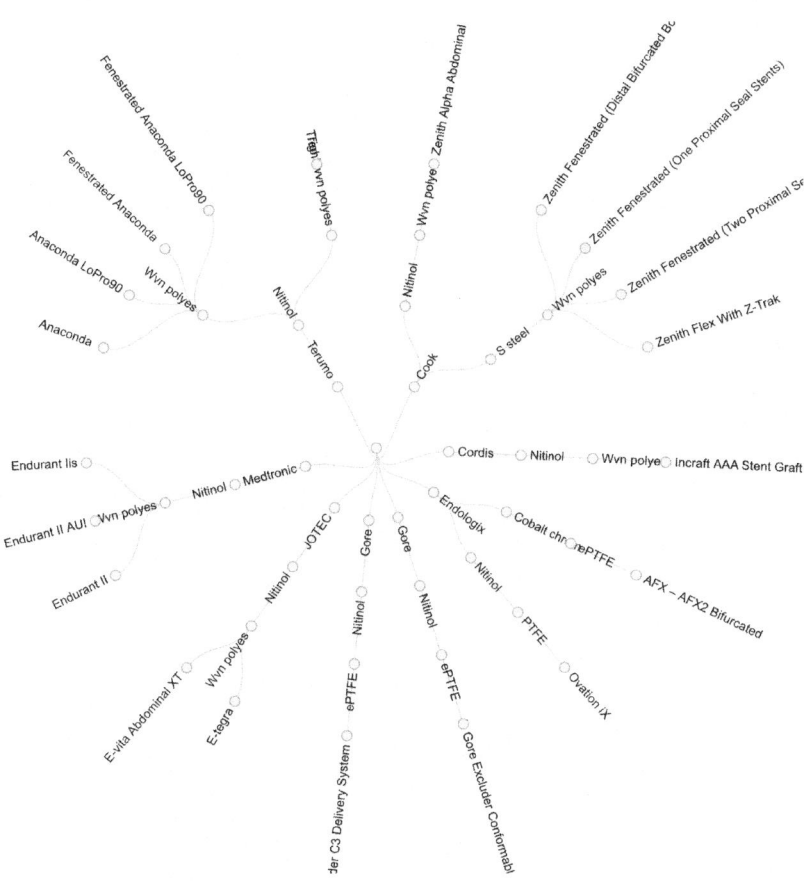

*Company, stent material, graft material, and device name

REFERENCES:

- Endovascular Tody. Device Guide. June 2020. URL: https://evto-day.com/device-guide/european

AAA Stent Grafts

GRAFT DIAMETER

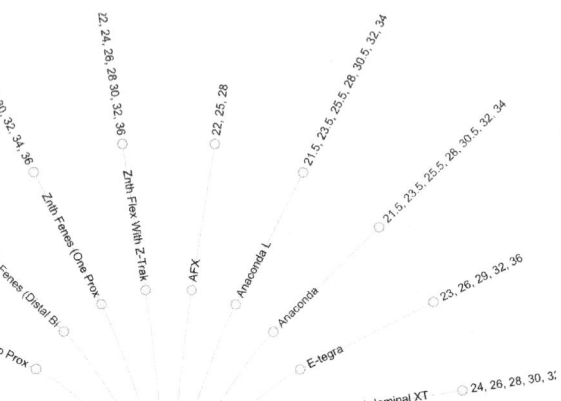
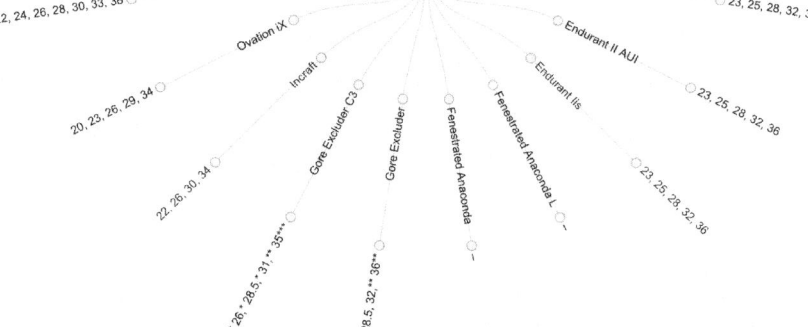

*Device name and Main Body Diameter (mm)

REFERENCES:

- Endovascular Tody. Device Guide. June 2020. URL: https://evto-day.com/device-guide/european

AAA Stent Grafts

Graft length

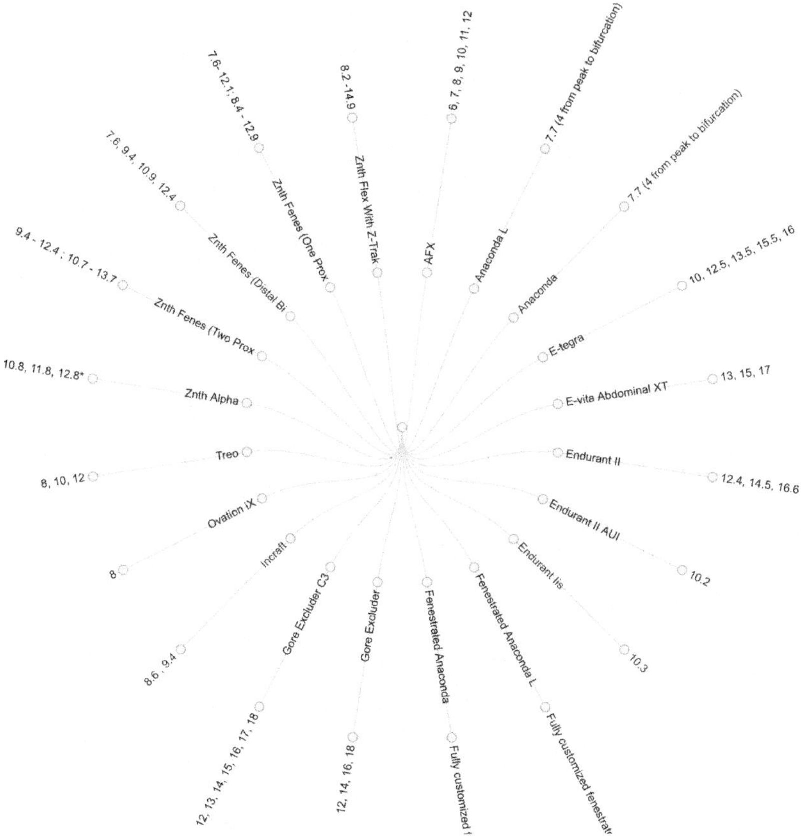

8.2 - 14.9
Znth Flex With Z-Trak
6, 7, 8, 9, 10, 11, 12
AFX
7.7 (4 from peak to bifurcation)
Anaconda L
7.7 (4 from peak to bifurcation)
Anaconda
10, 12.5, 13.5, 15.5, 16
E-tegra
13, 15, 17
E-vita Abdominal XT
Endurant II
12.4, 14.5, 16.6
Endurant II AUI
10.2
Endurant IIs
10.3
Fenestrated Anaconda L
Fully customized fenestrat
Fenestrated Anaconda
Fully customized f
Gore Excluder
12, 14, 16, 18
Gore Excluder C3
12, 13, 14, 15, 16, 17, 18
Incraft
8.6, 9.4
Ovation iX
8
Treo
8, 10, 12
Znth Alpha
10.8, 11.8, 12.8*
Znth Fenes (Two Prox
9.4 - 12.4 ; 10.7 - 13.7
Znth Fenes (Distal Bi
7.6, 9.4, 10.9, 12.4
Znth Fenes (One Prox
7.6- 12.1; 8.4 - 12.9

*Device name and Main Body Length (cm)

References:

- Endovascular Tody. Device Guide. June 2020. URL: https://evtoday.com/device-guide/european

AAA Stent Grafts

INTRODUCER SHEATH

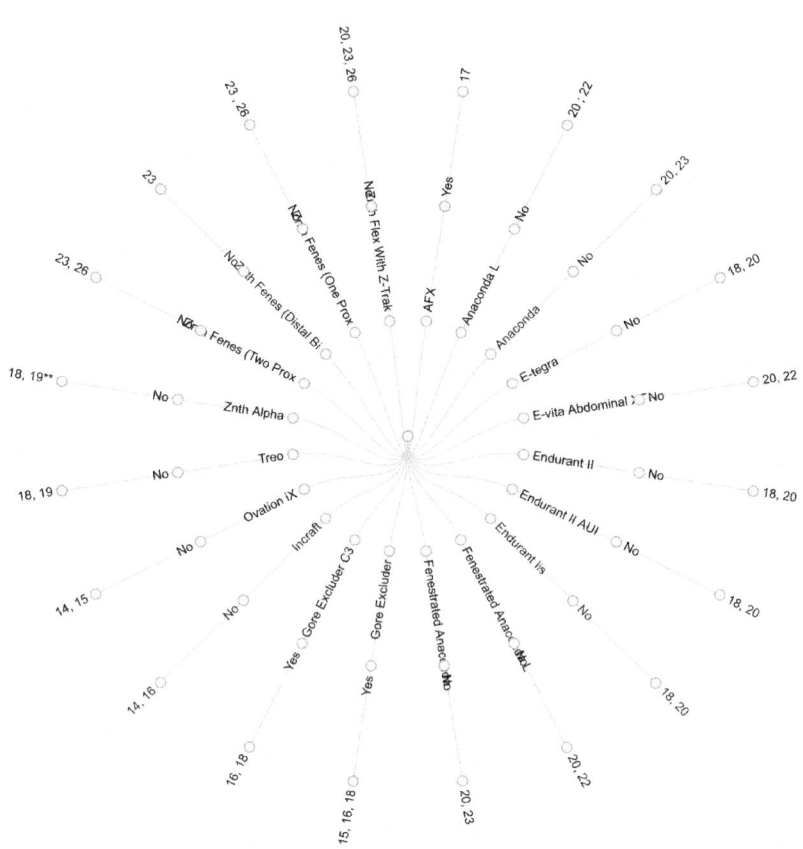

*Device name , Sheath Required for Delivery, and Delivery Sheath OD (F)

REFERENCES:

- Endovascular Tody. Device Guide. June 2020. URL: https://evto-day.com/device-guide/european

Thrombectomy and Thrombolysis

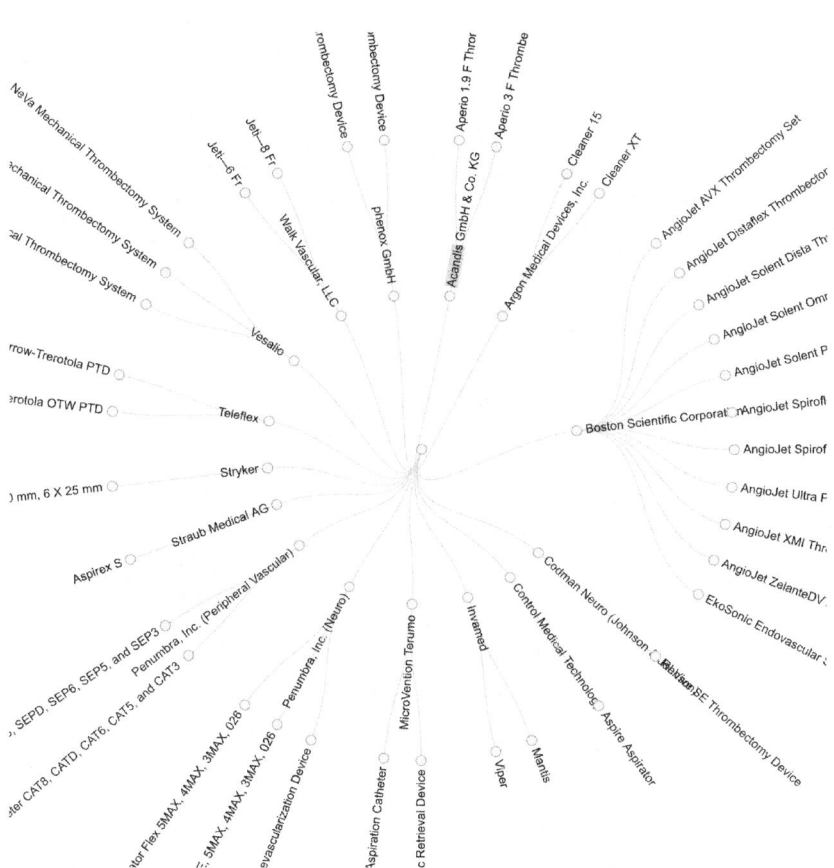

*Company name and Device name

REFERENCES:

- Endovascular Tody. Device Guide. June 2020. URL: https://evto-day.com/device-guide/european

Vein Endoablation

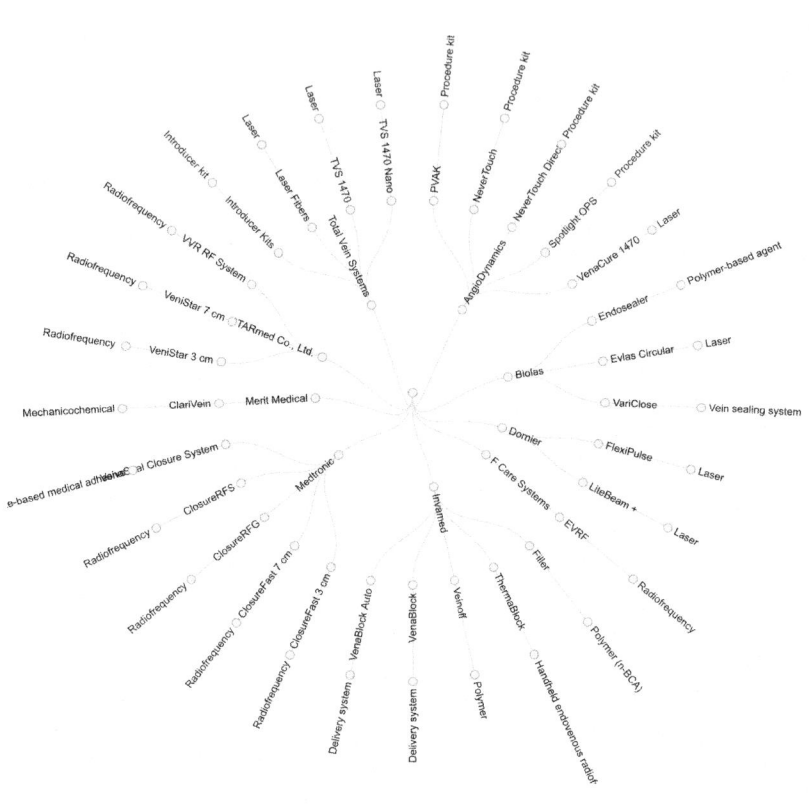

*Company name, Device name , and Technology used

REFERENCES:

- Endovascular Tody. Device Guide. June 2020. URL: https://evto-day.com/device-guide/european

Catheter Shape Analysis

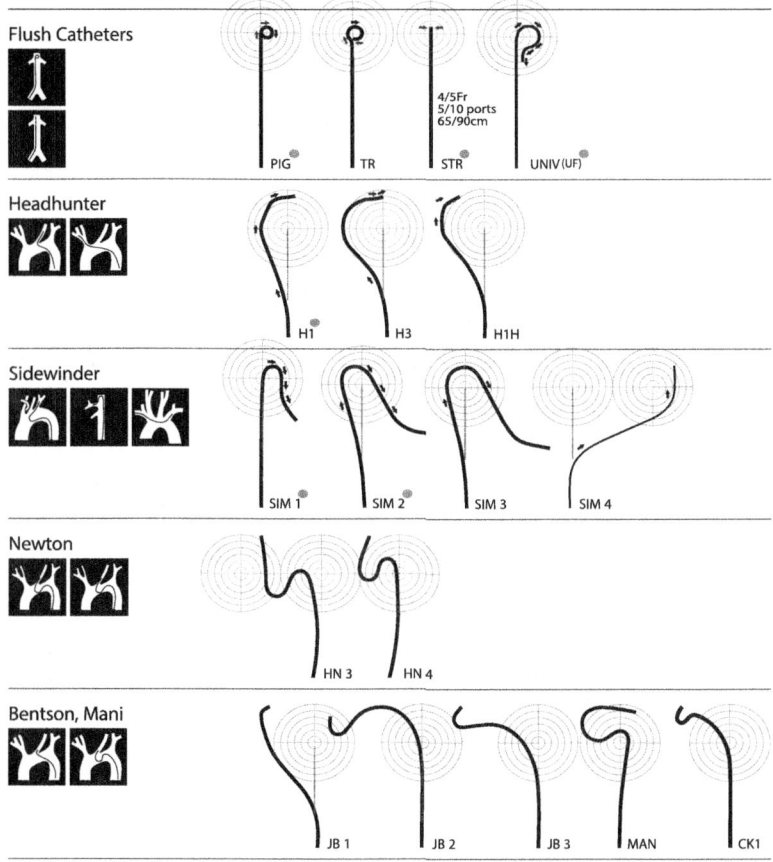

Flush Catheters

PIG   TR   STR   UNIV (UF)

4/5Fr
5/10 ports
65/90cm

Headhunter

H1   H3   H1H

Sidewinder

SIM 1   SIM 2   SIM 3   SIM 4

Newton

HN 3   HN 4

Bentson, Mani

JB 1   JB 2   JB 3   MAN   CK1

Catheter Shape Analysis

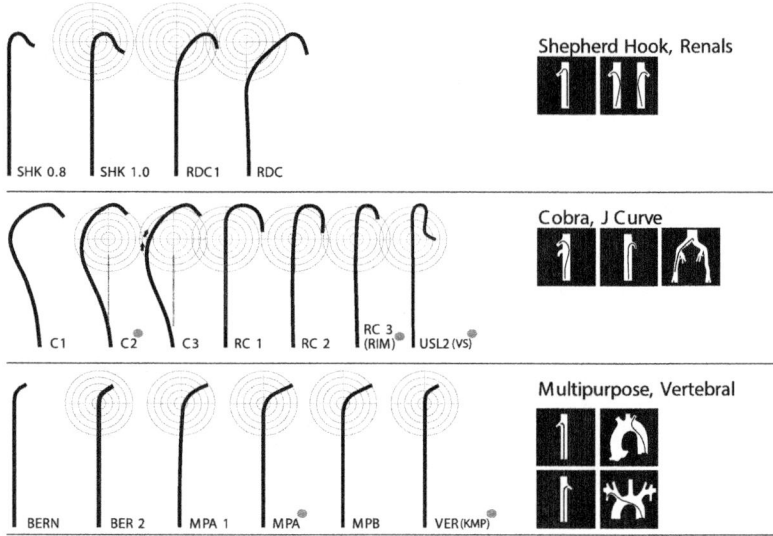

Shepherd Hook, Renals

SHK 0.8   SHK 1.0   RDC1   RDC

Cobra, J Curve

C 1   C 2   C 3   RC 1   RC 2   RC 3 (RIM)   USL2 (VS)

Multipurpose, Vertebral

BERN   BER 2   MPA 1   MPA   MPB   VER (KMP)

EVAR Preparation checklist

OTHER ACCESS SETUP

THORACIC AORTA

Multiplex

BONE MARKINGS

Complex

VISCERAL ARTERIES

Standard

Renal arteries

Caeliac

SMA

ILIAC ARTERIES

Access and risk of dissection

Landing Zones configurations

Diameters

Cannulation directions

Need for support wall stent/ conduit

ANEURYSM NECK

Length

Aorta-stent coupling area   Diameter

Effect of over-sizing

renal a. position

3D features   calcium hubs

Thrombus

Aneurysmal changes

Neck Angle   X-Ray

Behavior of Lindquest

Neck-iliac Exit Configuration

LUMBARS AND
SPINE PERFUSION

ANEURYSM SAC

expected stent graft body position

Expected c/l limb position vs cannulation

EVAR Planning

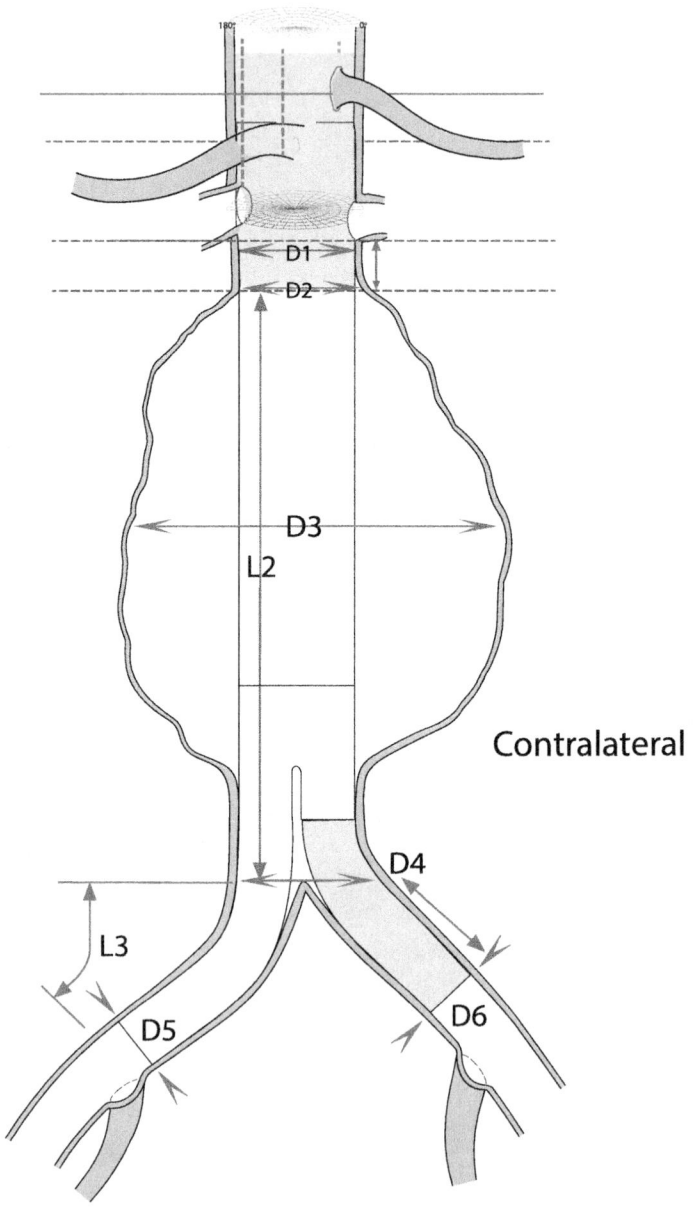

Contralateral

FEVAR PLANNING

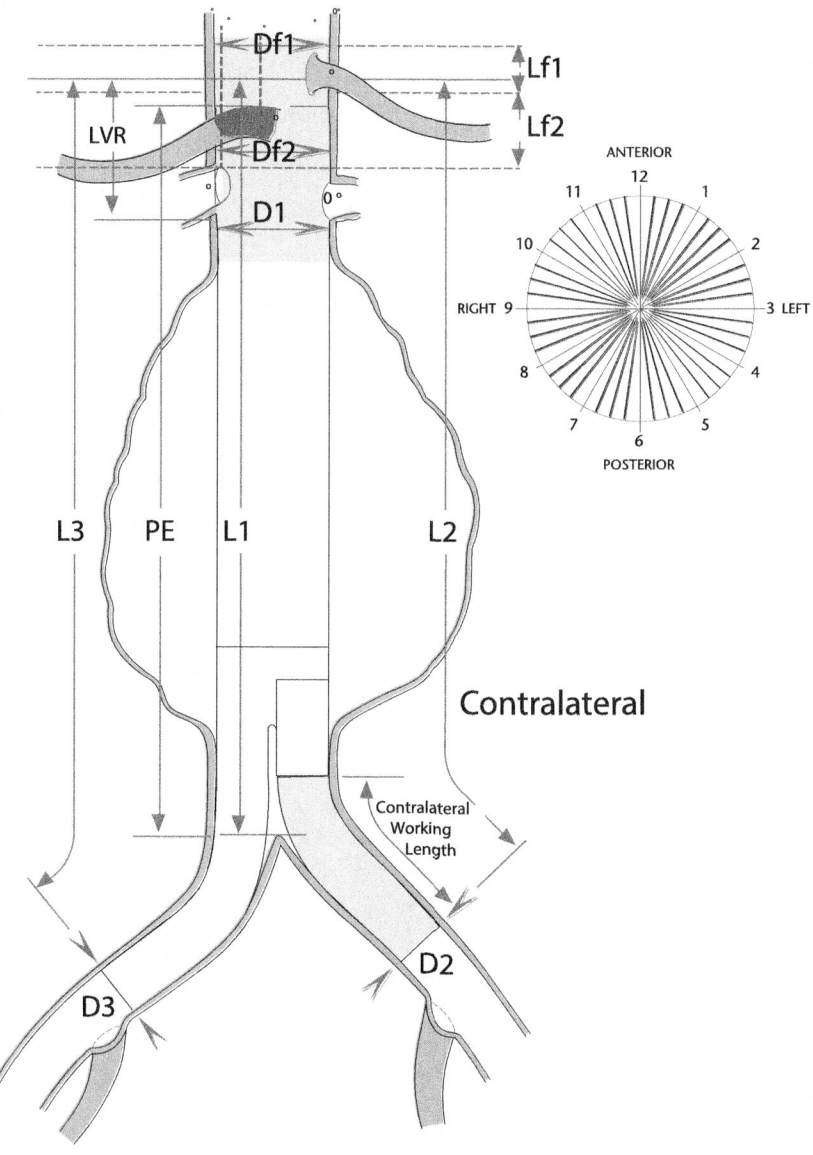

Endovascular Case Assessment Checklist

Case Assessment

Date: /   /2015 ID: _____
Indications-Procedure:

Allergies:
Weight:
Diabetic:
INR:
Creatinine/eGFR:

Renal protection:
Anticoagulant:
Antibiotics:
Max contrast (5 mL X weight [kg]/Creatinine):
Max Heparin dose (60U/kg):

Consent signed:

LESION:
Site:
Length:
Degree:
Inflow:
Outflow:
Calcium
Distal pressures/wave:

Proposed Access Site:
Site:
Location:
Hazards:

Resources:
  Sheaths:

  Wires:

  Catheters:

  Balloons:

  Others:

PROCEDURE:
Prepare, Access & Mark:

Crossing:

Anticoagulation:

Extras:
  Debulking:
  Filter:
  Embolisation:

Ballooning:

Stenting:

Completion:
  Retrieval of extra devices:
  Completion angio:
  Evaluation for distal emboli:
  Access site(s) management:

POSTPROCEDURE:
Evaluate:
  Access site
  Post-sedation status
  Distal pulses
  Total contrast volume/radiation dose:

Management:
  Access site:
  Anticoagulation/antiplatelate:

Communication:
  Nurses:
  Patient:
  Family:

OTHER NOTES:

Endovascular Tips and Tricks

VASCULAR ACCESS TIPS AND TRICKS:
The three principles for choosing access: a) Low risk of complications b) Easy conversion to endovasculr intervention c) Relative proximity to site of intervention
Aim at: a single perfect pass of the entry needle on every case.

TIPS & TRICKS for good access:
- It's not that complicated!
- Determine the likelihood of endovascular intervention prior to the puncture and take that into account when choosing a puncture site.
- Standardize your technique.
- Use Fluoroscopy for guidance.
- Don't be afraid to abandon the access and puncture elsewhere if the risk is too high.
- No one gets in every single time.
- If there is a problem, hold pressure for a few minutes.

- Special cases: 1) Pts on antiplatelates: keep unless other bleeding tendency expected. 2) Pts on warfarin: safe when using 4F sheath 3) Chronic renal failure: admit for overnight hydration. 4) Pts with allergy: consider hydrocortisone.

OPEN VS. PERCUTANEOUS ACCESS:
Size of access sheath > 10F (3.3mm): use open access

Size of access sheath <10F: consider percutaneous

BALLOON SIZING:
Abdominal aorta 8–18
Aortic bifurcation 6–10
Common iliac artery 6–10
External iliac artery 6–8
Superficial femoral artery 4–
Popliteal artery 3–6
Tibial artery 2–4
Renal artery 4–7
Subclavian artery 5–8
Dialysis graft 4–6
Infrainguinal graft 2–5

* Each arterial segment has a general range of appropriate balloon sizes from which to choose
* When kissing balloons are used at the aortic bifurcation, the diameters of the two balloons are additive. Kissing 10-mm balloons should be used only if the distal aorta can tolerate dilatation to 20 mm.

Endovascular Tips and Tricks

CIA Angioplasty

Requirements	Steps	Comments
Angio Set **Sheaths:** 4Fr (angiogram) or 5F (plasty) **Wires:** 0.035 standard J 0.035 Glidewire **Catheters** 4-5F / 65cm straight exchange **Balloons:** SFA 4-7; POP 3-6 TPT 2-4	**Access & Mark**	• **MAIN ACCESS** - LA inject/cut → Needle <u>in</u> → J wire <u>in</u> → Scr → Needle out → Sheath <u>in</u> → J Wire out → Run 1 • **EXTENDED ACCESS** - Str Catheter (±Glidewire) <u>in</u> →Scr → Run <u>1</u> (CFA/PFA/SFA)/<u>2</u> (SFA/Pop)/<u>3</u> (TPT)/±
	Crossing Lesion	• Glidewire <u>in</u> → Str Cath/Wire manipulation → **CROSSING** (Wire+Cath) → Wire out → **HEPARIN** (via sheath) → 0.018 wire <u>in</u> → Cath out
	Balloon Plasty	• Plasty Balloon <u>in</u> (Distal part first) → <u>In</u>flate (10-12 mmHg - 13-20 seconds) → Adjust/Inflate → No waisting: Baloon out • **FINAL CHECK** via sheath
	Haemostasis **Report**	

SFA Angioplasty

Requirements	Steps	Comments
Angio Set **Sheaths:** 4Fr (angiogram) or 5F (plasty) **Wires:** 0.035 standard J 0.035 Glidewire 0.018 **Catheters** 4-5F / 65cm straight exchange **Balloons:** SFA 4-7; POP 3-6 TPT 2-4	**Access & Mark**	• **MAIN ACCESS** - LA inject/cut → Needle <u>in</u> → J wire <u>in</u> → Scr → Needle out → Sheath <u>in</u> → J Wire out → Run 1 • **EXTENDED ACCESS** - Str Catheter (±Glidewire) <u>in</u> →Scr → Run <u>1</u> (CFA/PFA/SFA)/<u>2</u> (SFA/Pop)/<u>3</u> (TPT)/±
	Crossing Lesion	• Glidewire <u>in</u> → Str Cath/Wire manipulation → **CROSSING** (Wire+Cath) → Wire out → **HEPARIN** (via sheath) → 0.018 wire <u>in</u> → Cath out
	Balloon Plasty	• Plasty Balloon <u>in</u> (Distal part first) → <u>In</u>flate (10-12 mmHg - 13-20 seconds) → Adjust/Inflate → No waisting: Baloon out • **FINAL CHECK** via sheath
	Haemostasis	
	Report	

Endovascular Tips and Tricks

Puncture Site Pitfalls

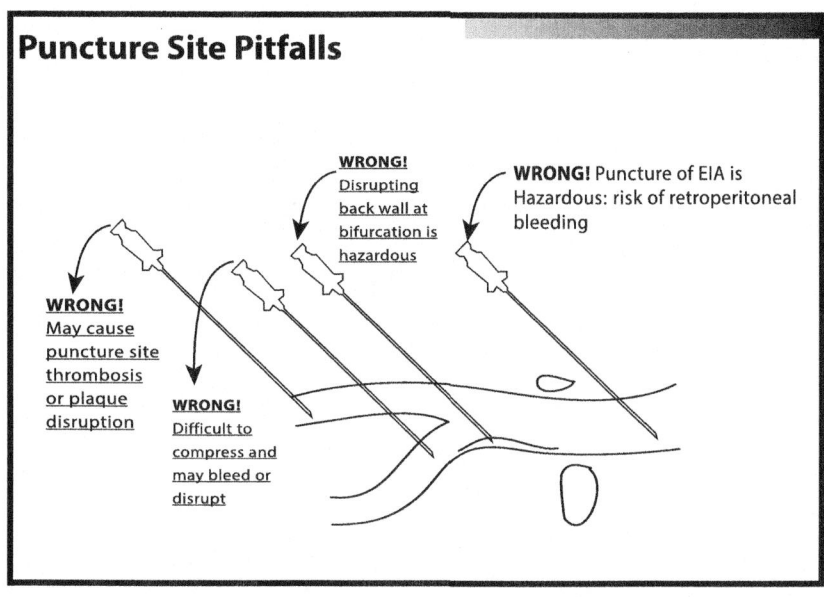

WRONG! Disrupting back wall at bifurcation is hazardous

WRONG! Puncture of EIA is Hazardous: risk of retroperitoneal bleeding

WRONG! May cause puncture site thrombosis or plaque disruption

WRONG! Difficult to compress and may bleed or disrupt

TIP: Guidewire NOT passing Beyond Needle

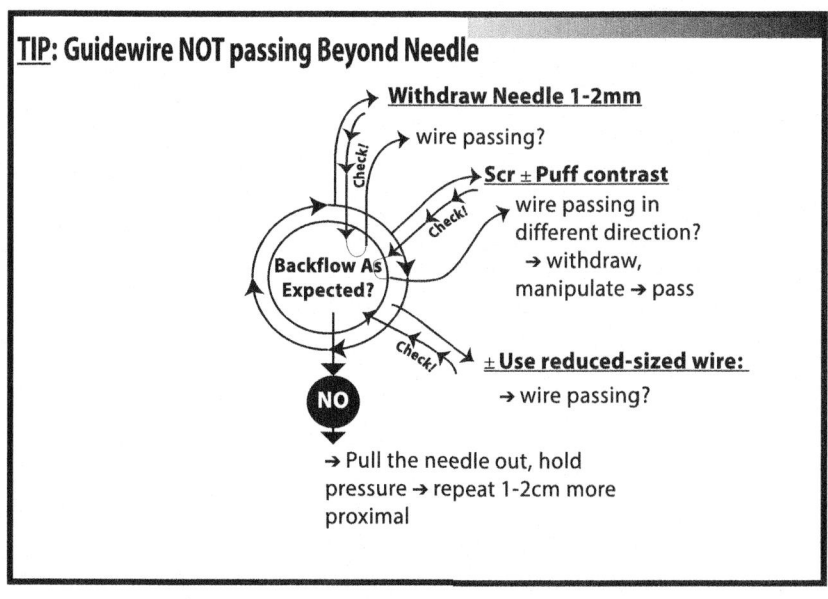

Withdraw Needle 1-2mm
→ wire passing?

Scr ± Puff contrast
→ wire passing in different direction?
→ withdraw, manipulate → pass

± Use reduced-sized wire:
→ wire passing?

Backflow As Expected?

Check!

NO
→ Pull the needle out, hold pressure → repeat 1-2cm more proximal

Endovascular Tips and Tricks

Puncture of Pulseless Femoral Artery
→ **Femoral artery is patent but pulsless**

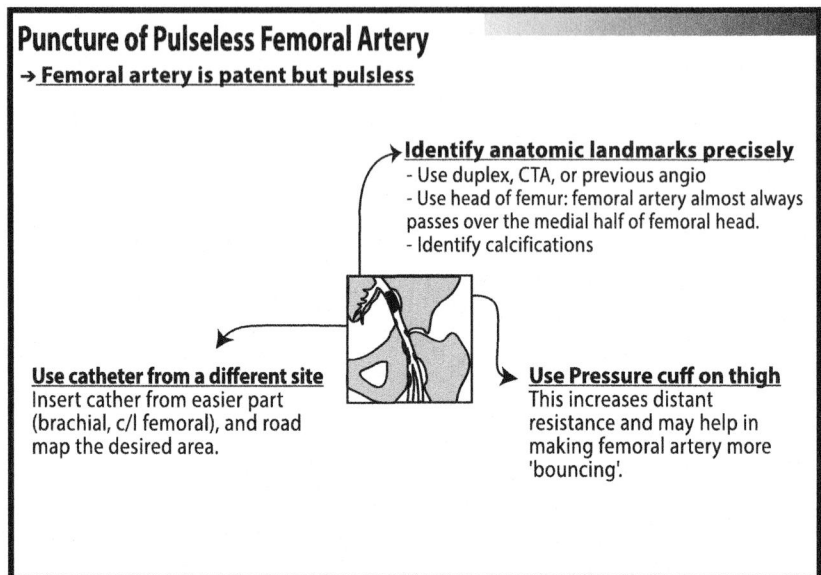

Identify anatomic landmarks precisely
- Use duplex, CTA, or previous angio
- Use head of femur: femoral artery almost always passes over the medial half of femoral head.
- Identify calcifications

Use catheter from a different site
Insert cather from easier part (brachial, c/l femoral), and road map the desired area.

Use Pressure cuff on thigh
This increases distant resistance and may help in making femoral artery more 'bouncing'.

Micropuncture Set

Needle: 21G (vs. 18G in normal set).
Guidewire: 0.018-in (vs. 0.035-in for normal set).
Access catheter: 4 Fr short
Complciation rate: decrease by ~10%

Special features:
Shelfless: No shelf between introducer and catheter.

Tips on use: After 21G needle is inserted, backflow is usually less than expected. Guidewire with 0.018-in floppy tip is introduced, and catheter (with small shlefless introducer) is inserted. Once established (and flushed), a 0.035-in guideire is inserted as required.

Endovascular Tips and Tricks

Access via Prosthesis Graft Tips and Tricks

- Administer antibiotics before access
- Dacron grafts are tight and may be challanging to puncture. considerable force is usually required to push the needle through.
- After inserting the guidewire, dilate the tract with 4-5F introducer BEFORE inserting the access catheter/sheath over the wire-introducer. If fibrous tissue still prevent access, a larger diameter (and stiffer 6Fr) dilator migth be required.
- Puncture needle into subcutaneously-situated graft should be inserted several millimeters in subcutaneous tissue BEFORE entering the graft @45 degrees. No skin incion should be made.
Use the smallest catheter required.

Index

Printed in Great Britain
by Amazon